Aromatherapy for Health Professionals

Commissioning Editor: *Claire Wilson*
Development Editor: *Fiona Conn*
Project Manager: *Sruthi Viswam*
Designer: *Kirsteen Wright*
Illustration Manager: *Bruce Hogarth*

Aromatherapy for Health Professionals

FOURTH EDITION

Edited by

Shirley Price Cert Ed, FISPA, HMIFA, FIAM (Aromatic Medicine)
Practitioner and Lecturer in Aromatherapy, Hinckley, Leicestershire, UK

Len Price MIT(Trichology), FISPA, HMIFA, FIAM(Aromatic Medicine)
Lecturer in Aromatherapy, Hinckley, Leicestershire, UK

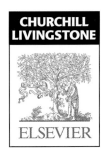

CHURCHILL
LIVINGSTONE

ELSEVIER

Edinburgh London New York Oxford Philadelphia St Louis Sydney Toronto 2012

ELSEVIER
CHURCHILL
LIVINGSTONE

© 2012 Elsevier Ltd. All rights reserved.

No part of this publication may be reproduced or transmitted in any form or by any means, electronic or mechanical, including photocopying, recording, or any information storage and retrieval system, without permission in writing from the publisher. Details on how to seek permission, further information about the Publisher's permissions policies and our arrangements with organizations such as the Copyright Clearance Centre and the Copyright Licensing Agency, can be found at our website: www.elsevier.com/permissions.

This book and the individual contributions contained in it are protected under copyright by the Publisher (other than as may be noted herein).

First edition 1995
Second edition 1999
Third edition 2007
Fourth edition 2012
    Reprinted 2012 (twice), 2013 (twice), 2014

ISBN 978-0-7020-3564-7

British Library Cataloguing in Publication Data
A catalogue record for this book is available from the British Library

Library of Congress Cataloging in Publication Data
A catalog record for this book is available from the Library of Congress

Notices
Knowledge and best practice in this field are constantly changing. As new research and experience broaden our understanding, changes in research methods, professional practices, or medical treatment may become necessary.

Practitioners and researchers must always rely on their own experience and knowledge in evaluating and using any information, methods, compounds, or experiments described herein. In using such information or methods they should be mindful of their own safety and the safety of others, including parties for whom they have a professional responsibility.

With respect to any drug or pharmaceutical products identified, readers are advised to check the most current information provided (i) on procedures featured or (ii) by the manufacturer of each product to be administered, to verify the recommended dose or formula, the method and duration of administration, and contraindications. It is the responsibility of practitioners, relying on their own experience and knowledge of their patients, to make diagnoses, to determine dosages and the best treatment for each individual patient, and to take all appropriate safety precautions.

To the fullest extent of the law, neither the Publisher nor the authors, contributors, or editors, assume any liability for any injury and/or damage to persons or property as a matter of products liability, negligence or otherwise, or from any use or operation of any methods, products, instructions, or ideas contained in the material herein.

 your source for books, journals and multimedia in the health sciences
www.elsevierhealth.com

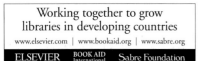

Working together to grow
libraries in developing countries

www.elsevier.com | www.bookaid.org | www.sabre.org

ELSEVIER   BOOK AID International   Sabre Foundation

The Publisher's policy is to use **paper manufactured from sustainable forests**

Printed in China

Book Contents

CD-ROM Contents

Appendix A   Essential Oils for General Use in Health-Care Settings

Appendix B   Indications for Uses of Essential Oils

Appendix C   Essential Oils to be Used with Caution

     1   Uterotonic oils which facilitate delivery
     2   Emmenagogic essential oils
     3   Disputed emmenagogic oils
     4   Toxic, neurotoxic and abortive oils not used in aromatherapy
     5   Neurotoxic and/or abortive oils occasionally used in aromatherapy
     6   Potential skin irritant oils
     7   Phototoxic oils
     8   Contact-sensitizing oils

Appendix D   General Properties of Essential Oils

Appendix E   Safety – A Summary

Appendix F   Essential oil: Definition for Aromatherapeutic Purposes

     References to Appendices

     Sources to Appendices

Contributors

Louise Anderson BSc (Hons) Cert Ed MIFPA MAR IFL Dip.
Holistic Aromatherapy and Massage, Dip. Reflexology, Dip. On Site
Massage Cert. Social Care
Curriculum Leader for Society, Care and Development,
Richmond Adult Community College, Richmond, UK

Angela Avis MBE MA RGN DN Cert PG Dip Ed PG Dip Advanced
Health Care Practice
Senior Lecturer, Oxford Brookes University, Oxford, UK

Elaine Cooper MIFPA LIAM
Clinical Lead and Manager, Complementary Therapy
Service NHS Walsall Community Health; aromatologist

Julia Fearon RGN RSCN BSc (Hons) Complementary
Therapy
Independent complementary therapist, Birmingham, UK

Jo Kellett TIDHA MIFPA CIMI
Holistic aromatherapist, Brighton, UK

Sandra A Oram MIFPA MIFA MBRA
Aromatherapist, Stratford-upon-Avon, UK

Carole Preen
Section Head, OCNLR Foundation Courses, Morley
College, London, UK

Penny A Price Cert Ed MED MIFPA
Aromatherapist & Aromatologist; Principal, Penny Price
Academy of Aromatherapy; Managing Director Penny
Price Aromatherapy, Hinckley, UK

Denise Raines RN
Aromatherapist & Aromatologist, The Algarve, Portugal

Robert Stephen FRSPH FRSA FIAM
Aromatology lecturer and Doctor of theology, Hinckley, UK

Sue Whyte RGN RM CertEd FE MIFPA
Former Macmillan lecturer practitioner; aromatherapy
practitioner, Oncology Unit Walsgrave Hospital,
Coventry, UK

International Contributors

Australia

Ron Guba Dip. Phytoaromatherapy
General manager, Essential Therapeutics, Victoria,
Australia

Belgium

Anny van Branteghem
Aromatherapist, Belgium

Sylvie Lenoir
Alternative therapist, Ross-on-Wye, UK

Philippe Gérard Pharm
Pharmacist, Phytotherapist, Aromatherapist; Director
Primrose Academy, Oostende, Belgium

Brazil

Vera L G O'Neill
Aromatherapist, Brazil

Canada

Marlene M Mitchell CA CRM
Principal, International Certified Aromatherapy Institute,
Canada

Tricia Eagle
Executive Director & Administrator, Canadian Federation
of Aromatherapists, Canada

China

Shaohua Lu
AromaValley Trading, China

Croatia

Zrinka Jezdić BSc Med Techn
Head teacher, AromaVita School for Aromatherapy,
Zagreb, Croatia

Finland

Ulla-Maija Grace LLSA IScB MIFA
Director and Principal Tutor, Aromatica Oy, Finnish College
of Aromatherapy

France

Rhiannon Harris FIFPA
Editor, International Journal of Aromatherapy; Director
Essential Oil Resource Consultants

Kuniko M Hadji-Minaglou BA DipAc DipMoxa, DipShiatsu,
Anma & Massage, CertPhyto & Aroma, CertCS, HMISIAM
Director of Zea Maïs Consultancy, Montauroux, France

Christian Busser
Lecturer in Phyto-aromatherapy, University of Paris;
Founder of Ecole Plantasanté, Obernai, France

Germany

Anna Maria Hoch
Director of Nursing, Stiftsklinik Augustinum, Munich,
Germany

Greece

Maria G Zorzou
Importer & Distributor of Penny Price Aromatherapy Ltd,
Kallithea, Greece

Iceland

Margrét Alice Birgisdóttir CPD Aromatherapy
Massage therapist, student of Institude of Integrative
Nutrition, Iceland

Ireland

Christine Courtney MIFPA, ITEC A&P, CertEd
Aromatherapy and reflexology tutor and practitioner,
Lucan, Ireland

Japan

Chieko Shiota MIFPA, MIFA
Aromatherapist, Fukuoka, Japan

Netherlands

Anneke Weigel-van der Maas
Aromatherapist, The Netherlands

Norway

Gry Fosstvedt Cand Mag
Founder, Aromedica (Norwegian School of Aromatherapy),
Norway

Päivi Renaa MNNH, Postgrad Dip Complementary Therapies in
Cancer Care
Registered Aromatherapist, Jevnaker, Norway

Portugal

Denise Raines RN
Aromatherapist, The Algarve, Portugal

Switzerland

Eliane Zimmermann
Author and lecturer, AiDA Aromatherapy International,
Ireland

Taiwan

Jen Chang Doctor of Psychology
Principal of Jen Aromatherapy Ltd, Principal of Deva Satya
Energy Essence School Ltd, Taichung City, Taiwan

USA

Lora Cantele RA, CMAIA, CSRT
President, Alliance of International Aromatherapists,
Colorado, USA

E Cristina CMP ACA
Certified massage practitioner, clinical aromatherapist,
Philadelphia, USA

Pam Conrad BSN PGd CCAP
Complementary Therapy Nurse Aromatherapist,
Indianapolis, USA

The health promoting aspect of aromatherapy has been in the ascendant since it began about 40 years ago and has progressed considerably during the last ten years. There is still inadequate training but minimum training standards have been set by professional associations (the Aromatherapy Consortium in the UK). Aromatherapy involves knowledge of a wide range of topics from botany, organic chemistry and essential oil understanding to massage, client care, aroma/mind effects, safety factors and more. Aromatherapy still remains as much an art as a science, which perhaps is not a wholly bad thing. Whilst aromatherapy as a complement to conventional medical treatment has recently made remarkable and significant progress, especially in hospitals, there still remains much to be discovered through research and experience.

Many books on the subject have been written in the past for the lay reader (not all of them completely reliable), each containing more or less the same information gathered from the two or three unreferenced aromatherapy books written before 1985. This has propagated many dubious and incorrect statements, which by repetition unfortunately became accepted. It is only in recent years that books have been written specifically as an aid for those health professionals wishing to practise *therapeutic* aromatherapy safely and effectively. For this reason it is advisable to say a few words on the quality of the information contained in this book.

The Aromatherapy Workbook (Price 1993, 2000) was one of the first aimed at helping student aromatherapists acquire some in-depth knowledge of the physiological and psychological effects of essential oils. The importance of accurately specifying the essential oils employed was stressed, by using the scientific name of the plant in preference to the common name alone. Fragrance and perfumery products were formerly widely used in 'aromatherapy' treatments and undoubtedly still are in some beauty salons, spas, etc. The properties attributed to essential oils were often confounded with plant properties given in old herbals (e.g. Culpeper, Gerard, Turner, Grieve) and these are not necessarily the same.

However, as physiotherapists, occupational therapists and nurses have become increasingly aware of the possibilities of using essential oils in many areas – hospices, hospitals, clinics, day care, residential and community care work – the Editors felt that the time was ripe for a book aimed specifically at health professionals. This feeling was confirmed at lectures and workshops given from 1992 to 1995 at many hospitals throughout Great Britain, S. Ireland and Switzerland where it became clear that many nurses were introducing essential oils into their hospitals without proper knowledge, not having attended an accredited training course. This problem may have arisen because so much aromatherapy course time is concerned with full-body massage, something that is seldom performed by professionals in health care situations because of the time factor. In response to this, the Editors devised an advanced, comprehensive course on aromatology which encompasses all aspects of essential oil use and this has been extremely successful; this is the way forward for professional aromatherapists. This book emphasizes the need to gain extensive knowledge of essential oils before using them on sick people to discourage the incorrect application of these powerful agents, which in some unfortunate instances has led to their use being limited and even banned in some health care settings.

It has been necessary to look at the many references on the properties and actions of essential oils researched in the past, mostly on animals, for the perfume and food industries – unfortunately not specifically for aromatherapy. There is a large body of such information available on some of the antiseptic, antibacterial, antiparasitic and even antiviral properties of essential oils and their effects on the skin but the information is by no means complete; the bulk of it concerns fragrance compounds and isolates and much more research needs to be done using unadulterated essential oils with aromatherapy and health problems in mind. Progress is being made thus it was thought necessary to bring out a fourth edition to

- update information on aspects of essential oils
- introduce recent references

- expand the information on aromatherapy worldwide
- give relevant, current information in the chapters in Section 3 which have been updated by practising aromatherapists and nurses (with aromatherapy training) using essential oils in their own particular field
- add a chapter on the effects of essential oils on grief

The bulk of research done in the past has been *in vitro* or on animals. There is a dearth of information on aspects such as (for example) analgesic and diuretic effects of essential oils, and when it comes to the effects of essential oils on conditions such as bronchitis, arthritis, depression, headaches, etc. there is realistically only anecdotal evidence available. Properly constructed and conducted trials are needed; unfortunately aromatherapists do not normally have the requisite training, the opportunity or the necessary finances to carry out this work.

Every aromatherapist is under pressure today to show efficacy and safety of essential oils and must at the same time care for the needs of clients. Although scientific proof is highly desirable many people needing help with health problems will choose to use complementary medicine despite the lack of it. There is no hard scientific evidence that essential oil therapy can ease the pain of arthritis but after decades of treating sufferers it is beyond question that aromatherapy does help. Clients accept this situation and are content to have pain relief on a daily basis; the fact that it is not scientifically proven does not bother them. Similarly, someone who now has a clear skin in place of a blotchy complexion does not pause to inquire if scientific trials have been carried out.

Empirically derived knowledge must be considered seriously: beneficial experiences repeated over a long period of time form the empirical basis for the therapeutic properties of plant volatile oils and should not be lightly dismissed. In our present day science-based society it is necessary to demonstrate that essentials oils do work but until the necessary proof is forthcoming it would be foolish to discontinue traditional practices.

For this book unreferenced consumer books on aromatherapy have not been used but anecdotal evidence of good quality – in our opinion – has been used where 'scientific' evidence is not available

- where it is in accord with our own experience obtained over four decades of practising and teaching

- from acknowledged sources, some of whom are medical practitioners

It is still true that 'We must be receptive to possibilities that science has not yet grasped. It is absurd not to use treatments that work, just because we do not yet understand them' (Siegel 1988).

There is now an increasing databank of research involving aromatherapy: double blind studies, though desirable, present a difficulty because the presence or absence of an aroma is obvious to the participants. Scientists rely on some animal testing yet is it possible to extrapolate to the human body the results of massive doses on small animals or the effects of essential oils on the entrails of sacrificed animals?

It is incumbent on aromatherapists to carry out such investigation as they are able to determine whether or not essential oils work in particular circumstances and to have a unified system of reporting and sharing information: at the present time this is not in place. Many more trials, projects and single case studies are needed to demonstrate unequivocally the efficacy of these holistic medicines before they can be generally accepted; although past clinical studies in this area were often defective in design and also in outcomes (Lis-Balchin 2010).

The value of anecdotal evidence is questionable due to various factors:

- many illnesses are self-limiting and spontaneously disappear
- the placebo effect
- some are only in the mind of the sufferer and such people are usually open to suggestion
- with some illnesses the sufferer has phases of feeling poorly alternating with phases of feeling well.
- there are also the unexplained 'miraculous' cures which do occasionally happen
- false 'good' results can occur

This book contains guidelines on the preparation of a professionally based policy and protocol to present to hospital management when applying for permission to use essential oils in a health care setting. In those hospitals where the use of essential oils has already been introduced on a correct footing, some trials and projects have been carried out. Although not constituting research in the accepted scientific sense of the word, such studies are extremely valuable for the future acceptance of aromatic medicine. It is hoped that by publicising some of them here, more health professionals will be encouraged to continue the good work.

This book undoubtedly falls short of its goals as do all written texts compiled in a changing world. It is hoped that it will lead those with a genuine interest in essential oils to a better understanding of their properties and possible uses and trust that this book will prove to be of value to all health professionals and their associates.

Shirley and Len Price

References

Lis-Balchin, M., 2010. Aromatherapy with essential oils. In: Baser, K.H.C., Buchbauer, G. (Eds.), Handbook of essential oils: science, technology and applications. CRC Press, Boca Raton, p. 571.

Price, S., 1993. Aromatherapy workbook. Harper Collins, London.

Siegel, B.S., 1988. Love, medicine and miracles. Arrow Books, London, p. 37.

Acknowledgements

The authors wish to thank not only Claire Wilson and Fiona Conn (at Elsevier) for their understanding and help with this 4th edition of their book, but also those who supplied the text for the different applications of aromatherapy in context, in Section 3.

We are indebted to all those enthusiastic people who supplied the text for Chapter 18 – Aromatherapy Worldwide; it was a mammoth task to find contacts in each country and we are only sorry that some countries are not represented – due to not being able to find someone who would know the answers, or was willing to provide them.

Further thanks are due to those aromatherapists who provided new case studies: Maria Zorzou, Nic Gerard, Alan Barker, Muriel Raynes, Debbie Moore, Jane Guscott, Maggie Slaney, Kate Nellist, Christopher Hassall, Sarah Wright, Rachel Clark, Gill Price, and Tracey Dickie. Thanks are also due to them for understanding that their cases were abbreviated and put into a standard format, without mentioning nutrition, etc. and the holistic relationship between client and patient (so necessary in complementary therapies). It has been done simply so that the aromatherapy interventions could be read more easily; no-one is more aware than the Editors that treatments should always aim to rebalance clients at a physical, mental and emotional level.

Section 1

Essential oil science

Section contents

The genesis of essential oils

1

Len Price

CHAPTER CONTENTS

Introduction

Aromatherapy is the use of essential oils, all of which are derived from plants. Anyone wishing to practise aromatherapy must gain as full an understanding of the plants concerned as possible, so that the oils can be used knowledgeably to their best effect. This chapter enables the practitioner to do this, looking beyond the oil in the glass bottle to the plant from which it was extracted, its growing environment and the family to which it belongs.

Botany for aromatherapists

What has botany to do with aromatherapy?

Everyone knows the quotation from Shakespeare's *Romeo and Juliet*: 'What's in a name? That which we call a rose by any other name would smell as sweet.'

What's in a name? The answer when dealing with essential oils is – *everything!*

To be an effective aromatherapist it is crucial to a good outcome that aromatherapeutic-quality essential oils pertinent to the particular client be employed, and to be able to do this the therapist must be able to discriminate between therapeutic-quality oils and those produced for other industries, which is the overwhelming bulk of essential oils produced. To be able to select such oils is not possible unless the therapist has a basic knowledge of some aspects of botany, and in particular the nomenclature used.

> That botany is a useful study is plain; because it is in vain that we know betony is good for headaches, or selfheal for wounds unless we can distinguish betony and self-heal from one another.
>
> John Hill, The Family Herbal (1808)

Taxonomy

In the early 18th century the identification of plants was in a chaotic state, for example John Tradescant brought spiderwort to England from North America and – including his own name after the fashion of the time – named it *Phalangum Ephenerum Virginianum Johannis Tradescanti*.

There was an obvious need for better naming of plants: names that were accurate, unambiguous, concise and part of a universally acknowledged and accepted system.

A good name is rather to be chosen than great riches.

The Bible, Proverbs 22:1

Then along came the Swedish naturalist Carl von Linné or Linnaeus (1707–1778) and changed everything. He devised the binomial system and applied it universally, making the precise nominal identification of plants possible (the spiderworts mentioned above are now known as *Tradescantia andersoniana*, a simple binomial title which is recognized the world over). Binomial means a two-name system; millions of people are differentiated by a family name and an individual personal name; in similar fashion plant names are made up of a generic name and an individual specific descriptive name. Binomials are written in italics and may be followed by the name (perhaps abbreviated) of one or more persons, e.g. *Panax quinquefolius* L: the L stands for Linnaeus, the author of this name for American ginseng. Sometimes there is a double citation (a second botanist) and this means that the plant has been reclassified, the original author being put first, in parentheses; although not essential, this does give an abbreviated bibliographical reference. Over the years the Linnaean system of classifying organisms in groups according to their similarities has been subject to much modification but is still at the core of the international taxonomic system used today.

What is taxonomy? It is a study devoted to producing a system of classification of organisms which best reflects the totality of their similarities and differences. The word taxonomy comes from two Greek words (*taxis* – arrangement and *nomia* – method). Major taxonomic groups of the plant kingdom include categories as follows, and several subgroups:

Kingdom: Plantae
Division: Tracheophyta
Subdivision: Spermatophyta
Class: Dicotyledons
Subclass: Asteridae
Order: Lamiales
Family: Lamiaceae

Genus: *Lavandula*
Species: *angustifolia*

In aromatherapy it is sufficient for identification purposes to know:

- **The family** that the plant belongs to (all family names end in -aceae).
- **The genus:** generic names are based on structural characteristics and are always written in italics with an initial capital letter and can be used alone.
- **The species:** these are adjectival, describing the genus, and are never written with a capital letter, even when it is after a person, e.g. *smithii*: the whole word is in lower-case italics and cannot be used by itself.

Lavender must therefore be referred to by the genus name *Lavandula* and the descriptive adjective *angustifolia* to identify the particular plant (and its essential oil).

However, there are further divisions below this level, such as:

- **Subspecies:** often denotes a geographic variation of a species.
- **Variety:** indicates a rank between subspecies and forma. They are named by adding 'var.' in Roman font and the italicized variety name, e.g. *Citrus aurantium* var. *amara*. The label 'var.' is used to indicate a major subdivision of a species, or a variant of horticultural origin or importance (although these are now labelled cultivar). Many names of horticultural origin reflect the historical use of the variety rank.
- **Forma:** denotes trivial differences.
- **Cultivar:** indicates a cultivated variety, and a rank known only in horticultural cultivation. These names are non-Latinized and in living languages (usually the name of, or chosen by, the originator, in the following case Monsieur Maillette). They are not italicized, and appear within quotation marks, e.g. *Lavandula angustifolia* 'Maillette'.
- **Chemotype:** indicates visually identical plants but having different, perhaps significantly so, chemical components, resulting in different therapeutic properties. Chemotypes occur naturally in plants grown in the wild, some species throwing up many chemical variations; they can be propagated by cuttings for cultivation and they are named by the abbreviation 'ct.' followed by the chemical constituent, e.g. *Thymus vulgaris* ct. thujanol-4, T. *vulgaris* ct.

geraniol, *T. vulgaris* ct. carvacrol, etc. Chemotypes are plants that look the same from the outside, but have different chemical constituents inside. (By contrast, **phenotypes** are plants that look different on the outside but are chemically similar inside.)

- **Hybrid:** indicates natural or artificially produced crosses between species. The name contains 'x' (in Roman font) which means the plant is a hybrid produced by sexual crossing, e.g. *Mentha* x *piperita*, which is a cross between *Mentha aquatica* and *Mentha spicata*.

When procuring and prescribing essential oils therapists must take care to identify precisely the plants from which they are derived, and this means giving not only the generic and specific names but also specifying, where necessary, the chemotype, variety, etc.

Note on pronunciation: aromatherapists are sometimes worried about how to pronounce the Latinized names, but there are no strict rules and almost anything goes! The same names are used throughout the world, but there is a wide variation in pronunciation from country to country, and indeed by individuals within a country.

The genesis of essential oils

Plants are capable of transforming the electromagnetic rays from the sun into energetic substances including a major group of compounds, the terpenes. According to Harborne (1988) more than 1000 monoterpenes and possibly 3000 sesquiterpenes have so far been identified. The phenylpropenes constitute another much smaller but significant group: they always consist of a 3-carbon side chain having a double bond attached to an aromatic ring. In essential oils most of the components belong either to the terpene group, based on the mevalonic acid pathway, or to the phenylpropene group, formed through the shikimic acid pathway.

Synthesis of volatile oils

Photosynthesis is the process by which green plants use the electromagnetic energy of sunlight, absorbed by the chlorophyll in the plant, to drive a series of chemical reactions leading to the formation of carbohydrates. The plant takes up water and minerals from the soil through its roots and carbon dioxide from the air, mainly through its leaves. This whole process is called photosynthesis, and because it is essential to the life of the plant it is termed primary metabolism. All animals, including humans, depend on this photosynthesis because it is the method by which the basic food, sugar, is created.

During the complex reactions of the first, *light reaction* stage of photosynthesis, light energy is used to split water (H_2O) into oxygen (O_2), protons (hydrogen ions H^+) and electrons; the oxidation of water gives rise to free oxygen, a waste product for the plant. In the second, *dark reaction* stage, no light is required and the protons and electrons are used to reduce carbon dioxide, which enters the plant through the stomata, to carbohydrates in the form of simple sugars, providing food for the plant's growth. A complex series of chemical changes occurs, which can be represented by the equation

$$6CO_2 + 12H_2O \rightarrow C_6H_{12}O_6 + 6O_2 + 6H_2O$$

(in this example the formation of glucose).

Simple sugars that provide energy for the plant are stored as starch; glucose is released from starch as and when energy is required.

The elements in sugar (carbon, hydrogen and oxygen) are the same as those in essential oils, but differently grouped, and hundreds of chemicals are produced by the decomposition/glycolysis of sugars with aid of enzymes: enzymes are highly specific and assist in only one particular reaction (as they do in humans). Mevalonic acid goes through phosphorylization, decarboxylation and dehydration to become five-carbon isoprene units, which are the basic building blocks for the terpenes found in essential oils (Fig. 1.1). The phenols are arrived at via a different route – the shikimic acid pathway.

Chemicals produced by plants that do not have an obvious value to the producer plant are known as secondary metabolites; the array of secondary metabolites, which of course includes volatile oils, is enormous (Waterman 1993 p. 31). Secondary metabolism products include alkaloids, bitters, glycosides, gums, mucilages, saponins, steroids, tannins and essential oils, which are not necessary for the vital functions of the plant (see Fig. 1.1), and of these secondary metabolites the essential oils have the greatest commercial significance, being used in many industries (Verlet 1993). Volatile oil secondary

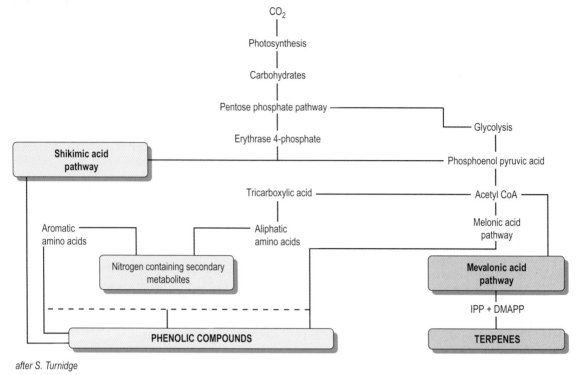

after S. Turnidge

Figure 1.1 • Secondary metabolite synthesis within the plant.

metabolites vary widely in chemical structure and their purpose and function in the plant is little understood.

With genetic techniques, it is now possible to intervene in these pathways and change both the quality and the quantity of essential oils – a prospect which brings new dimensions into the natural balance (Svoboda 2003).

Why does a plant contain essential oil?

Before seeing how an essential oil comes into being, it is worth reflecting on what value essential oils have for plants. This has been debated for many years and there is as yet no definitive answer. However, conjecture on the subject has thrown up many possible reasons:

- To prevent attack by herbivores: both mono- and sesquiterpenes are involved in various ways, such as acting as insect hormones to interfere with the development of the feeding

insects, or having a straightforward repellent action. Essential oils and other secondary metabolites can render plant tissue bitter and unpalatable.

- To prevent attack from insects: it has been shown that the number of oil glands in a plant increases when it is under attack by insects (Carlton 1990, Carlton, Gray & Waterman 1992).
- To prevent attack by bacteria, fungi and other microorganisms: there is ample proof available from studies done in vitro on the antifungal and bactericidal properties of herb volatile oils (see section on aromatograms in Ch. 4).
- To aid pollination by attracting bees and other insects such as moths and bats (Harborne 1988).
- To help in the healing of wounds inflicted on the plant itself.
- To act as an energy reserve.
- To help survival in difficult growth conditions: for instance by the production of allelopathic

compounds, such as 1,8-cineole and camphor, which are freely given off from the plant and find their way to the soil, where they prevent other plants from growing (Deans & Waterman 1993).

- To prevent dehydration and afford some degree of protection in hot dry climates by surrounding the plant with a haze of volatile oil, thus helping to prevent water loss from its foliage. Leaves with a dense covering of glandular hairs can help trap the water molecules that evaporate through the stomata. One of the oldest plants in the world, the leaves of which can be as much as 10% oil by weight, is the eucalyptus. Living root stock of this plant has been found dating back thousands of years to the Ice Age (Dr Mike Crisp, Australian National Botanic Gardens, unpublished information 1986). The free oil vapour emanating from other ancient plants, e.g. pine trees, can be smelt easily when walking in pine forests on a sunny day.

Whatever else essential oils may do, they do give the plant its aroma and flavour and often have a significant physiological effect on people.

Secretory structures

Essential oils and their mixtures with resins and gums are commonly found in special secretory structures. Secretory structures in plants are divided into two main types: those occurring on the plant surfaces, which usually secrete substances directly to the outside of the plant (exogenous secretion), and those which occur within the plant body and secrete substances into specialized intercellular spaces (endogenous secretion) (Svoboda 2003).

Essential oils are synthesized and stored in different sites; they may be found in the leaves, seeds, petals, roots, bark, etc. Sometimes different oils occur in more than one site in a plant; for example, two different oils are produced by the cinnamon tree (bark, leaf), and three different oils by the orange tree (leaf, blossom, peel). The type of secretory structure is a characteristic of a plant family and it is possible to place secretory structures into the following categories:

- Oil cells and resin cells
  - Lauraceae (e.g. cinnamon)
  - Zingiberaceae (e.g. cardamom, ginger, turmeric)
  - Piperaceae (e.g. black pepper)
  - Myristicaceae (e.g. nutmeg)
  - Illiciaceae (e.g. star anise)
- Cavities, sacs, oil reservoirs (schizolysigenous)
  - Rutaceae (e.g. orange)
  - Myrtaceae (e.g. clove, eucalyptus)
- Oil or resin canals, ducts
  - Apiaceae (e.g. dill)
  - Pinaceae (e.g. pine, cedarwood)
  - Burseraceae (e.g. myrrh)
- Glandular hairs, trichomes
  - Lamiaceae (e.g. lavender, rosemary, sage)
  - Asteraceae (e.g. elecampane)
  - Geraniaceae (e.g. geranium)
- Internal hairs
  - Orchidaceae (e.g. vanilla)
- Epidermal cells
  - Essential oils obtained from flowers such as roses are usually not secreted by glandular hairs, but by the actual epidermal cells of the petals. The amount of essential oil in flowers (*Rose, Acacia, Jasminum* sp.) is very low, usually between 0.02 and 0.08% (v/w).
- Isodiametric cells
  - Orchid flower epidermal tissues called osmophores secrete the volatile substances.
- Stigmata
  - Many flowering plants also secrete volatile oils, lipids, sugars and amino acids.
- Tree buds
  - Such as horse chestnut, alder, poplar, cherry, and buckthorn, secrete sticky substances (mucilages); similar tissues also occur on the stipules and the edges of their young leaves (Svoboda 2003).

Chemical variation within species

Chemotype is a term applied to plants of the same genus and species which have the same external appearance but differ, sometimes considerably, in their internal chemical composition. These chemotypes usually occur naturally in plants growing in the wild, and can result partly from cross-pollination. The place and manner of a plant's growing will also promote internal changes: many essential-oil-bearing plants, e.g. rosemary and thyme, are prone to this kind of change owing to genetic and environmental factors. They become resistant to local pests and diseases and have adapted to make the best use of the soil and other surrounding conditions. Such plants are termed 'landrace', and strains which yield specified chemical constituents are sought and selected for propagation by cloning: that is to say, cuttings are taken and then cultivated to produce the specific oils required. Included in this category are the thymes and lavenders flourishing wild on the sunny dry hills of Provence, which are extensively cloned and then grown commercially.

Thyme chemotypes

The thyme plant is particularly prolific in spontaneously producing strains bearing essential oils of different compositions. Some of these are described below:

- *Thymus vulgaris* ct. thymol. The thymol-bearing thyme is strongly antiseptic and aggressive to the skin owing to the presence of the phenol thymol. Cut in the spring, the essential oil contains 30% thymol (Fig. 1.2) plus *para*-cymene (also written *p*-cymene), a monoterpene hydrocarbon. When the same plant is cut in the autumn the essential oil may be found on analysis to contain 60–70% thymol and less *p*-cymene (Table 1.1).
- *Thymus vulgaris* ct. carvacrol. This variant behaves in the same way as the thymol chemotype of thyme, but the phenol involved is carvacrol

Table 1.1 *Thymus vulgaris* chemotypes – variation with season

Chemotype	Spring	Autumn
Thymol	γ-Terpinene + *p*-cymene	Thymol
Carvacrol	γ-Terpinene + *p*-cymene	Carvacrol
Geraniol	Geranyl acetate	Geraniol

(Fig. 1.3). In the spring the essential oil contains 30% carvacrol, which increases to 60–80% in the autumn (Table 1.1).

- The thymol and carvacrol chemotypes do not flourish at high altitudes but are cultivated in the valleys. Both of these phenolic chemotypes are often, although inaccurately, referred to as red thymes (because the now obsolete iron still imparted a red colour to the oil) and they are major anti-infective agents with a wide range of action (Belaiche 1979). For the thyme chemotypes, the harvesting time is crucial in order to obtain the required composition of an essential oil, as the internal chemistry of the plant changes with the seasons (see also Fig. 1.11). Concerning the thymol and carvacrol chemotypes, *p*-cymene is the precursor of both thymol and carvacrol (Table 1.2); at the beginning of the season, in the spring, the plants contain γ-terpinene (Fig. 1.4) and *p*-cymene (Fig. 1.5), but as the season progresses these precursors are transformed into either carvacrol or thymol, so that plants harvested in the autumn yield essential oils containing phenols. Proven by aromatogram, the bacteriostatic effect is useful in avoiding the long-term use of antibiotics, thereby minimizing serious problems: thyme oil, having both bactericidal and bacteriostatic

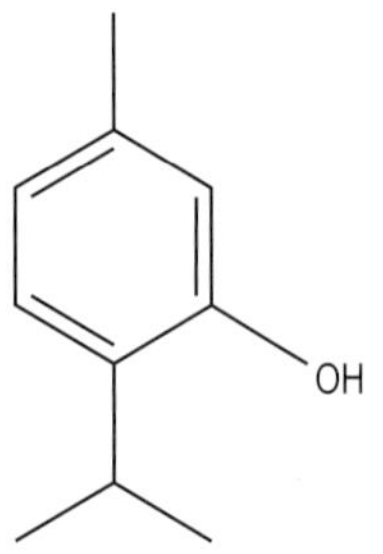

Figure 1.2 • Thymol.

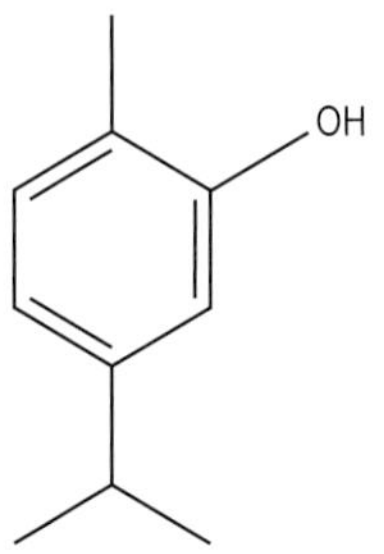

Figure 1.3 • Carvacrol.

Table 1.2 *Thymus vulgaris* chemotypes – variation with stage of growth

	Stage of growth		
	Bud	Flower	End of flowering
Carvacrol	22.8	35.9	53.7
Thymol	5	10.7	13.7
p-Cymene	32.1	22.4	17.8
γ-Terpinene	13.5	7.4	0.9

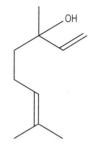

Figure 1.6 • Linalool.

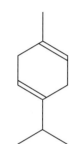

Figure 1.4 • γ-Terpinene

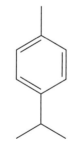

Figure 1.5 • *p*-Cymene.

properties, is in effect a complete antibiotic (Scimeca & Tétau 2009 p. 14).

- The alcohol-containing chemotypes below are commonly referred to as yellow or sweet thymes. These chemotypes do not have the aggressive effects of the red thymes (thymol and carvacrol) and can be used safely on Pénoël Pénoël children, sensitive skins and mucous surfaces (Roulier 1990 p. 305).
- *Thymus vulgaris* ct. linalool. The linalool-bearing thyme has a herbaceous smell and (like the thujanol and terpineol thymes) is grown at high

altitudes. It contains the alcohol linalool (Fig. 1.6) and the ester linalyl acetate, therefore the essential oil from the linalool thyme is gentle in action. This chemotype is antibacterial, fungicidal (e.g. against *Candida albicans*), viricidal, parasiticidal and vermifugal, as well as neurotonic and uterotonic (Franchomme & Pénoël 2001 p. 403).

- *Thymus vulgaris* ct. thujanol-4. In contrast to all the other chemotypes of thyme, the thujanol-4 type does not show seasonal variation in the constitution of the essential oil, but is the same all year round, with a content of 50% of the alcohol *trans*-thujanol-4 (Fig. 1.7), 15% approximately of terpinen-4-ol and 15% approximately of *cis*-myrcenol-8. It is found only in the wild because it has so far resisted all attempts to cultivate it – cloning has not yet been successful, except on a very small scale. It has a floral smell. The oil is anti-infectious, bactericidal (against *Chlamydia*) and a powerful viricide. It stimulates the immune system (by augmenting IgA) and the circulation. It is described as neurotonic, balancing to the nervous system, hormone-like and antidiabetic (Franchomme & Pénoël 2001 p. 432). According to Roulier (1990 p. 305) this oil is a notable hepatic regenerator and is non-irritant.
- *Thymus vulgaris* ct. α–terpineol. The oil from this chemotype contains the ester terpenyl acetate

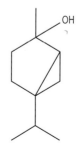

Figure 1.7 • Thujanol-4.

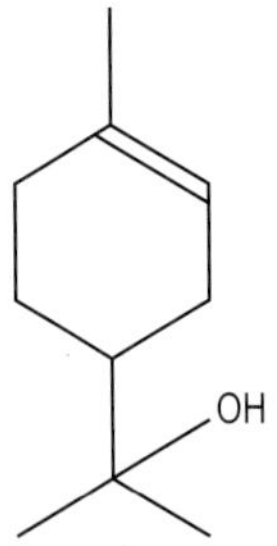

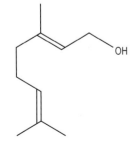

Figure 1.8 • α-Terpineol.

(more so in the spring) and the alcohol α-terpineol (Fig. 1.8) (80–90% free and esterified). The smell is slightly peppery.

- *Thymus vulgaris* ct. geraniol. The geraniol thyme grows at high altitude and the oil contains the ester geranyl acetate and the alcohol geraniol (80–90% in free and esterified forms) (Fig. 1.9); again there is a seasonal variation: the thyme chemotype which produces geraniol in the autumn contains geranyl acetate in the spring and geraniol in the autumn (see Table 1.1). This thyme is very assertive, and when grown in a field of mixed thymes it gradually comes to predominate. It has a lemony smell. (It is interesting to note that the wild *Thymus serpyllum* [creeping thyme] which is found everywhere in the hills, also has a somewhat lemony smell because the geraniol chemotype is dominant and is gradually taking over.) The properties are antiviral, antifungal and antibacterial, also uterotonic, neurotonic and cardiotonic (Franchomme & Pénoël 2001 p. 431). Other *Thymus vulgaris* chemotypes also exist. The cineole-bearing plant has 80–90% 1,8-cineole. According to Franchomme and Pénoël (2001 p. 431), the *p*-cymene chemotype is analgesic when applied to the skin, a notable anti-infectious agent and useful for rheumatism and arthritis.

Figure 1.9 • Geraniol.

Altitude and light

The lower the altitude at which the thyme plant is grown, the more pronounced are the following effects:

- The essential oil becomes more aggressive – more phenolic and antiseptic.
- The colour of the essential oil also changes, from a light straw to a deeper hue.
- The structure of the main component molecule changes from an open chain to a monocyclic chain to an aromatic ring base.

These effects are due in part to the quality of light available to the plant. At high altitudes (above 1000 metres) there is a relatively high amount of free ultraviolet, whereas at low altitudes there is less ultraviolet and a proportional increase in the more penetrating infrared frequencies. The plant responds to the quality of light falling on it (and to other growing conditions) and produces different chemicals accordingly (see Fig. 1.11). Another influencing factor is the latitude of the country of origin. The further north the plant grows, the more phenols are produced – for instance *Thymus vulgaris* grown in Finland produces up to 89% phenol (von Schantz et al. 1987).

More changes may be expected in oil-bearing plants in the future because of chlorofluorocarbon damage to the ozone layer. Higher levels of ultraviolet radiation are expected to reach the surface of the earth, and research carried out to test the possible effects of this on plant growth suggests that alpine species will be least affected by increased ultraviolet radiation. These tests involved *Aquilegia canadensis* and *A. caerulea*. The first normally grows at low altitude and showed less growth during the test, but the second (alpine) plant was not affected in this way: it even grew extra leaves (Gates 1991).

Rosemary chemotypes

Rosemary has three main chemotypes, all of which are used in aromatherapy:

- *Rosmarinus officinalis* ct. camphor (camphor 30%) (Fig. 1.10a) with the properties: mucolytic, cholagogic, diuretic, circulatory decongestant/stimulant (vein), emmenagogic (non-hormonal), muscle relaxant.
- *Rosmarinus officinalis* ct. cineole (1,8-cineole 40–55%) (Fig. 1.10b) whose properties are anticatarrhal, mucolytic, expectorant, fungicidal

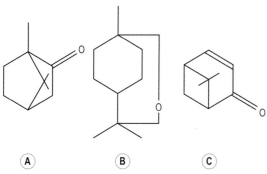

Figure 1.10 • (A) Camphor; (B) 1,8–cineole; (C) verbenone.

(e.g. *Candida albicans*), bactericidal (*Staphylococcus aureus* and *S. alba*).

- *Rosmarinus officinalis* ct. verbenone (Fig. 1.10c) (verbenone 15–40%, α-pinene 15–35%). It is anticatarrhal, expectorant, mucolytic (Roulier 1990 p. 298), antispasmodic, cicatrizant and an endocrine system regulator (Franchomme & Pénoël 2001 p. 431).

In this book the camphor and cineole chemotypes are classed together as having similar effects because more often than not rosemary oil contains similar quantities of cineole and camphor.

Other chemotypes

Some further examples of the many other plants with different chemotype forms are:

- *Artemisia dracunculus* [tarragon] ct. estragole, ct. sabinene (Tucker & Maciarello 1987).
- *Ocimum basilicum* [basil] ct. linalool, ct. estragole, ct. eugenol (Sobti et al. 1978).
- *Salvia officinalis* [sage] ct. thujone, ct. cineole (there is also a thujone-free chemotype) (Tegel 1984, Tucker & Maciarello 1990).
- *Valeriana officinalis* [valerian] ct. valeranone, ct. valeranal, ct. cryptofuranol (Bos, van Putten & Hendricks 1986).
- *Melissa officinalis* [lemon balm] ct. citral, ct. citronellal (Lawrence 1989).

See also Figs 1.11a and 1.11b

Lavender

Three lavenders are described below:

- *Lavandula angustifolia* contains mainly alcohols and esters. It is a calming oil recommended to

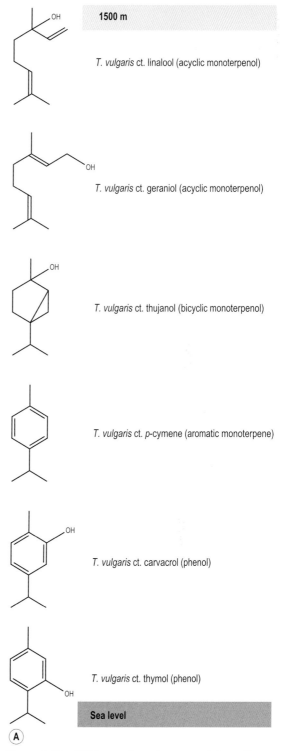

1500 m

T. vulgaris ct. linalool (acyclic monoterpenol)

T. vulgaris ct. geraniol (acyclic monoterpenol)

T. vulgaris ct. thujanol (bicyclic monoterpenol)

T. vulgaris ct. p-cymene (aromatic monoterpene)

T. vulgaris ct. carvacrol (phenol)

T. vulgaris ct. thymol (phenol)

Sea level

(A)

Figure 1.11 • (A) Thyme chemotypes – variation with altitude. Courtesy of J Lamy.

Continued

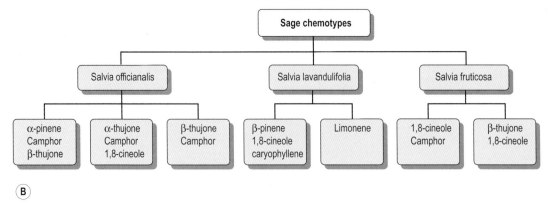

Figure 1.11, cont'd • (B) Sage chemotypes. After Franz and Novak 2010.

induce sleep. However, an overdose has the opposite effect – another pointer to the importance of using these potent oils correctly. It has been recommended for respiratory ailments, asthma, spasmodic cough (whooping cough), influenza, bronchitis, tuberculosis and pneumonia (Valnet 1980) on account of its anti-inflammatory properties.

- *Lavandula latifolia* [spike lavender] (syn. *L. spica*) is a much bigger plant, with larger florets than true lavender. It contains very few esters and is slightly lower in alcohol content also, containing instead about 30% of the oxide 1,8-cineole and about 15% of the ketone camphor. It is an efficient expectorant and is also indicated for severe burns (Franchomme & Pénoël 2001 p. 392) because it is well tolerated on all parts of the skin surface. It is especially useful in chest and throat infections, whether for children or for adults (Roulier 1990 p. 276).

- *Lavandula stoechas* contains about 75% ketones, of which almost two-thirds are fenchone. It shares some properties with the previous two, being anticatarrhal, anti-inflammatory and cicatrizant. This plant, sometimes known as Spanish lavender, sometimes as French lavender, is believed to be the one used by the Romans in their baths which gave rise to the name lavender, but has never been cultivated commercially (Meunier 1985). It is not easily available, which is perhaps fortunate because it is sometimes confused with true lavender (*L. angustifolia*) which is almost free of ketones. The effects of *L. stoechas* can be found in many other, safer oils.

Clones of lavender and lavandin

True lavender grown from seed is properly called *Lavandula angustifolia* Miller (syn. *L. officinalis*, *L. vera*). When grown from seed it is described as 'population'. Many cultivated lavender plants are cloned, i.e. not grown from seed but grown from cuttings selected from the hardiest, healthiest, most colourful and biggest plants with a high yield of good-quality oil, the name of probably the most popular clone nearest to true lavender being *L. angustifolia* 'Maillette'.

Unlike population plants, which being grown from seed are much richer in their array of constituents, clones contain only the constituents found in the source plant, and this lack of complexity of composition renders them more liable to disease. For aromatherapy purposes the volatile oil is of a lesser quality, although perhaps the oil from cloned plants is of a more consistent quality from year to year.

Lavandins

Lavandin is the natural hybrid between *L. angustifolia* Miller and *L. latifolia* Medicus. The resulting plant has been given many taxonomical classifications, such as *Lavandula x burnatii* 'Briq.', *Lavandula spica–latifolia* 'Albert', *Lavandula x hortensis* 'Hy', *Lavandula x leptostachya* 'Pau', etc. All these are in common use along with other names – Duraffourd (1982 p. 77) calls it *Lavandula fragrans*. This confused state of affairs prompted Tucker (1981) to research the situation and he reported that the correct name for lavandin is *Lavandula x intermedia* 'Emeric' ex 'Loiseleur', which covers all the lavandin cultivars, and *Lavandula* x *intermedia* is the name used in this book. The 'x' in the names above indicates that the plant is a hybrid or cross-pollinated plant and should not be mistaken for a variety of true lavender. Lavandin plants occur naturally, but cultivators have attempted for many years to find a plant that combines the oil yield of *L. latifolia* with the aromatic quality of *L. angustifolia*. As a result hundreds of lavandins have been created, many with little or no benefit, and there are numerous cultivars currently grown, including *L.* x *intermedia* 'Abrialis', *L.* x *intermedia* 'Super', *L.* x *intermedia* 'Grosso' and *L.* x *intermedia* 'Reydovan'. Although the Abrialis clone is deteriorating after long use, other cultivars are now producing large quantities of lavandin oil. All cultivated lavandin plants are grown from cuttings – they are all clones.

When lavandin is used, especially in clinical trials, it is imperative to specify the particular clone. The two clones of lavandin most used in aromatherapy are:

- *L.* x *intermedia* 'Reydovan': principally antibacterial, antifungal and antiviral, it is also a nerve tonic and expectorant.
- *L.* x *intermedia* 'Super' (sometimes known under other names): this is calming, sedative and anti-inflammatory. It seems to display many of the properties of true lavender and it is widely produced. It was this oil which was used by Buckle (1993) along with true lavender in tests on cardiac patients; the oil from this cultivar of lavandin was found to be more effective than oil of lavender in this instance.

Human factors in plant change

It is not only nature that brings about changes in the chemicals produced in a plant: farmers have an influence too. The use of chemicals in the form of artificial fertilizers influences some of the plant's secondary metabolites, but has little effect on the essential oils. These are composed in the main of carbon, hydrogen and oxygen, whereas fertilizers are made up of nitrogen, phosphates and potassium. However, as fertilizers cause an increase in plant growth, there may be an overall gain in the yield of essential oil.

Herbicides, pesticides and heavy metals are absorbed by the plant, and the more pesticides are absorbed, the more they appear as residue. A safe level of residue may be regarded as 2 mg (per) 1 kg of dry material. Some safe herbicides are decomposed in the plant, but still add to the residue levels. In Europe, toxic pesticides are prohibited, but unfortunately they are still manufactured and sent to developing countries (Wabner 1993). Although heavy metals do not pass over in the steam distillation process many herbicide and pesticide molecules are similar in size to volatile oil molecules and can end up in essential oils, although it is not clear how many are taken into distilled oil. Toxic residues are easily transferred to expressed oils, absolutes and vegetable oils, which makes it necessary to know the source and the manner of growing of such oils before using them therapeutically.

Wabner (1993) concludes that 'aromatherapy is much safer than eating' because 'no clear-cut correlation has been established between pesticide residues in oils and detrimental effects on the human organism' and 'essential oils are used in much smaller quantities and much less frequently than food products'. This article emphasizes the fact that health professionals should purchase their oils for therapeutic use from a trusted supplier, who knows where to procure high-quality, pesticide-free, unadulterated essential oils and fixed vegetable oils, especially the latter, as they normally make up 95% or more of any blend for use on the skin.

Yield of essential oils

Many factors affect the yield, in terms of both quantity and quality, of an essential oil. Some are under the control of the farmer, e.g. time of harvest, chemicals used and plant selection, and others are more or less beyond control, e.g. available light, altitude, temperature and rain (although drought can be remedied by use of a watering system).

Essential oils are not spread equally throughout all parts of the plant, and the quantity of essential oil varies throughout the growing season to such a degree that the time of harvesting, even to the time of day, can have a critical effect on the quantity and quality of the essential oil derived (Fig. 1.12).

The farmer may have to face the fact that the time of maximum yield of essential oil may not coincide with the quality required. This is especially so when the oils are intended for therapeutic use, when compromise on quantity against quality cannot be accepted.

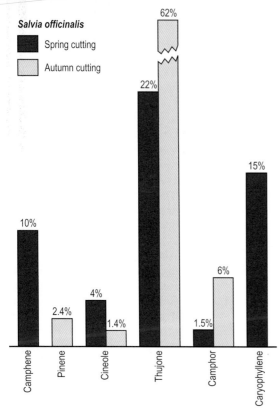

Figure 1.12 • Variation in sage oil constituents with season.

Plant families which produce essential oils

Plants are divided into families, and it is generally recognized that familial therapeutic characteristics may be ascribed to many of the individual plants in a particular family, e.g. the beneficial influence on the digestive system of the citrus oils, or the warming action of oils from the ginger family. There can also be toxic familial effects, as with the Solanaceae and Apiaceae. Several hundred plant essential oils have been identified worldwide. Many are not commercially available, either because the yield of distilled oil is so small that the cost is prohibitive (as in the case of lime blossom oil) or because there is no commercial demand for them. Between 40 and 60 essential oils are normally used by the professional aromatherapist, and most suppliers offer in the region of 70–80. These oils generally belong to just a few of the many plant families, and the families dealt with below include the majority of plants harvested for the production of essential oils.

In the text below, the common names have been used, since to name each species or variety is not necessary when giving general familial characteristics. The botanical name will be used when talking about a specific essential oil. Where only one oil from a family is used in aromatherapy, no family characteristics will be given, only the therapeutic properties of that individual oil. Where there are several oils in a family, only the family properties will be given. The list is not comprehensive – the main purpose in this book is to make health professionals aware of the principal beneficial essential oils. Specific individual properties, indications and composition of about 100 essential oils can be found in Appendix A (see CD-ROM).

Reference sources for the properties and effects of the essential oils mentioned below are as follows: Bardeau (1976), Bernadet (1983), Duraffourd (1982), Franchomme & Pénoël (2001), Lautié & Passebecq (1984), Mailhebiau (1989), Roulier (1990), Willem 2002, Scimeca & Tétau 2009. Other references are mentioned individually.

Angiospermae

Because they bear seeds, all the plants used to obtain essential oils belong to the Spermatophyta subdivision. The vast majority also belong to the class Angiospermae, or flowering plants.

Anonaceae

This family consists of only one species, *Cananga odorata*, with two varieties, of which ylang ylang is one (*C. odorata* forma *genuina*). Distillation is carried out in several stages, and the resulting oils (superior, extra and grades one, two and three) each have a slightly different make-up and aroma and consequently a variation in effect. It is not easy to procure the complete oil, which would be preferable for the holistic aspect of aromatherapy (Price 2000). *C. odorata* is anti-inflammatory, antispasmodic, hypotensive, sedative and a tonic to the pancreas.

Apiaceae

Examples include aniseed, caraway, coriander, dill and fennel. In this family the oils are usually extracted from the seeds, which are renowned for their digestive properties. They have been used in digestive and aperitif drinks and consumed for centuries with bread, and as an accompaniment to cheeses such as Munster. Apiaceae therapeutic qualities are aromatic, carminative, stimulating, tonic and warming when grown naturally in dry regions. It should be noted that this family is also known as the hemlocks. If grown in the shade or humid regions a narcotic principle can develop (particularly so for green anise), and many of the oils in this family are neurotoxic because of the presence of particular ketones or phenolic ethers.

Asteraceae

Examples include *Calendula officinalis* (only available macerated in a fixed oil), the chamomiles, tagetes and tarragon. The essential oils from plants in the Asteraceae are taken from the flower heads. In the case of calendula they are macerated in a fixed oil – not distilled, so the fixed oil also contains larger non-volatile plant molecules, including some coloured molecules. Two of the main characteristics of essential oils in this family are their anti-inflammatory and antiseptic actions on the skin and digestive tract, notably oils from the chamomiles. Many toxic oils come from this family, e.g. the artemisias, which contain a high percentage of ketones or phenolic ethers. *Tagetes glandulifera* also contains a ketone (tagetone) at 50% and should be used with caution.

Burseraceae

Examples include frankincense (olibanum) and myrrh. These two are available as distilled oils and as resinoids, but the distilled oils are required for therapeutic use. The family has cicatrizant properties, indicating their use for scar tissue, ulcers and wounds. They are also expectorant, and useful in catarrhal conditions. *Boswellia carteri* [frankincense] is also indicated in the treatment of depression, immune system deficiency and perhaps cancer (Franchomme & Pénoël 2001 p. 356).

Cupressaceae and Pinaceae

Examples include cypress, juniper (Cupressaceae), pine and cedar (Abietaceae). The chief common characteristics of essential oils derived from plants in these two families of the conifer order are their good general hygienic qualities, particularly in the air and on the skin. Cedar, cypress and juniper also have specific individual properties for urinary tract infections, the circulatory system and scalp maladies (Rouvière & Meyer 1983 p. 7). Thuja belongs to the Pinaceae, but is not used in aromatherapy because of its toxic high ketone content. These two families are noted for their beneficial effects on the respiratory system.

Geraniaceae

The oil utilized from this small family comes from one or two species belonging to the genus *Pelargonium*. The essential oil of *Pelargonium graveolens* [geranium] has anti-inflammatory, astringent, cicatrizant and haemostatic properties and is antidiabetic (Valnet 1980 p. 133).

Gymnospermae

The Gymnospermae display their seeds directly, rather than hiding them within a structure of petals. The important oil-bearing plants of this class belong to the order Coniferae (cone-bearing plants).

Lamiaceae

This is by far the biggest family from which essential oils are gained; examples include basil, clary, hyssop, lavandin, lavender, marjoram, melissa, origanum, patchouli, peppermint, rosemary, sage, savory and thyme. Of all the families in the plant kingdom none offers a greater array of healing aromatic plants than the Lamiaceae. These plants are strongly aromatic owing to the volatile essence stored in special glandular trichomes, which are found principally on the leaves. In general the Lamiaceae produce both relaxing and stimulating essential oils, which bring vigour and energy to the whole body (or sometimes to just one system in particular, e.g. the respiratory system). They have remarkable antiseptic and antispasmodic properties and some are also emmenagogic and sudorific. Oils derived from the Lamiaceae are generally safe, with one or two possible exceptions such as *Salvia officinalis* [sage] and *Hyssopus officinalis* [hyssop], both of which contain ketones (thujone and pinocamphone, respectively) and could theoretically be neurotoxic in overdose. Ingestion of large quantities of these two oils can lead to serious disorders, as pointed out by the Centre Anti-poisons de Marseille (Rouvière & Meyer 1983 p. 6).

Many of the plants in this family have been in constant culinary use for thousands of years, not only to add flavour but for their preservative and health-giving properties as well. The use and ingestion of herbs and their essential oils in small doses over such a long period of time proves their fundamental safety.

Lauraceae

Examples include cinnamon and camphor. Members of this family generally have a pleasant aroma, sometimes strong and penetrating, a warm pungency, and are sometimes bitter. All the oils are considered to be uplifting in their effects (Rouvière & Meyer 1983 p. 7). However, the majority of the family are highly toxic (e.g. cassia, laurel and sassafras), and they will not be recommended in this book because similar therapeutic properties can be found in other, safer oils. Even when they are not actually dangerous, these oils all need expertise and extra care in use.

Myrtaceae

Examples include cajuput, eucalyptus, niaouli, clove and tea tree. The essential oils from this family are contained in cells in the body of the leaf. They are powerful antiseptics (especially to the respiratory system) as well as being antiviral, astringent, stimulant and tonic.

It is advisable to use them with caution as they can be irritant. This is particularly so of clove and adulterated niaouli. It is worth mentioning that the latter oil is adulterated more often than not and will not have the desired therapeutic effect unless effort has been made to obtain a genuine oil. Rectified *Eucalyptus globulus* [Tasmanian blue gum] is irritant because the natural balance has been destroyed. It can be identified because the rectification process renders it clear, and unfortunately very little of the eucalyptus oil harvest escapes this fate.

Oleaceae

Jasminum officinale is a well-loved oil, but a steam-distilled essential oil does not exist and the absolute is subject to the most deplorable adulteration. 'A large number of synthetic materials, some of them chemically related to the jasmones...are of great help... to reproduce the much wanted jasmine effect at a much lower cost.... Jasmine absolute is frequently adulterated. Its high cost seems to tempt certain suppliers and producers beyond their moral resistance' (Arctander 1960 pp. 310–311). This makes jasmine absolute unsuitable for use on the skin, and if it is to be used therapeutically at all (it is sometimes used as a relaxant on account of its aroma) then only the finest quality should be procured. Jasmine extracts are not used by the authors.

Piperaceae

Examples include black pepper and cubeb. *Piper nigrum* is the more used of the two oils and possesses analgesic, anticatarrhal, expectorant, stimulant and tonic properties.

Poaceae

Examples include citronella, lemongrass, palmarosa and vetiver. Most of this family have anti-inflammatory and tonic properties, *Vetivera zizanioides* [vetiver] also being stimulating to the immune system (Franchomme & Pénoël 2001 p. 433). Oils from this family, together with lemon and/or grapefruit oil, are used to make cheap 'melissa' oil.

Rosaceae

The only essential oil utilized from this family is rose otto, whose aroma is less sweet than the absolute oil obtained by solvent extraction. Strictly speaking, only the distilled oil should be used by health professionals (see comments on *J. officinale* above, which also apply to rose otto). Rose otto has astringent, antihaemorrhagic, cicatrizant, hormonal and neurotonic properties.

Rutaceae

Citrus oils are derived from three different sites in the plant. These are:

• **Peel:** bergamot, grapefruit, lemon, mandarin and orange; to obtain citrus peel oils for aromatherapy the rinds are not distilled, but mechanically expressed. They are therefore not strictly essential oils and are more properly described as essences. They contain large molecules which would not come over in distillation, including colour and waxes, and the latter can precipitate if the oils are stored incorrectly or kept for a long time; the waxes do no harm and may be removed by filtration. Citrus essences are especially susceptible to oxidation and the precious active aldehydes may degrade into acids; to help prevent this nitrogen gas is used to displace the air as the oil is decanted. For small bottles, the air can be displaced with tiny glass beads as the level of the oil goes down with use. Expressed oils from the citrus family have a refreshing aroma and are antiseptic, stimulating and tonic, having significant effects on the whole of the digestive tract. This is especially true of bergamot and bitter orange, which are stomach antispasmodics. These two are also sedative to the nervous system.

- **Leaf:** petitgrain essential oils, mainly from the bitter orange, but occasionally from other citrus trees. Petitgrain bigarade from the bitter orange tree (bigarade means 'bitter') is indicated for infected acne.
- **Flower:** neroli, mainly from the bitter orange tree for therapeutic purposes: neroli bigarade is indicated for varicose veins and haemorrhoids, and is also a hypotensor. (NB neroli is expensive; beware of cheaper substitutes.)

Both leaf and flower oils from *Citrus aurantium* [orange] are obtained by distillation and their aroma is sweeter and more floral than that of the peel oils. The best leaf and flower oils are obtained from the bitter orange, *C. aurantium* var. *amara*: both of these oils are effective on the nervous system, relieving irritability and promoting sleep (Mailhebiau 1989 pp. 269–270).

Styracaceae

The only extracts from this family which are of interest to aromatherapists are the resinoids from *Styrax tonkinensis* and *S. benzoin* (both have the common name benzoin). This resinoid is anticatarrhal and expectorant. It is also cicatrizant, promoting healing on cracked and dry skin. Care should be taken when purchasing this oil: some sources abroad still use benzene as a solvent (forbidden in Europe), and a high proportion of benzene may remain in the final product.

Valerianaceae

Examples include valerian and spikenard. The general family effects are calming and sedative, and they are helpful in the reduction of varicose veins and haemorrhoids. The true oil is very difficult to obtain.

Verbenaceae

Aloysia triphylla (= *Lippia citriodora*) [lemon verbena] is rarely obtainable; like jasmine it is frequently grossly adulterated, and *Thymus hiemalis* is often sold in its place as Spanish verbena (Arctander 1960 pp. 648–649).

Summary

Traditionally, plants have been the main source of materials to maintain health and prevent ill health, and it is only comparatively recently that they have been replaced by synthetics. The study of plant structure and function should not be regarded simply as an interesting but inessential requirement for aromatherapy. The more knowledgeable therapists are about the exact botanical derivation of the oils used, the more effective they can be in practice.

References

Arctander, S., 1960. Perfume and flavour materials of natural origin. Elizabeth, New Jersey Published by the author.

Bardeau, F., 1976. La médecine aromatique. Laffont, Paris.

Belaiche, P., 1979. Traité de phytothérapie et d'aromathérapie vol.1, Maloine, Paris, p. 93.

Bernadet, M., 1983. La phyto–aromathérapie pratique. Dangles, St–Jean–de–Braye.

Bos, R., van Putten, F.M.S., Hendriks, H., 1986. Variations in the essential oil content and composition in individual plants obtained after breeding experiments with a Valeriana officinalis strain. In:

Brunke, E.J. (Ed.), Progress in essential oil research. W de Gruyter, Hamburg, pp. 223–230.

Buckle, J., 1993. Does it matter which lavender essential oil is used? Nurs. Times 89 (20), 32–35.

Carlton, R.R., 1990. An investigation into the rapidly induced responses of Myrica gale to insect herbivory.

University of Strathclyde Unpublished PhD Thesis.

Carlton, R.R., Gray, A.I., Waterman, P. G., 1992. The antifungal activity of the leaf gland oil of sweet gale (Myrica gale). Chemecology 3, 55–59.

Deans, S.G., Waterman, P.G., 1993. Biological activity of volatile oils. In: Hay, R.K.M., Waterman, P.G. (Eds.), Volatile oil crops. Longman, Harlow, pp. 100–101.

Duraffourd, P., 1982. En forme tous les jours. La Vie Claire, Périgny.

Franchomme, P., Pénoël, D., 2001. L'aromathérapie exactement, third ed Jollois, Limoges.

Franz, C., Novak, J., 2010. Sources of essential oils. In: Başer, K.H.C, Buchbauer, G (Eds.), Handbook of essential oils: science, technology and applications. CRC Press, Boca Raton, p. 43.

Gates, P., 1991. Gardening in tomorrow's world. Gardener's World (July), 4.

Harborne, J.B., 1988. Introduction to ecological biochemistry. Academic Press, London.

Hill, J., 1808. The family herbal. Brightly & Kinnersley.

Lautié, R., Passebecq, A., 1984. Aromatherapy. Thorsons, Wellingborough.

Lawrence, B.M., 1989. Progress in essential oils. Perfumer and Flavorist 14 (3), 71.

Mailhebiau, P., 1989. La nouvelle aromathérapie. Vie Nouvelle, Toulouse.

Meunier, C., 1985. Lavandes et lavandins. Edisud, Aixen–Provence.

Price, S., 2000. The aromatherapy workbook. Thorsons, London, pp. 119–120.

Roulier, G., 1990. Les huiles essentielles pour votre santé. Dangles, St–Jean–de–Braye.

Rouvière, A., Meyer, M.C., 1983. La santé par les huiles essentielles. M A Editions, Paris.

Scimeca, D., Tétau, M., 2009. Votre santé par les huiles essentielles. Alpen Editions, Monaco.

Sobti, S.N., Pushpangadan, P., Thapa, R.K., Aggarwal, S.G., Vashist, V.N., Atal, C.K., 1978. Chemical and genetic investigations in essential oils of some Ocimum species, their F1 hybrids and synthesised allopolyploids. Lloydia 41, 50–55.

Svoboda, K., 2003. Secrets of plant life. Essence 2 (2), 6–11 Autumn.

Tegel, C., 1984. Morphologische und chemische Variabilität sowie Anbau und Verwendung von Salvia sp (Salbei). Technical University of Munich Unpublished MSc Thesis.

Tucker, A.O., 1981. The correct name of lavandin and its cultivars (Labiatae). Baileya 21, 131–133.

Tucker, A.O., Maciarello, M.J., 1987. Plant identification. In: Simon, J.E., Grant, L. (Eds.), Proceedings of the first national herb growing and marketing conference. Purdue University Press, West Lafayette, pp. 341–372.

Tucker, A.O., Maciarello, M.J., 1990. Essential oils of cultivars of Dalmatian sage (Salvia officinalis L). Journal of Essential Oil Research 2, 139–144.

Valnet, J., 1980. The practice of aromatherapy. Daniel, Saffron Walden.

Verlet, N., 1993. Commercial aspects. In: Hay, R.K.M., Waterman, P.G. (Eds.), Volatile oil crops. Longman, Harlow, p. 144 Ch. 8.

von Schantz, M., Holm, Y., Hiltunen, R., Galambosi, B., 1987. Arznei– und Gewürzpflanzenversuche zum Anbau in Finnland. Dtsch. Apoth. Ztg. 127, 2543–2548.

Wabner, D., 1993. Purity and pesticides. Int. J. Aromather. 5 (2), 27–29.

Waterman, P.G., 1993. The chemistry of volatile oils. In: Hay, R.K.M., Waterman, P.G. (Eds.), Volatile oil crops; their biology, biochemistry and production. Longman Scientific, Harlow.

Willem, J.P., 2002. Les huiles essentielle: médicine de l'avenir. Dauphin, Paris.

Bibliography

Bailey, L.H., 1963. How plants get their names. Dover, New York.

Foster, S., 1979. Latin binomials: learning to live with the system. Well–Being 48 (Dec), 41–42.

Foster, S. (Ed.), 1992. Herbs of commerce. American Herbal Products Association, Austin.

Foster, S., 1993. Herbal renaissance. Gibbs Smith, Salt Lake City International Code of Botanical Nomenclature.

Jeffrey, C., 1977. Biological nomenclature. Crane Russack, New York.

Stern, W.T., 1983. Botanical Latin. David & Charles, Newton Abbot.

Tippo, O., Stern, W.L., 1977. Humanistic botany. Norton, New York.

Chemistry of essential oils

2

Len Price

CHAPTER CONTENTS

Introduction

For the optimum practice of aromatherapy it is desirable to have at least a basic understanding of the chemistry of the essential oils so as to select their use in a safer, more effective way – not randomly or indiscriminately. Such understanding reveals that while isolated chemicals have certain effects, there is no simple relationship between the effects of isolated components and the effects of the synergistic totality of the complete oil. These complex relationships are little understood because hundreds, even thousands, of different chemical compounds are involved, and many of them are unidentified. Until such time as more is discovered about the interaction of the plant chemicals within the human body, suffice it to say that knowledge of the basic composition of each oil contributes to the overall knowledge of aromatherapists, thereby promoting confidence and aiding selection of the oils to be used. Adams and Taylor (2010) write that 'based on the wealth of existing chemical and biological data on the constituents of essential oils and similar data on essential oils themselves, it is possible to validate a constituent based safety evaluation of an essential oil. Fundamentally it is the interaction between one or more molecules in the natural product and macromolecules (proteins, enzymes, etc.) that yield the biological response'. In order to reap the benefits of essential oils it is not essential to know chemistry, but some understanding of their composition will enable more effective use, and often a little knowledge of chemistry will enable aromatherapists to respond to health professionals with a technical background who will inevitably pose questions.

The list of the physiological and pharmacological properties of aromatic molecules encompasses almost all the organs and all the functions of the organism, from skin conditions to psychological disturbances. Chemists have identified more than 3000 different molecules found in essential oils, and new ones are continually being discovered. Fortunately, these molecules are gathered in main groups, with a general relationship between the chemical function and the pharmacological activities. Although we use whole essential oils and not isolated molecules, it is necessary to undertake the study not only of the classes of molecules but also of a few important individual molecules and possible actions.

Essential oil components

It is not the intention to give a lesson in organic chemistry in this book, but a brief explanation of the building blocks which go to make up essential oils will be helpful to the therapist. Carbon, hydrogen and oxygen are essential to life itself, and these three atoms are contained in every essential oil. They combine naturally in countless numbers of ways to make up terpenic and terpenoid compounds such as hydrocarbons, alcohols, aldehydes, ketones, acids, phenols, esters, coumarins and furanocoumarins. The name terpene here conveys the meaning of a compound made up entirely of carbon and hydrogen atoms, and the name terpenoid means a molecule which includes the oxygen atom in addition.

Terpene compounds

All terpenes are hydrocarbons that consist only of carbon and hydrogen atoms, and they are almost always easily recognizable from their name: all end in -ene. Terpenes, so named by Kekulé because of their occurrence in turpentine oil (Kubecka 2010), are hydrocarbons arranged in a chain, which can be either straight, perhaps with branches, or cyclic. Within the plant, the starting point for the terpenes is acetyl coenzyme A (acetyl coA) from which is formed six-carbon mevalonic acid. This is then modified to the five-carbon unit commonly known as the isoprene unit (Fig. 2.1), which occurs in two unsaturated forms: IPP (isopentenyl pyrophosphate)

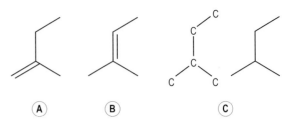

Figure 2.1 • Isoprene unit. (A) IPP; (B) DMAPP; (C) isoprene carbon skeleton.

(Fig. 2.1a) and DMAPP (dimethylallyl pyrophosphate) (Fig. 2.1b). This isoprene unit comprised of five carbon atoms does not exist on its own but is the basic building block for terpenes and is shown diagrammatically as a saturated chain (Fig. 2.1c) for the sake of simplicity, as used later in the book, but it must be borne in mind that it is in fact unsaturated.

Monoterpenes

Two isoprene units joined together head to tail form the basis of all monoterpenes (therefore monoterpene hydrocarbons have 10 carbon atoms arranged in a chain) (Fig. 2.2a). Sometimes a chain can, as it were, loop round on itself (Fig. 2.2b) and give the appearance of a ring, although it is still a 10-carbon chain. When this looping occurs, the terpene is said to be monocyclic, because one circle has been created, and therefore the complete description is monocyclic monoterpene. More than one circle can arise in a chain, so that it is possible to have bicyclic and tricyclic monoterpenes. If they do not form a circle at all (i.e. if they form a straight chain) they are said to be acyclic (as in

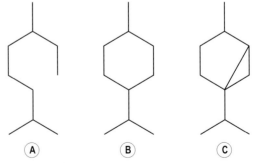

Figure 2.2 • Monoterpenes: two isoprene units join to form a monoterpene. (A) An acyclic monoterpene; (B) a monocyclic monoterpene; (C) a bicyclic monoterpene (thujane).

Fig. 2.2a). Not enough is yet understood about the pharmacological effects of these compounds in essential oils in order to know how these variations in structure may modify the effect. Further complexity arises when double bonds are added (by oxidation) or subtracted (by reduction).

Monoterpenes constitute the most commonly oc-curring kind of terpene in plant volatile oils and are formed, as stated above, from two isoprene units and so contain 10 carbon atoms; sesquiterpenes are formed from three isoprene units and have 15 carbon atoms; and diterpenes are made up of four isoprene units with 20 carbon atoms. Molecules larger than this do not occur in essential oils because the molec-ular weight exceeds the limit imposed by the distill-ation process.

Generally speaking, terpenes are the least active, albeit the most numerous, of all components which occur to a lesser or greater (usually) degree in all in essential oils, and they tend to be regarded by some as being merely inert fillers. While it is true that the effects of terpenes on the human system are not very great, that is not to say that specific molecules do not have their uses, and a few examples are given below.

Effects of monoterpenes

They are all slightly antiseptic, bactericidal, and may also be analgesic, expectorant and stimulat-ing (Franchomme & Pénoël 2001 pp. 239–244, Roulier 1990 p. 51), and they may also play an important part in the quenching effect mentioned earlier, thus making fragrance quality oils which have had the terpenes partially or totally removed (deterpenated oils) unsuitable for aromatherapeutic purposes.

The limonene found in citrus oils quenches the skin-irritant properties of the citrals, as can readily be seen by the fact that deterpenized lemon oil is four or five times as irritant to the skin as whole lemon oil; others are recently thought to be possible antitumour agents, some stimulate the circulation, etc., and it is undeniable that pine oils, with their rich content of terpenes, are good as air antiseptics, etc.; moreover pine oils appear to have a hormone-like effect on the suprarenal glands. The aromatic monoterpene *p*-cymene occurs in numerous essential oils and is known to be analgesic on the skin. The essential oil of *Cupressus sempervirens*, which may be up to 70%

monoterpenes, is an anti-inflammatory agent by immunomodulating action (Franchomme & Pénoël 2001 p. 243).

Sesquiterpenes

Three isoprene units provide the basic structure for the larger molecules known as sesquiterpenes (sesquiter-pene hydrocarbons have 15 carbon atoms) (Fig. 2.3).

As well as the antiseptic and bactericidal proper-ties mentioned above, the sesquiterpenes as a class are said to be anti-inflammatory, calming, and slight hypotensors; some are analgesic (e.g. germacrene) and/or spasmolytic.

Diterpenes

Four isoprene units joined together are called diter-penes (diterpenic hydrocarbons have 20 carbon atoms) (Fig. 2.4), and are not often met with in steam-distilled oils because they are almost too heavy to come over in the distillation process – only a very few manage it.

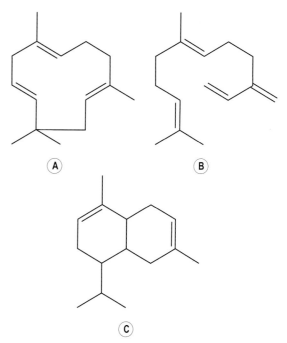

Figure 2.3 • Sesquiterpenes: three isoprene units join to form a sesquiterpene. (A) An acyclic sesquiterpene (α-humulene); (B) a monocyclic sesquiterpene (*trans*-β-farnesene); (C) a bicyclic sesquiterpene (α-cadinene).

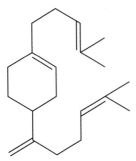

Figure 2.4 • Diterpenes: four isoprene units join to form a diterpene. This figure shows a monocyclic diterpene (α-camphorene).

Diterpenes are believed to have the further properties of being expectorant and purgative, and some are antifungal and antiviral.

Terpenes have a reputation for causing skin irritation (perhaps this is unjust, as so many oils are adulterated with turpentine, polyethylene glycol, white spirit, isolated terpenes etc., and not everyone is as careful as they should be when procuring their essential oils), but if irritation does occur then application of a fixed oil brings swift relief.

Terpenoids

When hydrocarbons – molecules consisting of only carbon and hydrogen – have oxygen added they are described as being terpenoid. With the addition of various oxygen-containing active groups to a compound, numerous alcohols, ketones, aldehydes and esters are formed and the effects produced in aromatherapy use are much more evident.

Nomenclature

The naming of molecules for a precise definition can be difficult, and here the terms used above may be used for a full description, i.e. the type of chain, the kind of terpene or the term 'aromatic' (ring based) should be included when describing a particular chemical constituent of an essential oil. Here are some examples:

- Myrcene – an acyclic monoterpene
- Limonene – a monocyclic monoterpene
- Cadinene – a bicyclic sesquiterpene
- Patchoulol – a tricyclic sesquiterpenol

- Citronellal – an acyclic monoterpenal
- Cinnamic aldehyde – an aromatic aldehyde
- Geranic acid – an acyclic monoterpenic acid
- Cinnamic acid – an aromatic acid.

Therapeutic effects

In the chemical 'families' discussed below, some of the general therapeutic properties attributed to each of the families are based on a theory (set out in detail in Franchomme & Pénoël 2001 pp. 107–131) which associates certain properties with the esters, alcohols, etc., taking into account the electronegative/-positive nature of the molecules coupled with their polar/apolar properties. Although this information is a useful general guide to the probable properties of the chemical families discussed, the information given does not hold true for each and every compound (e.g. alcohols are given the familial characteristic of being stimulating, but the alcohol linalool shows as a sedative – see Table 4.9 – when tested on mice, although the results obtained in animal testing do not necessarily extrapolate directly to humans). In any case, aromatherapists do not use isolated compounds but whole essential oils, and although it is both important and interesting to study the effects of single compounds, it is worth repeating the statement made above that there is not necessarily any simple direct relationship between the therapeutic effect of any one constituent and that of the whole essential oil.

Alcohols

When a hydroxyl group (or hydroxyl radical as it is sometimes called) consisting of one oxygen atom and one hydrogen atom (—OH) joins on to one of the carbons in a chain by displacing one of the hydrogen molecules, an alcohol (Figs 2.5, 2.6, 2.7) is formed: a monoterpenic alcohol, sesquiterpenic alcohol or diterpenic alcohol, depending on whether the chain to which it attaches itself has two, three or four isoprene units. The name of the alcohol so formed always ends in -ol, e.g. geraniol. There are alternative names which are in current use for these alcohols: monoterpenic alcohol is also called monoterpenol, sesquiterpenic alcohol is known also as sesquiterpenol and diterpenic alcohol as diterpenol and also diol.

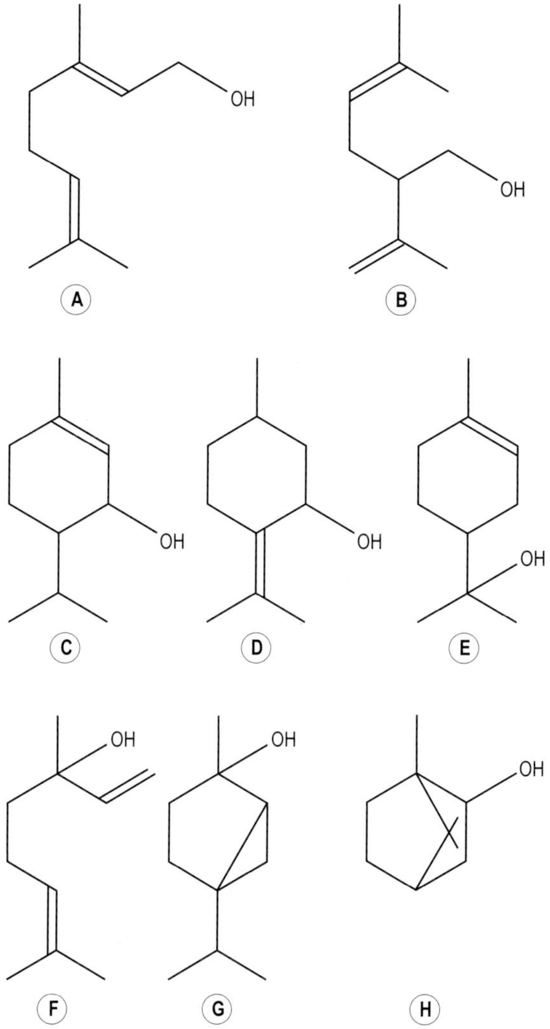

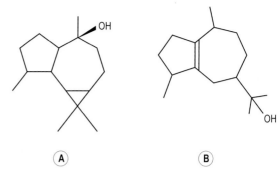

Figure 2.6 • Alcohols – sesquiterpenols (15 C). (A) A bicyclic sesquiterpenol (viridiflorol); (B) a bicyclic sesquiterpenol (guaiol).

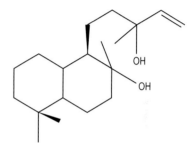

Figure 2.7 • Alcohols – diols (20 C). This figure shows a bicyclic diol (sclareol).

e.g. the diterpenic alcohol sclareol in *Salvia sclarea* [clary], as does the sesquiterpenic alcohol viridiflorol in *Melaleuca viridiflora* [niaouli]: borneol is given as a cholagogue and analgesic, cedrol is phlebotonic and spathulenol is fungicidal – as is sclareol (Beckstrom-Sternberg & Duke 1996 pp. 384, 416, Franchomme & Pénoël 2001 pp. 133, 135).

The aromatic ring

The second building block for the volatile molecules found in distilled plant oils occurs when six carbon atoms join together in the form of a ring, which is not formed from isoprene units, giving a completely different structure from that of the terpenes. Energy transference across the aromatic ring is much greater (due to conjugation) than in the terpenes, making them much more reactive, therefore the effects of aromatic compounds on the body can be quite remarkable, making care in use essential. Note that the term 'ring' is reserved for this six-carbon unit C_6H_6, which has three names in common use:

Figure 2.5 • Alcohols – monoterpenols (10 C). (A) An acyclic monoterpenol (geraniol); (B) an acyclic monoterpenol (lavandulol); (C) a monocyclic monoterpenol (piperitol); (D) a monocyclic monoterpenol (pulegol); (E) a monocyclic monoterpenol (α-terpineol); (F) an acyclic monoterpenol (linalool); (G) a bicyclic monoterpenol (thujanol-4); (H) a bicyclic monoterpenol (borneol).

Effects of alcohols

Alcohols as a group are anti-infectious, strongly bactericidal, and antiviral as well as being stimulating to the immune system; they are generally non-toxic in use and do not cause skin irritation (Roulier 1990 p. 53). The thujanol-4 molecule is a liver stimulant, as is menthol. Some of the heavier alcohols appear to have a balancing effect on the hormonal system,

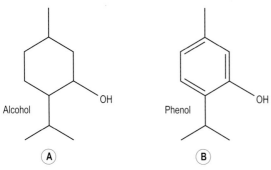

Figure 2.8 • Alcohol vs phenol. (A) A hydroxyl group (—OH) attached to a chain gives an alcohol (menthol); (B) a hydroxyl group (—OH) attached to a benzene ring gives a phenol (thymol).

1. Aromatic ring, because many of the substances based on it are pleasant smelling.
2. Benzene ring, because the basic ring of six carbon atoms and six hydrogen atoms is known as benzene.
3. Phenyl ring, because phenols are formed from this base.

As seen above, when the hydroxyl group —OH is attached to a chain it is an alcohol (Fig. 2.8a); but when the same group is attached to a benzene ring (see below) it is a phenol (Fig. 2.8b). Thus both aliphatic and aromatic aldehydes, ketones and organic acids (involving both chain and ring building blocks) are to be found occurring naturally in essential oils.

Phenols – the other alcohols

When the hydroxyl group attaches itself to a carbon in an aromatic (also phenyl also benzene) ring, the resulting molecule is known as a phenol (Fig. 2.9),

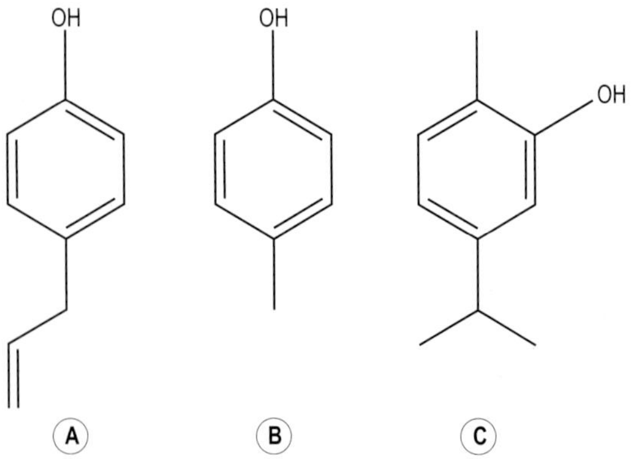

Figure 2.9 • Phenols. (A) Chavicol; (B) p-cresol; (C) carvacrol.

which may also be termed an aromatic alcohol, and has strong effects. Phenols also have names which end in '-ol', e.g. carvacrol; to discriminate between the two classes it is necessary to learn the names of the most important members in each group.

Phenols, like alcohols, are antiseptic and bactericidal and because they stimulate both the nervous system (making them effective against depressive illness) and the immune system, they activate the body's own healing process. However, because the —OH is attached to a ring rather than to a chain molecule, aromatic phenols, unlike the aliphatic alcohols, can be toxic to the liver and irritant to the skin if used in substantial amounts or for too long a time (Roulier 1990 pp. 51–52). 'Some oils – for example, thyme and origanum – owe their value in the pharmaceutical field almost entirely to the antiseptic and germicidal properties of their phenolic content' (Guenther 1949). Eugenol is an effective antispasmodic (Franchomme & Pénoël 2001 p. 134).

Valnet (1980 p. 67) states that phenols have the property of attaching themselves to the amino acids which cause the destruction action of numerous microbial germs or their secretions, as well as tissual waste in wounds, burns and skin conditions. The resulting products (amino-phenols) are well known for their antiseptic action: alcohols behave in a similar fashion, producing amino-alcohols.

Methyl ethers

These generally are more complicated structures than the phenols: precursors (phenylalanine, tyrosine, cinnamic acid) of these molecules act to form compounds that include a six-carbon benzene ring attached to a short (three-carbon) chain. Even though this type of molecule occurs much less frequently in essential oils than do terpenes, they can have a great impact on the aroma, flavour and therapeutic effect. They have various forms of name, as seen in the following examples: safrole, methyl chavicol, eugenol methyl ether and asarone (which may cause confusion owing to the similarity to the ketone name ending); other examples are estragole in tarragon oil, cinnamaldehyde in cinnamon bark oil, anethole (Fig. 2.10a) in aniseed oil and apiole (Fig. 2.10b) in fennel seed oil.

Some occur in two forms, as in *trans*-anethole and *cis*-anethole, the latter being the more toxic of the two (Witty 1993 personal communication).

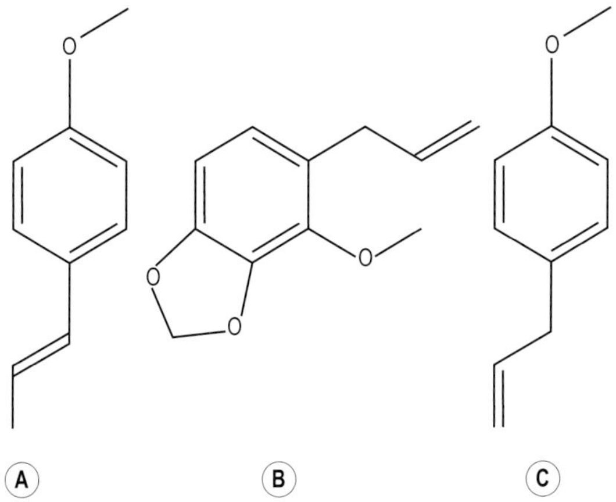

Figure 2.10 • Methyl ethers. (A) *trans*-Anethole; (B) apiole; (C) chavicol methyl ether.

Effects

These molecules have powerful effects on the body and essential oils containing them should always be used with great care. Several of them are amphetamine-like and may be neurotoxic if present in large amounts in an essential oil; thus such oils should be used only in the short term and in low concentration. Whereas the phenols are aggressive to the skin and mucous surfaces, in the phenyl methyl ethers it seems that the methylation of the phenol function negates this aggressive aspect and these compounds are well tolerated on the skin. They are, as a class, strong antispasmodics: anethole (*para*-anol methyl ether) is oestrogen-like (see also Hormone-like, Ch. 4 p. 96) and β-asarone (asarol trimethyl ether) is sedative; safrole relieves pain and myristicin has anaesthetic and hallucinogenic properties (Beckstrom-Sternberg & Duke 1996 p. 406).

Ethers rarely, if ever, occur alone in essential oils, but their relationship to phenyl methyl ethers is close, and their antidepressant, antispasmodic and sedative properties echo those of the phenolic ethers, as do those of esters (see below) (Roulier 1990 p. 53).

Aldehydes

An aldehyde is formed when the carbonyl radical (=O) together with a hydrogen atom (—H) attaches itself to one of the carbon atoms in the basic structure, forming a —CHO group (Fig. 2.11). It is easy to recognize an aldehyde from its name, as it either ends in -al, e.g. citral, or the name aldehyde is stated, as in cinnamic aldehyde (may be shortened to cinna-mal). Benzaldehyde is one of the three constituents of vitamin B_{17}. They usually have powerful aromas, making them important to the perfumer, and are very reactive, which means that they must be used with care in aromatherapy.

Effects

The beneficial properties of aldehydes are that they are antiviral, anti-inflammatory, calming to the nervous system, hypotensive, vasodilatory, air antiseptic and antipyretic; their negative properties – when used incorrectly or ill advisedly – include skin irritation and skin sensitivity (Franchomme & Pénoël 2001 pp. 231–236, Roulier 1990 p. 53). Aldehydes, with their lemon-like aroma, are reputed to calm the tension that follows nicotine withdrawal in those who are giving up smoking. Cinnamaldehyde is a general tonic and stimulates peristalsis and uterine contractions; cuminal, on the other hand, is sedative and calming.

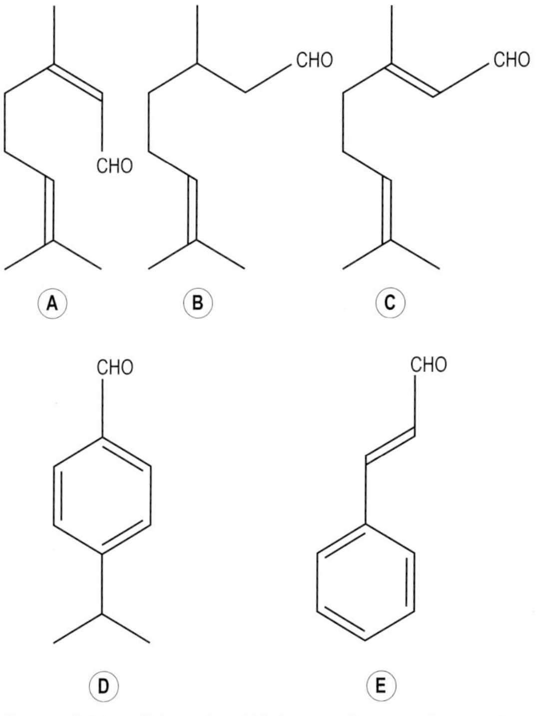

Figure 2.11 • Aldehydes. (A) An acyclic monoterpenal (neral); (B) an acyclic monoterpenal (citronellal); (C) an acyclic monoterpenal (geranial); (D) an aromatic aldehyde (cuminal); (E) an aromatic aldehyde (cinnamal).

Ketones

When the carbonyl group (=O) attaches itself (without a hydrogen atom this time) to a carbon on a chain structure, an aliphatic ketone (Fig. 2.12) is formed; aromatic ketones hardly ever occur in essential oils. The ketone names normally end in -one, but look out for false friends such as asarone, mentioned above, which is a phenolic ether and not a ketone.

As with all molecules, the ketone molecules are not flat, two-dimensional structures but occupy space in three dimensions. This means that changes in molecular spatial shape can take place. Hence differently

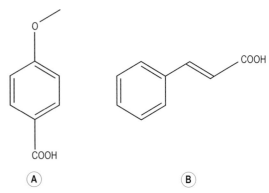

Figure 2.13 • Organic acids. (A) Anisic acid; (B) cinnamic acid.

shaped molecules made up of the same atoms do occur and their seemingly insignificant differences can alter the effect that these molecules have on the body. For example, (−)-carvone and (+)-carvone are two examples, one being less toxic than the other. Opdyke (1973, 1978) suggests that α-thujone and β-thujone may have differing effects on the body, but research along these lines is yet to be carried out.

Effects

Generally speaking, ketones are cicatrizant, lipolytic, mucolytic and sedative; some are also analgesic, anticoagulant, anti-inflammatory, digestive, expectorant or stimulant. They need to be used with care, particularly by pregnant women (Franchomme & Pénoël 2001 p. 212, Roulier 1990 p. 53).

Organic acids and esters

Unlike the above there is no active radical group whose presence creates an ester. This type of compound is formed by the joining together of an organic acid (Fig. 2.13) with an alcohol, the formula being:

organic acid + alcohol = ester + water

It has been suggested that this chemical reaction may be capable, in vivo, of flowing the other way too, which could result in interchanges from acids to esters and back again. Perhaps this is why esters (Fig. 2.14) are useful for normalizing some emotional and bodily conditions which are out of balance. To recognize an ester from its name is not difficult: it usually ends with -ate, e.g. linalyl acetate, or else the word ester is included.

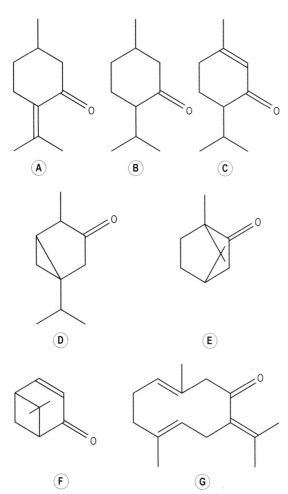

Figure 2.12 • Ketones. (A) A monocyclic monoterpenone (pulegone); (B) a monocyclic monoterpenone (menthone); (C) a monocyclic monoterpenone (piperitone); (D) a bicyclic monoterpenone (thujone); (E) a bicyclic monoterpenone (camphor); (F) a bicyclic monoterpenone (verbenone); (G) a monocyclic sesquiterpenone (germacrone).

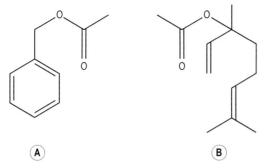

Figure 2.14 • Esters. (A) Benzyl acetate; (B) linalyl acetate.

Effects

Esters generally are believed to be antifungal, anti-inflammatory, antispasmodic, cicatrizant and both calming and tonic (adaptogenic), especially to the nervous system (Buchbauer, Jirovetz & Jäger 1992, Buchbauer et al. 1993). Like alcohols, they are gentle in action, and being free from toxicity they are 'user friendly'. The exception is methyl salicylate, which comprises over 90% of both wintergreen oil and birch oil (neither of which is used in the current British style of aromatherapy).

Oxides

The only oxide (Fig. 2.15) known well in aromatherapy is 1,8-cineole, which is otherwise known as eucalyptol; it may also be regarded as a bicyclic ether (Buchbauer 1993).

Effects

Eucalyptol is stimulant to mucous glands and is expectorant and mucolytic, its unwanted effect being skin irritation, especially on young children. Another

oxide, ascaridole, is an anthelmintic, and linalyloxide and piperitonoxide have antiviral properties ascribed to them.

Lactones

Important members of this family occurring in essences are the coumarins and their derivatives (Fig. 2.16). They occur only in the expressed oils and some absolutes, e.g. jasmine, because the molecular weight is too great to allow distillation. They are sometimes called circular esters because the ester group is incorporated in the structure.

Effects

Lactones are reputed to be mucolytic, expectorant and temperature reducing, their negative aspects being skin sensitization and phototoxicity (Franchomme & Pénoël 2001 p. 222). Lactones are neurotoxic when ingested and some oils containing lactones are toxic

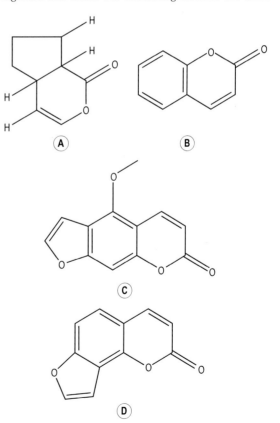

Figure 2.16 • Lactones, coumarins. (A) Nepetalactone; (B) coumarin; (C) bergapten; (D) angelicin.

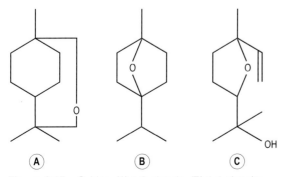

Figure 2.15 • Oxides. (A) 1,8-cineole; (B) 1,4-cineole; (C) linalool oxide.

on the skin, but the risk is slight as there is usually a very low content of lactones in an essential oil.

Coumarins

Coumarins, which number probably almost 1000, are present only in very low concentration in essential oils, but their presence has an undoubted effect.

Effects

Coumarins are anticoagulant hypotensors; they are uplifting and yet at the same time sedative (Buchbauer, Jirovetz & Jäger 1992, Franchomme & Pénoël 2001 p. 225). Lavender is known for its sedative properties and this is partly due to the synergistic presence of coumarins, albeit very low; unfortunately, the coumarins appear only after longer distillation than is usually commercially viable, so unless the lavender has been distilled especially for aromatherapy then the full sedative potential is not realized.

Furanocoumarins are known mainly for their phototoxicity, and oils containing these should not be used immediately prior to sunbathing (or using sunbeds) owing to their ability to increase the sensitivity of the skin to the sun, the main culprits in aromatherapy being psoralen and bergapten, found in the citrus essences. Some are antiviral and antifungal.

There are too many individual essential oil components (several thousand) to name here, but knowledge of the different chemical families will aid recognition of new constituents if they are encountered in a listing from a gas chromatography report (see below).

Stereochemistry

The word 'stereo' comes from the Greek meaning solid, and here refers to the spatial arrangement of atoms within a molecule. The same kind and number of atoms in different molecules can occupy different relative positions, giving the molecules variations in shape which have an influence – perhaps slight, perhaps significant – on the chemical activity.

Isomers

In essential oils many compounds share the same molecular formula and thus are made up of precisely the same number and kind of atoms, but occupy different spatial arrangements: these are known as isomers. For example, many monoterpene hydrocarbons are made up of 10 carbon atoms and 16 hydrogen atoms, having the same molecular formula $C_{10}H_{16}$, but many different structures are made from these same atoms, each having differing properties. The difference between these structural isomers may lead to slight or great variations in characteristics.

Optical isomers

Some molecules are able to rotate plane-polarized light and are classed as either dextrorotatory or laevorotatory, indicating their capability to rotate light in a particular direction. Molecules that divert the light to the right are known as dextrorotatory, written as (+)-, and molecules that turn the light to the left are known as laevorotatory, written as (−)-.

Carvone, a ketone, is one such molecule and exists in two forms, (−)-carvone (Fig. 2.17a) being present in spearmint, where it has the aroma of spearmint, and (+)-carvone (Fig. 2.17b) in caraway, where it has the aroma of caraway, showing that quite a small change in the spatial arrangement of atoms within the molecules can have a significant effect on the perceived aroma; Craker (1990) says that the stereochemical form of the molecule will determine the odour and flavour attributes of the oil.

Menthol, $C_{10}H_{20}O$, is also optically active but only the (−) form is found in nature, particularly in peppermint oils.

These optical isomers, sometimes called 'mirror molecules', are mirror images of each other, rather like a pair of hands which appear to be the same but in fact are different (gloves cannot be exchanged) and this is known as chirality (from the Greek word for hand). The majority of both mono and sesquiterpenic compounds in any given essential oil are to be found in

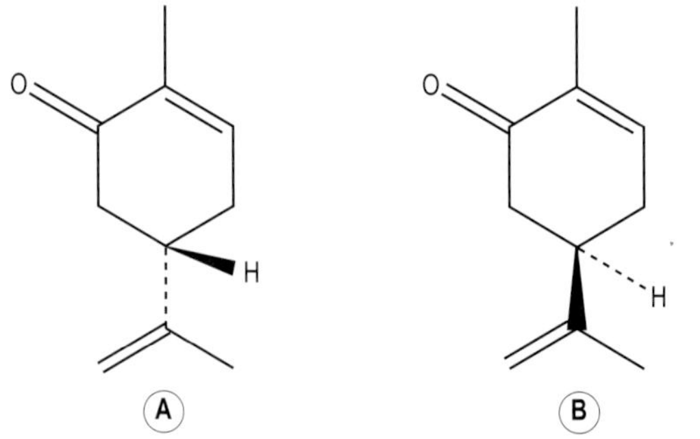

Figure 2.17 • Isomers – molecules in the mirror. (A) (−)-carvone; (B) (+)-carvone.

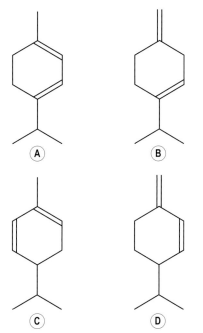

Figure 2.18 • Isomers. (A) α-terpinene; (B) β-terpinene; (C) α-phellandrene; (D) β-phellandrene.

one stereochemical form. A mixture of dextrorotatory and laevorotatory forms of a molecule is termed racemic.

The terpene pinene occurs in two slightly different forms (distinguished nominally by the Greek letters α and β), with only a change in the position of the double bond (Fig. 2.18).

Geometric isomers

The aldehydes geranial and neral are very similar in structure and are said to be geometric isomers (Fig. 2.19). The prefixes *cis*- and *trans*- are used to describe the positioning of groups on either side of a

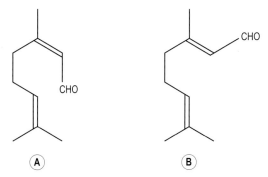

Figure 2.19 • Geometric isomers. (A) *cis*-Citral (neral); (B) *trans*-citral (geranial).

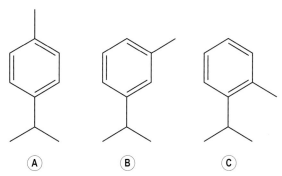

Figure 2.20 • Isomers. (A) *para*-Cymene; (B) *meta*-cymene; (C) *ortho*-cymene.

double bond. Neral is a *cis*- isomer and geranial a *trans*-isomer, and because they often occur together and it is difficult to discriminate between the two during analysis, the mixture of these two isomers is called citral.

The aromatic terpene cymene is an example of a molecule that has three isomers, *para*-, *meta*- and *ortho*-, respectively, denoting the positions of side groups attached to the benzene ring (Fig. 2.20).

Functional isomers

Both molecules shown here have the same molecular formula, C_2H_6O, but because of their arrangement have different functional groups. One is an ether and the other is an alcohol, and so they have quite different characteristics despite being composed of the same atoms.

$$CH_3-O-CH_3 \quad CH_3-CH_2OH$$
Ether   Alcohol

Because the different physical structures of isomers can give widely different physical properties such as boiling point, relative density etc., it is probable that the structural shape of the molecules also has an influence on therapeutic properties, as was the case with the drug thalidomide (see also Hormonal, Ch. 4 p. 96).

Chemical variability

It is important to recognize that, because of the variability of both climate and soil, no natural chemical will be present in any essential oil in exactly the same proportion at each distillation. Further variations are produced according to the time the plant is harvested. For instance, sage plants cut early in the season contain a much lower percentage of ketones than do those harvested late (Lamy 1985). Constituents can vary sometimes from 20% to 70% in a genuine oil, and suppliers must have obtained an oil from a specific plant grown in the right place and harvested at the right time to ensure the correct proportion of whatever component is required. If this is not the case then the oils may have been adulterated before they reach the buyer, unless bought from source. Even a gas–liquid chromatograph carried out by an independent authority cannot always be relied upon completely. More than one test is needed when checking the purity of an oil, and not all distributors are able to afford such an expensive procedure as this for each batch. A certificate showing that an oil is of a required standard is no guarantee unless it refers specifically to the batch currently being traded.

Testing oils for quality

Gas chromatography (GC)

This is sometimes called gas–liquid chromatography (GLC). The gas chromatograph consists of a coiled, temperature-controlled, tubular column into which a minute amount (say 1 μL) of essential oil is injected and volatilized. It then passes through the column, which may be 10–50 m long and contains a liquid phase and a gas phase. At the other end is a flame ionization detector and a pen recorder, which plots a trace (Fig. 2.21) of each component of the essential oil as it exits the column. The smaller, lighter molecules have the shortest retention time and appear after the shortest time, and so are recorded first on the trace. These are followed by successively larger molecules, the heaviest having the longest retention time and being recorded last. From the resulting trace the percentage of each constituent present in the oil being tested can be calculated. As the reading will always differ for each batch of any one essential oil, a trace for each named essential oil is retained as a standard, to which all future batches are compared. It can be seen that this test is comparative rather than absolute, and although the GC does not directly identify the constituents present, this can be done by comparing the results obtained with known standards.

Mass spectrometry

The GC is a valuable test but is not the only one. At the forefront of modern technology is the gas chromatography–mass spectrometry (GC-MS), a more expensive process that is capable of analysing and identifying the

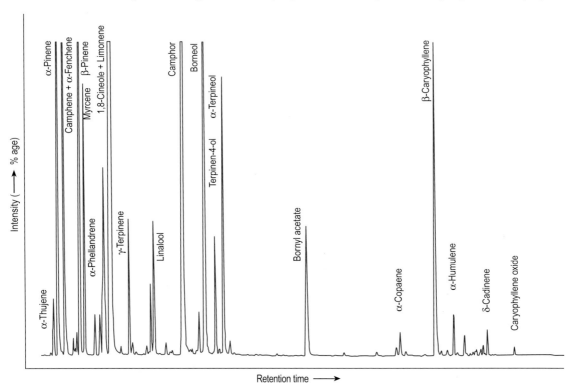

Figure 2.21 • Gas chromatograph trace (rosemary).

individual components of essential oils. The mass spectrometer is interfaced to the gas chromatograph apparatus described above, and as the molecules emerge from the GC column they are bombarded with high-energy electrons, which fragment them. There is a characteristic fragmentation pattern for each molecule, and for identification it is compared by computer with patterns held in a library. Using this technique it is possible to identify each component in a complex mixture such as an essential oil.

Optical rotation

Some molecules are optically active and have the capacity to rotate plane-polarized light; the sense and degree of rotation are measured by an instrument called a polarimeter, and the angle through which the light is rotated is an important physical characteristic by which an essential oil may be recognized.

The optical rotation of a whole essential oil is dependent on the mix of molecules within it, and this results in the oils being what is termed 'optically active', with the ability to bend plane-polarized light. When plane-polarized light is passed through a sample of the essential oil the direction and degree of rotation, as measured by a polarimeter, is an indication as to whether or not an essential oil has been adulterated. Table 2.1 gives some physical characteristics of essential oils by which their quality may be judged.

Refractive index

When light passes through a liquid it is refracted, and this refraction is easily measured to give consistent figures for a particular oil. This refractive index (Table 2.1) is quite consistent for a given oil and is another aid in verifying the authenticity of that oil.

Table 2.1 Physical characteristics of some essential oils

Essential oil	Family	Optical rotation	Refractive index	Specific gravity
Cananga odorata (flos) [ylang ylang]	Annonaceae	−23.44 to −31.45	1.5041–1.5065	0.960–0.986 (20°)
Carum carvi (fruct.) [caraway]	Apiaceae	+74 to +80	1.485–1.492	0.902–0.912 (20°)
Cedrus atlantica (lig.) [Atlas cedarwood]	Pinaceae	+34 to +53.8	1.515–1.523	0.953–0.9756 (20°)
Cinnamomum zeylanicum (cort.) [cinnamon bark]	Lauraceae	0 to −2	1.573–1.500	1.000–1.040 (20°)
Citrus aurantium var. amara (per.) [orange bigarade]	Rutaceae	+94 to +99	1.472–1.476	0.842–0.848 (20°)
Citrus bergamia (per.) [bergamot]	Rutaceae	+8 to +24	1.465–1.4675	0.875–0.880 (20°)
Citrus limon (per.) [lemon]	Rutaceae	+57 to +65	1.474–1.476	0.849–0.858 (20°)
Citrus reticulata (per.) [mandarin]	Rutaceae	+65 to +75	1.475–1.478	0.854–0.859 (15°)
Coriandrum sativum (fruct.) [coriander]	Apiaceae	+8 to +12	1.462–1.472	0.863–0.870 (20°)
Cymbopogon flexuosus (fol.) [lemongrass]	Poaceae	−3 to +1	1.485–1.4899	0.889–0.911 (25°)
Eucalyptus globulus (fol.) [Tasmanian blue gum]	Myrtaceae	0 to +10	1.458–1.470	0.905–0.925 (20°)
Foeniculum vulgare var. dulce (fruct.) [fennel]	Apiaceae	+5 to +16.30	1.5500–1.5519	0.971–0.980 (20°)
Juniperus communis (fruct.) [juniper berry]	Cupressaceae	−15 to 0	1.4740–1.4840	0.854–0.871 (20°)
Lavandula angustifolia [lavender]	Lamiaceae	−5 to −12	1.457–1.464	0.878–0.892 (20°)
Melaleuca alternifolia (fol.) [tea tree]	Myrtaceae	+6.48 to +9.48	1.4760–1.4810	0.895–0.905 (15°)

Continued

Table 2.1 Physical characteristics of some essential oils—cont'd

Essential oil	Family	Optical rotation	Refractive index	Specific gravity
Melaleuca leucadendron (fol.) [cajuput]	Myrtaceae	+1 to −4	1.464–1.472	0.910–0.923 (20°)
Mentha x piperita (fol.) [peppermint]	Lamiaceae	−16 to −30	1.460–1.467	0.900–0.912 (20°)
Myristica fragrans (sem.) [nutmeg EI]*	Myristicaceae	+8 to +25	1.475–1.488	0.883–0.917 (20°)
Myristica fragrans (sem.) [nutmeg WI]*	Myristicaceae	+25 to +45	1.467–1.477	0.854–0.880 (20°)
Nardostachys jatamansi (rad.) [spikenard]	Valerianaceae	−20	1.5078	0.9649−0.9732 (17°)
Ocimum basilicum (fol.) [basil]	Lamiaceae	−7.24 to −10.36	1.4821–1.4939	0.912–0.935 (20°)
Origanum majorana (fol.) [sweet marjoram]	Lamiaceae	+14.2 to +19.4	1.4700–1.4750	0.890–0.906 (25°)
Pelargonium graveolens (fol.) [geranium]	Geraniaceae	−7.0 to +13.15	1.461–1.472	0.888–0.896 (20°)
Piper nigrum (fruct.) [black pepper]	Piperaceae	−7.2 to +4	1.480–1.492	0.864–0.907 (20°)
Pogostemon patchouli (fol.) [patchouli]	Lamiaceae	−47 to −70	1.506–1.513	0.955–0.986 (20°)
Santalum album (lig.) [sandalwood]	Santalaceae	−15.58 to −20	1.505–1.510	0.971–0.983 (20°)
Syzygium aromaticum (flos) [clove bud]	Myrtaceae	−1.5	1.528–1.537	1.041–1.054 (20°)
Vetiveria zizanioides (rad.) [vetiver]	Poaceae	+19 to +30	1.514–1.519	0.9882–1.0219 (30°)
Zingiber officinale (rad.) [ginger]	Zingiberaceae	−28 to −45	1.4880–1.440	0.871–0.882 (20°)

*EI = East Indies; WI = West Indies.

Essential oils also undergo other checks on their physical characteristics, which must be within the accepted tolerances for the given oil. These checks include specific gravity, solubility in alcohol, colour, ester content and so on.

Infrared test

When electromagnetic radiation in the infrared region is passed through a sample of essential oil, the spectrum produced (Fig. 2.22) is a fingerprint from which the level of some of the components can be estimated. Some forms of adulteration can readily be seen by this method, depending to some extent on the skill and knowledge of the person who has carried out the adulteration.

The nose

In addition to all this, possibly the finest tool for some purposes is a well-trained 'nose' (an expert perfumer, perhaps 20 years in the training) who can make an organoleptic assessment of the oil. The trained nose can identify the presence of certain molecules at extremely low levels that would be almost impossible for a mechanical device, although 'sniffing' technology is available (but expensive).

The distillation process

Distilling as we know it today can involve efficient cooling systems, electronic control gear to regulate the temperature and pressure of the process, energy-saving steam generators and so on. Some thousands of years ago, to obtain the essential oil, the plant material, (for example cedarwood pieces, was placed with water in a clay vessel with a lid made of woollen fibres. The vessel was heated over a wood fire, and as the volatile molecules from the water and the cedarwood escaped they were trapped in the wool. Later they were squeezed out by hand, and the aromatic water and essential oil, being of different densities, separated and so could be collected. Over the centuries methods

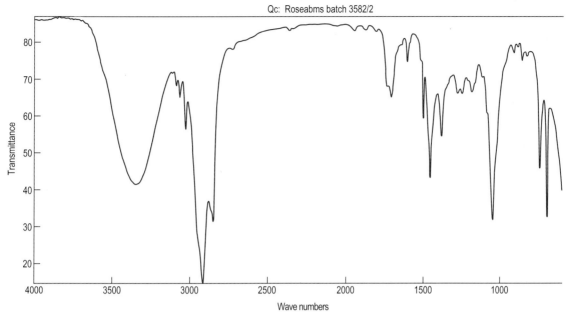

Qc: Roseabms batch 3582/2

Figure 2.22 • Example of an infrared spectrum (rose absolute).

of distillation gradually improved, and 4th century Chinese and 10th century Islamic scientists developed methods of obtaining the distillate. Since then, apart from minor improvements, distillation has remained very much the same in principle up to the present day. The availability of modern materials and resources, such as stainless steel and electricity, has permitted much greater control over the whole process, and there is a dramatic increase in the quality of the essential oils produced today compared with that in former times. Oils produced in previous centuries, and even during the middle of the last century, cannot be compared with some of the very high-quality products we have available for aromatherapy today (assuming they are not adulterated after distillation).

Rectification

Some essential oils are put through a rectification process; rectification means to put right, and this process is carried out to clean up an essential oil which has been contaminated with undesirable volatile plant products produced by careless distillation procedures. These undesirable products may be due to the decomposition of plant constituents, and although they occur mainly in the water, giving a smell which is rather 'off', they can also appear in the essential oil itself as, for example, unwanted

aldehydes or bad-smelling sulphur compounds. Sometimes a dark colour appears in the oil due to non-volatiles such as plant dust, and rectification separates out any such material. Rectified essential oils are not normally suitable for aromatherapy use.

Fractional distillation

This is a process which separates the volatile oil into its various fractions having different boiling points. This process is usually carried out under vacuum to keep temperatures involved low and hence prevent degradation of the essential oil; it is a dry distillation: this means that no water or steam is used. Fractionated essential oils are not normally suitable for aromatherapy use.

Percolation, hydrodiffusion

This method of extraction is like usual distillation but upside down! – in that the steam enters the alembic from the top and percolates down through the plant material. This has been used on a small scale and, when successful, excellent oils are produced at a much lower cost, because the time of extraction is only a few minutes, saving man-hours and fuel. There is a drawback in that sometimes an inseparable emulsion is produced which cannot be used, and so this method of extraction has not been widely adopted.

Carbon dioxide

This is a solvent extraction method using supercritical CO_2, by which a wider range of molecules can be extracted from the plant material than is possible by distillation. CO_2 is injected into a stainless steel tank containing the plant material, and under pressure the CO_2 liquefies and acts as a solvent, extracting molecules from the plant; the CO_2 later returns to a gaseous state and unlike other solvents is easily and completely removed. The process is a selective method of extraction without distillation, yielding chemicals which are pure and stable; the solvent, CO_2, is colourless, odourless and tasteless The whole process is performed without heat, which means that molecules are not degraded, thereby producing a material which is new, and there is no doubt that CO_2-extracted oils will be of use to aromatherapists in the future. The oils produced by this method contain a different molecular mix, and until more is known about their particular therapeutic and possible toxic effects, aromatherapists may be best advised for the time being to use only steam-distilled essential oils and expressed essences. These have been proved to be therapeutically effective by traditional use over time and by research.

Complexity of essential oils

During the 19th century the first analyses were carried out on essential oils and attempts made to isolate and identify the various components, some of the terpenes, alcohols and aldehydes being among the first to be named. This was followed by successful attempts to synthesize the individual components; for example, eugenol found naturally in clove bud oil, was synthesized in 1822 (Valnet 1980 p. 28).

The complexity of essential oils should be borne in mind when referring to the therapeutic qualities of a given oil; it helps to explain why one oil (lavender) can be listed as being at the same time 'analgesic, anticonvulsive, antidepressant, antimicrobial, antirheumatic, antiseptic, antispasmodic, antitoxic, carminative, cholagogic, choleretic, cicatrizant, cordial, cytophylactic, deodorant, diuretic, emmenagogic, hypotensive, insecticidal, nervine, parasiticidal, rubefacient, sedative,

stimulant, sudorific, tonic, vermifuge, vulnerary'. This staggering array of properties (Lawless 1992) perhaps overstates the case, but demonstrates what the author describes as the 'shotgun' holistic approach, which sprays all sorts of benefits (wanted side effects), in contrast to the 'single synthetic bullet' symptomatic approach aimed at a particular site, mostly with unwanted side effects.

This complexity underlines the fact that only genuine essential oils should be used therapeutically, even though there is natural variation in the oils. It needs to be emphasized that for perfectly valid reasons the fragrance industry requires essential oils which are standardized by one means or another, and that most (if not all) essential oils in the general marketplace may have synthetic or natural additions or fractions removed. As well as these already-mentioned cautions, it is also true that some oils are not obtained from natural plants at all, for stainless steel plants do play their part! These laboratory creations are known as reconstructed oils (RCO) and lack many tiny and as yet unidentified components which could well be important to the overall effect of the natural oil.

Summary

The requirements of the food and perfume industries differ dramatically from those of aromatherapy. Essential oils are very complex by nature, and careful selection and extensive testing are needed to obtain oils of therapeutic quality. When altered in any way, essential oils will probably not be of a quality suitable for aromatherapy, since the synergy of the natural mix of components in the whole oil will have been destroyed. It goes without saying that they should be obtained only from a reliable and knowledgeable source. The therapist must have at least a basic knowledge of the chemistry of the molecules found in essential oils to:

- be able to appreciate fully the nature of plant volatile oils
- increase their understanding of how essential oils may be used to best therapeutic advantage
- be able to communicate with other health professionals
- increase confidence in their own ability to treat clients.

References

Adams, T.B., Taylor, S.V., 2010. Safety evaluation of essential oils: a constituent-based approach. In: Başer, K.H.C., Buchbauer, G. (Eds.), Handbook of essential oils: science, technology and applications. CRC Press, Boca Raton, pp. 185–208.

Beckstrom-Sternberg, S., Duke, J.A., 1996. CRC handbook of medicinal mints. CRC Press, Boca Raton.

Buchbauer, G., 1993. Biological effects of fragrances and essential oils. Perfumer & Flavorist 18, 22.

Buchbauer, G., Jirovetz, L., Jäger, W., 1992. Passiflora and lime blossoms: motility effects after inhalation of the essential oils and some of the main constituents in animal experiments. Archiva Pharmaceutica (Weinheim) 325, 247–248.

Buchbauer, G., Jirovetz, L., Jäger, W., Plank, C., Dietrich, H., 1993. Fragrance compounds and essential oils with sedative effects upon inhalation. J. Pharm. Sci. 82 (6), 660–664.

Craker, L.E., 1990. Herbs and volatile oils. Herb, Spice and Medicinal Digest 8 (4), 1–5.

Franchomme, P., Pénoël, D., 2001. L'aromathérapie exactement. Jollois, Limoges.

Guenther, E., 1949. The essential oils. In: Van Nostrand, New York, p. 499 vol. 2.

Kubecka, K.H., 2010. History and sources of essential oil research. In: Başer, K.H.C., Buchbauer, G. (Eds.), Handbook of essential oils:science, technology and applications. CRC Press, Boca Raton.

Lamy, J., 1985. De la culture à la distillerie: quelques facteurs influant sur la composition des huiles essentielles. In: Chambre d'Agriculture de la Drôme, Valence, p. 5.

Lawless, J., 1992. The encyclopaedia of essential oils. In: Element, Shaftesbury, p. 118.

Opdyke, D.L.J., 1973. Monographs on fragrance raw materials: laevo-carvone. Food and cosmetics toxicology. In: Pergamon Press, Oxford, p. 1057 vol. 11.

Opdyke, D.L.J., 1978. Monographs on fragrance raw materials: dextro-carvone. Food and cosmetics toxicology. In: Pergamon Press, Oxford, p. 673 vol. 16.

Roulier, G., 1990. Les huiles essentielles pour votre santé. Dangles, St-Jean-de-Braye.

Valnet, J., 1980. The practice of aromatherapy. Daniel, Saffron Walden.

Quality and safety

3
(Part I)

Len Price

CHAPTER CONTENTS

Introduction

The dangers of essential oils have often been exaggerated, usually based on insufficient evidence and inappropriate comparisons. This chapter shows that these powerful substances, used knowledgeably and with due caution, pose no threat to health. The highest possible quality of medicament is always required in therapy, and this chapter shows that aromatherapy is no exception to the rule. The main chemical groups found in essential oils are outlined, along with an account of methods of testing for quality.

Background

It is remarkable that the safety record of essential oils is as good as it undoubtedly is, bearing in mind that:

- essential oils are powerful mixtures and have physiological, psychological and pharmacological effects, both desirable and undesirable, when applied to the body;
- in most countries, including the UK, these oils are freely available and there is no restriction on their sale and use;
- the majority of people who buy essential oils are members of the general public, who do not have expert knowledge of their nature and use.

Despite this good record, statements are sometimes made which sensationalize aromatherapy or exaggerate unwanted effects of the oils. More to the point would be to educate both the supplier and the general user in the appropriate and safe use of essential oils. That way lies a safe and sound future for the popular use of aromatherapy.

The food industry is the greatest user of essential oils, where they are used at low levels as flavourings and when used in this way there are none that could be expected to pose any significant risk to health (Adams & Taylor 2010). Chronic studies using animals, sponsored by the National Toxicity Program, have been performed on more than 30 major components of essential oils at much higher intake levels than the daily intake dose, and the majority showed no carcinogenic potential (Smith et al. 2005). Obviously, when consumed in higher quantities some plant extracts do exhibit toxicity, e.g. hemlock (used as a poison) and pennyroyal (toxic side effects), which underlines the need for adequate training.

Essential oil quality

Genuine aromatherapeutic essential oils

For therapeutic purposes the quality and wholeness of any essential oils used are of paramount importance, irrespective of cost, whereas when used in the flavour and fragrance industries the price, taste and aroma are the most important considerations; for them, standardized essential oils are necessary to ensure repeatability and a consistent quality.

Quality variation

Variation in the quality of an essential oil may be natural or due to human intervention. Wine is a commodity which is expected to have a different taste and character from year to year, although harvested, processed and bottled at the same vineyard and from the same vines. Plants are subject to varying amounts of sunshine, frost, rain, heat or cold each year, and it is these factors, plus the composition of the soil, which are responsible for the variations in quality and composition (and therefore the aroma) of the plant extracts, occurring naturally from year to year.

Synthetic materials, adulteration

Traders in essential oils may add cheaper oils or synthetics to the genuine oils, in order to maintain the same standard taste, aroma and price level for successive repeat deliveries to the same customer. The needs of the flavour and food industries are today so great that there are scarcely enough natural products in the world to meet the demand, and even where available some products are just too expensive for their purposes compared with synthetics. The aromatherapist, however, needs above all to acquire the natural physicochemical characteristics, whatever the variation from harvest to harvest.

Essential oils are made up of a vast array of natural chemicals, most of which are found in more than one oil. It is a fairly simple matter for the chemist to remove a desired constituent from a cheap oil and add it to an expensive oil, or to sell a modified 'pure' oil to an unsuspecting customer for a high price. Adulteration also takes place when a synthetic isolate is added, especially to one of the costly oils such as rose otto, when synthetic phenyl ethyl alcohol (occurring naturally in rose otto) is used as the adulterant. 'Nature identical' products are manufactured in a laboratory and are simply synthetic copies of ingredients found in nature. Alcohol, and occasionally a small amount of vegetable oil, which are both good solvents of essential oils, are used to adulterate, stretch or cut Nature's gifts, and many descriptive words are used to justify the standardization sometimes necessary in the fragrance and food industries. 'Certain suppliers with highly developed imagination will even use the term "ennobling" for the disfiguration of an essential oil' (Arctander 1960). With some oils it is almost standard practice to adulterate, e.g. the use of PEG (polyethylene glycol) to extend lavender essential oil.

Imitations

Expensive essential oils such as *Melissa officinalis* [melissa] and *Aloysia triphylla* [lemon verbena] are often imitated by the perfume industry by using blends of cheaper oils to simulate the aroma; to the perfumer, the aroma is the most important asset of an 'essential oil', not whether it is natural, adulterated or synthetic. Tisserand and Balacs (1995 p. 177) say that *Aloysia triphylla* should not be used in therapy, but this advice is based on tests carried out at 12% using fragrance quality oils (Opdyke 1992). Most oils named lemon verbena are blends of lemon, citronella, lemongrass etc., as the genuine oil is expensive; these 'made up' verbena oils are likely to be phototoxic and also skin sensitizers because of the high citral content in the oils from which they have been constructed. However, the genuine oil, which has a similar concentration of citral to the above oils, does not

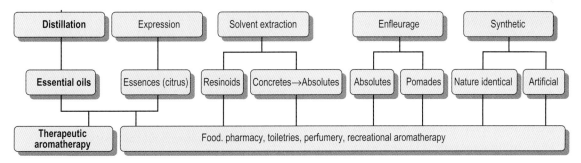

Nature identical – a manmade copy of a natural product   Artificial – a product devised and manufactured by man

Figure 3.1 • Aromatic products and their uses.

irritate the skin (Schnaubelt 1998 p.117) – a good reason for not using industrial quality essential oils therapeutically!

Deterpenized oils

Essential oils used in the fragrance industry often have their terpenes partly or wholly removed on account of their insolubility in alcohol, which would result in cloudiness – a distinct commercial and aesthetic disadvantage in a perfume! The deterpenized oil is incomplete and contains in higher proportions the remaining constituents of the oil, for example the deterpenization of peppermint increases the content of the possibly hazardous ketone menthone. In aromatherapy there is no necessity for this and it is imperative not to interfere with the natural balance of the essential oil. Some therapists purchase bergapten-free bergamot oil, as this constituent (a furanocoumarin) can be responsible for phototoxicity of the skin in sunlight, but this is unnecessary (see Ch. 3 Part II).

Contaminants

The majority of essential oils are produced for use by the food and fragrance industries which, generally speaking, are not concerned whether or not fertilizers, pesticides or herbicides may be present in the oil. Stewart (2004 p.10) says that herbicides, fungicides and pesticides are intrinsically toxic and inevitably end up as contaminants in the oils, directly affecting their efficacy and safety.

Commercial grade oils can present toxic effects as a result of adulteration, folding, stretching etc. to which they are subjected in order to have:

- a standardized product which can be repeated at any time, which is impossible with naturally grown plants;
- a product at a price compatible with their marketing strategy (often meaning cheap).

The various types of aromatic product available are shown in Figure 3.1. For therapeutic use aromatherapists use only distilled essential oils and expressed essences, although some occasionally make exception to the rule by using jasmine absolute or benzoin.

Procurement of genuine, authentic essential oils

Of the many factors involved in the safe use of therapeutic essential oils, not least is the specification of the oil itself. Knowledge of factors such as where it is grown, whether it is cloned by cuttings or grown from seed, the plant variety, how it is grown (wild, organic, or with chemicals), the part of the plant used and the chemotype is important for safe usage.

The need for the use of genuine essential oils in therapeutic treatments is illustrated perfectly by the following case cited by Valnet:

A patient being treated for a fistula of the anus by the instillation of pure and natural drops of lavender and who was beginning to recover, had to go on a journey. Having forgotten his essential oil, he purchased a further supply from a chemist. Unfortunately, this essence was neither pure nor natural; one single instillation resulted in such severe inflammation that the patient was unable to sit down for over two weeks.

Valnet (1980 p. 27)

The overriding consideration must be consumer safety and to this end genuine, authentic essential oils must be procured, genuine in this case meaning of known plant origin and authentic meaning not standardized: note that the word natural does **not** necessarily mean unadulterated or safe.

It is not easy to procure such oils, for many and varied reasons, some of which follow:

1. High quality at the time of harvesting can diminish due to distillation, rectification, fractionation, adulteration, transportation, storage and time.
2. The bulk of essential oils comes from faraway countries, only 3–5% coming from Europe.
3. Availability is influenced by various factors including war (vetiver, patchouli) and changing climate (ambrette seed).
4. The trade has very limited knowledge of scientific names and it is vital for aromatherapy to use the scientific name, because the use of local common names for the plants leads to confusion. More than one name may be given to the same plant, or the same common name can be given to different plants (such as marjoram, which might be *Origanum majorana* or *Thymus mastichina*). Cedarwood oil may be any of the following, since all are traded simply as cedarwood: *Cedrus atlantica* [Atlas cedarwood], *Cedrus deodora* [deodar or Himalayan cedarwood], *Cedrus libani* [cedar of Lebanon], *Chamaecyparis lawsoniana* [western white cedar], *Cryptomeria japonica* [Japanese cedar], *Juniperus procera* [east African cedarwood], *Juniperus mexicana* [Texas cedarwood], *Juniperus virginiana* [red cedarwood], *Thuja occidentalis* [white cedar], *Thuja plicata* [western red cedar]. The common name oregano is applied to more than 43 different species and 18 hybrids belonging to five different families (Skoula & Harborne 2002).
5. A supply problem exists because the market for herbal medicines is increasing and more oils are being used in aromatherapy.
6. Wild plants are sometimes collected by an unsupervised, unskilled labour force paid by weight of plant collected, and who are not always able to identify the required plant, resulting in indiscriminate harvesting.

Accurate identification

The importance of knowing what material is being used in a treatment is obvious, therefore it is imperative that the oil is precisely identified. This fact escapes the attention of many people treating others, and even of some carrying out scientific trials. Before embarking on a trial using essential oils it is of primary importance that a specified oil from a known source is used, and to have as a minimum a GC (gas chromatography) analysis of the oil actually used in the test. The scientific botanical name of the plant should be used and oil from the same harvest batch should be used throughout the test(s).

In many cases it is not sufficient merely to specify the genus and species (and the variety if applicable): it is also necessary to designate the chemotype (explained in Ch. 1) and the part of the plant used for extraction. An example is the cinnamon tree, where the oil from the bark consists principally of an aldehyde, whereas the oil from the leaf is mainly a phenol, with different effects and uses. The oil from the thuja or white cedar tree, *Thuja occidentalis* (responsible for the restriction on cedarwood oils in France), is taken from the leaves, but other 'cedarwoods' are taken from the wood. In the Apiaceae family, the seed oils can be significantly different from oils extracted from other parts of the same plant, e.g. in the case of *Angelica archangelica* the root oil is phototoxic, whereas that from the seed is not. Therapists need to be aware of this; it is their responsibility to ensure that inappropriate treatment is not given.

Some oils that are sold do not exist, and Dürbeck (2003) calls them phantom oils; some examples are:

- Peru balsam from El Salvador and tolu balsam are both standardized or synthesized in Europe.
- Sandalwood from South India (Mysore) is not available yet continues to be sold.
- Rosewood oil from the Amazon is not available because the industry is now finished.
- The same situation exists with *Copaiba balsam*.
- Tea tree – there is three times more sold in the world than is produced in Australia; tea tree oil is a comparatively simple essential oil comprising only about 30 compounds (*cf.* ylang ylang, with about 1200) and so is easy to reconstruct; also the 'natural' oil is often 'regulated' at source.
- Sumatran *Patchouli* may be relabelled Malaysian *Patchouli*.
- Barrème lavender (a lavender high in linalyl acetate) has not been produced for many years but unbelievably still appears on some sales lists.

Pharmacopoeia

About 60 different standards exist for the chemical composition of essential oils, yet there are only 16 essential oils listed in the *New European Pharmacopoeia* (Dürbeck 2003). Current pharmaceutical formulae demonstrate that essential oils and oleoresins derived from spices and herbs are valued not only as flavouring agents but also for other properties they possess; for instance, they:

- stimulate the appetite by increasing salivation
- act as carminatives to relieve gastric discomfort and flatulence
- counteract the griping action of purgatives
- contribute as mild expectorants in cough mixtures and pastilles
- check profuse secretion and relieve congestion of the bronchioles when used in inhalants
- act as counterirritants and rubefacients, for the chest in bronchitis and pleurisy, and for the relief of rheumatic pain, when formulated as ointments, creams and liniments.

As flavouring agents, essential oils are acceptable for repeated dosage, e.g. in tablets to be chewed and for repeated usage in such products as toothpaste. As perfumes they are present in a variety of cosmetics which are used daily over long periods of time.

Some essential oils listed in the *British Pharmacopoeia* (BP) are stocked in hospital pharmacies, but oils prepared to BP standards may not be suitable for use in aromatherapy. One reason for this is that many plants, for example thyme, *Thymus vulgaris*, exist in the wild as many different chemotypes, each chemotype producing quite a different essential oil in makeup and therapeutic action (see Ch. 1 p. 8) and such differences are not always reflected in the pharmacopoeia. Another reason is because the specification is either too broad or incomplete and does not reflect the natural materials currently available; some oils listed are folded, which alters their composition: such essences are not used in aromatherapy.

Storage and shelf life

Factors that affect the storage of aromatherapy products are:

- Air – oxidation can be a problem and essential oils keep best when bottles are full, with as little air as possible. Oxidation – the combining of free oxygen with compounds in the essential oils – affects some oils particularly, altering their therapeutic effects, e.g.
  - ○ the aldehydes in citrus oils (e.g. lemon) can turn to acids
  - ○ oils with a significant monoterpenes content can lead to the formation of sensitizing hydroperoxides (e.g. turpentine)
  - ○ some oils high in the terpenes limonene and pinene may react with oxygen; the antibacterial activity of lemongrass oil is diminished when oxidized (Orafidiya 1993)
  - ○ once a bottle is opened, air enters to replace any essential oil used, which poses no problem if used within a reasonable time. The degradation process is accelerated by the other two factors, heat and light
- Temperature – heat speeds up the oxidation process and a cool temperature is best for extending the shelf life, especially for blends of essential/carrier oils and carrier oils. Sudden changes in temperature appear to be more harmful than a slow seasonal change.
- Light – essential oils should be stored in dark-coloured glass bottles – dark amber, green or black for best results. Blue glass does not protect the oil from some harmful light rays and nor does clear glass.

If products are not stored under the best conditions possible there can be a change in molecular composition and therefore there may be different therapeutic effects, perhaps adding undesired effects such as skin irritation or even sensitization.

Essential oils

Distilled oils which have not been adulterated generally have a shelf-life of many years because the small molecules of which they are composed are relatively stable. Experience shows that, with few exceptions, most essential oils have a very long shelf-life under the right conditions. One writer (Stewart 2004 p. 446) states that the shelf-life is not known but that it is measured in millennia, not months; with personal experience the author is inclined to agree with this, and it is reasonable to expect a shelf-life of several years, but there are exceptions, as indicated above. Essential oils are flammable and must be protected from naked flame; some aroma 'burners' are not safe in some situations.

Expressed oils

It is often recommended that expressed citrus oils be stored under refrigeration, which extends their shelf-life by up to a year if the bottle is unopened. Once opened, half a year is a reasonable life to expect, assuming conditions are not extreme. These expressed oils under cool conditions will precipitate their natural waxes; this does not affect their therapeutic value and so the oil can be used as normal; the only drawback is that the wax may clog the dropper.

Blended oils

The shelf life of a blend of essential oils in a vegetable carrier oil is not as long as that of single or blended essential oils, depending as it does on the ratio of the mix – a 5% dilution will not last as long as a 50% dilution. The fatty oils contain unstable compounds (proteins, polypeptides, amino acids) which can break down. These blends go rancid because of the fatty acids, but storage in a fridge will slow down this effect, giving a shelf life of perhaps 2 years. There is an easy test to verify the blend: if it smells rancid it is unusable; if it smells good, then it is suitable for use.

Summing up, to maintain aromatherapy products in good condition:

- essential oil bottles should be of amber or black glass, not plastic
- the bottles should be full and airtight
- storage is best in a dark place, temperature maintained at about 10–15°C.

Safety

Tradition and experience

Centuries of experience with many essential oils worldwide have shown them to be effective and safe:

- The Egyptians proved the antiseptic powers of aromatics in the mummification process.
- Hippocrates fought the plague in Athens by using aromatic essences for fumigation.
- St Hildegard of Bingen was using lavender oil in the 12th century.
- Hungary water (a lotion scented with rosemary) began its 600-year life in the 14th century.
- By the year 1500, oils of benzoin, calamus, cedarwood, cinnamon, frankincense, myrrh, rose, rosemary, sage, spikenard and turpentine were known to and used by pharmacists.

Essential oils were first mentioned in an official pharmacopoeia around the year 1600 in Germany (Price 2000 p. 6). Borneo camphor (an alcohol) was mentioned in Schröder's pharmacopoeia of 1689 as a 'prodigious alexipharmic' or antidote to poison. For other oils there is little historical evidence, and for almost all essential oils, although there is ample proof of their antiseptic powers in vitro, clinical trials are lacking. While this may be due in part to shortage of research funds, it is also attributable to the difficulty (even impossibility) of conducting blind trials with aromatic substances.

Animal testing

Although toxicological tests have been performed on humans, aromatherapists should be aware that the majority have been carried out on animals – normally rabbits for dermal toxicity and rats for oral toxicity. However:

- Animal physiology cannot be compared with that of a human being: it is not possible to extrapolate the results of animal testing to human physiology: basil and tarragon oils may contain estragole (methyl chavicol) in high amounts and this compound has been implicated by research on animals as being a strong carcinogen. The carcinogenicity is due to the metabolite 1-hydroxyestragole, but estragole presents little hazard to humans at normal food usage levels of 1 μg/kg per day (Howes, Chan & Caldwell 1990).
- Absorption is usually higher through animal skin than human skin (Hotchkiss 1994) but for the aromatic amines the reverse is true: 13% of MDA (methylenedioxy-amphetamine) permeated the skin in rats compared to 33% in human skin, while for MbOCA (methylene bis[orthochloroaniline]) the figures were 2% and 6%, respectively; for (+)-limonene the figures are 6% (rat) and 3% (human) (Hotchkiss 1994).
- Many tests were carried out using isolated components, which is not relevant to whole oils as used in aromatherapy.
- RIFM administered relatively massive overdoses to determine lethal toxicity.

Huge sums are spent on research, clinical trials and licensing for each orthodox medicine, pill or tablet which appears on the market to help alleviate suffering and disease, but despite all the care and time spent on research there are still many serious side effects. Essential oils have not been clinically tested in this way because it would cost billions, not millions, of pounds to test each oil and synergistic mix for each therapeutic effect of which it is capable. In the absence of scientific proof, orthodoxy finds it difficult to accept aromatherapy, which is still more art than science; yet in the recent past clinical tests on animals have allowed the creation of drugs that have had disastrous effects on humans, e.g. thalidomide, opren. There is room for more than one approach in the healing arena and natural ways need to be included too.

The book *Essential Oil Safety* (Tisserand & Balacs 1995) is not universally accepted because most of the information is based on tests carried out using perfume grade oils.

> This book is not recommended for use by people who use good quality therapeutic grade oils because it does not contain any information relevant to such oils ...it is a book on commercial grade oils. ...If you are using cheap perfume grade oils, such as those in most retail stores, then you may need to read and heed this book (Stewart 2004 p. 21). Such commercial quality oils are used in candles, soaps, shampoos, toothpaste, fragrancers etc. and this is recreational aromatherapy, not therapeutic aromatherapy.
>
> (Stewart 2004 p. 11).

The book is an excellent guide in itself, although the authors themselves say that 'this text is largely an extrapolation of toxicological reports from the Research Institute for Fragrant Materials' (RIFM). In the absence of specific information on therapeutic oils, there is a useful body of knowledge on fragrance materials as used on the skin by the perfume industry, thanks to impressive work carried out by RIFM (established in 1966). RIFM has published over 1000 monographs on fragrance materials, almost 200 of these concerning aromatic materials derived from plants, including essential oils, absolutes and resins. The International Fragrance Association (IFRA) makes recommendations to the perfume industry for the safe use of such materials based on the published findings of RIFM, and these may be useful guides to aromatherapists when applying essential oils to the skin.

Isomers and safety

The activity of an essential oil molecule depends on its shape, and it is necessary to be aware of the existence of isomers, where one name (e.g. thujone) can apply to different molecular shapes each having different activities. Thujone is a ketone and should not to be treated lightly whenever and wherever it occurs. The thujone molecule has four possible shapes, and it is not known

whether they all have the same toxic potential or whether they ought to be avoided. Tyman (1990) suggested that there are probably differences in effect between α- and β-thujone, and others have suggested that the same is true for *cis*- and *trans*-anethole isomers. The thujone in the whole essential oil of *Thuja occidentalis* (up to around 80%) is definitely toxic. One frequently repeated statement is that all forms of ketone are neurotoxic, but this is not so: some are neurotoxic but not all; the author has found the intelligent use of sage oil (*Salvia officinalis*) containing the ketone thujone to be problem free.

There is a variation of opinion on the safety of carvone isomers, viz. the (+)-carvone molecule in caraway oil and the (−)-carvone in spearmint oil. *Carum carvi* [caraway] is considered to be a safe oil in all respects by Tisserand and Balacs (1995 p. 204) (despite noting it as a mucous membrane irritant), but Winter (1999 p. 113) states that both (+)-carvone and the (−)-carvone have no known toxicity. The seed oil of *Anethum graveolens* [dill] contains 40–60% of ketones including (+)-carvone and is considered neurotoxic by Franchomme and Pénoël (2001 p. 351). There are many anomalies to be found in aromatherapy books and training courses. In some circumstances the so called 'toxic' molecules are the very ones that are needed for beneficial results, such as the phenol thymol in *Thymus vulgaris* ct. thymol, an extremely effective antiseptic and antifungal agent (Mills 1991).

Toxicity depends not only on the nature of the main component, but also on the relationships and synergy (see below) between it and some of the smaller (perhaps as yet unidentified) constituents, which are known to lessen or nullify undesirable effects in some cases. This may illustrate why certain oils high in ketones are not considered toxic, and why a few oils considered toxic by some people do not appear to be so (see Synergism below). It should be remembered that a great deal of good has been effected by qualified aromatherapists in the UK since the 1960s, and no serious harm has so far been recorded.

Synergism

> Essential oils are complex substances, and there is no simple direct relationship between the effects of any single component of an essential oil and the effects of the complete natural essential oil – essential oils are synergistic mixes.
>
> Price (1990b)

Single oils

A whole essential oil has a natural synergistic power where the combined action of disparate individual molecules within an essential oil has a total effect greater than the sum of their individual effects. The word is derived from the Greek *syn* = together, *ergon* = work.

As discussed in Ch. 2, essential oils are complex mixtures, some containing from a few dozen to several hundreds of different molecules which act in synergy to produce their healing effect, but if the composition is altered then the natural synergy of the remaining constituents is diminished or destroyed. An isolated component generally needs much greater care in use as unwanted side effects may be produced. When that same constituent is present in the whole oil, other constituents act as 'quenchers' of these unwanted effects (see Quenching, below), enabling the oil to be used without harmful effect. Complete essential oils have been found in practice to be more effective than their isolated principal constituent(s) and without side effects on account of this synergistic effect (Hall 1904).

Very rarely an oil consists largely of only one component and then the effects of the oil may be closely correlated with that component, so that the effect of the oil and that of the main component are the same (wintergreen oil is almost wholly methyl salicylate, 98% or 99%). Usually, however, the essential oil consists of many components creating a synergy, and so it is not possible to ascribe the effects of the whole oil to one particular component, even a major one. Constituents present in very small amounts (e.g. furanocoumarins) are often found to be as active as, or even more active than, the principal constituent.

> ' ... minor components of essential oils can modify the activity of main components, reaffirming the importance of chemically characterizing essential oils in order to understand the overall bioactivity'
>
> Nunes et al. (2010)

Similarly, in herbal medicine research has been done on isolated chemical constituents of *Echinacea* in an attempt to determine the active principle within the plant. This has proved illusive, and the conclusion drawn is that the medicinal effect is most likely to be as a result of the unique interplay of the naturally occurring substances within the living plant (Raynor 1999).

The synergism of many commercial essentials oils is destroyed during the production process, e.g. rectification and fractionation, as illustrated by the case of eucalyptus. Most eucalyptus products generally found commercially have routinely been redistilled, rectified and refined, which means that some molecules have been left behind in the redistillation process following the rectification of the crude oil, e.g. the rare phenol australol (Pénoël 1993, personal communication).

Antimicrobial synergy

Tests carried out on individual components from *Eucalyptus citriodora* revealed that they were relatively inactive; however, a combination of the three isolated major components in the same ratio as found in the natural oil produced a fourfold increase in antimicrobial activity against *Staphylococcus aureus* (Low, Rawal & Griffin 1974).

Antioxidant synergy

In tests to measure the antioxidant activity of essential oils, nutmeg, pepper and thyme oils, among others, were found to be effective and to have beneficial effects on lipid metabolism (Simpson 1994). Thyme oils are known to be biologically active in the antibacterial, antifungal and antioxidant areas. Nine of the constituent components of thyme oil were shown to have antioxidant properties (linalool, thujone, camphene, thymol, carvacrol, γ-terpinene, β-caryophyllene, borneol and myrcene, listed in descending order of activity), but it was noted that antioxidant activity for the whole oil was greater than that of the most active single component linalool (Deans et al. 1993).

Enhanced synergistic effect of blends

Apart from the synergy produced by the components of a single oil, there is also an enhancement of effect when two or more whole oils are mixed together. For example, the combined bactericidal effect of several oils together is greater than the effect of any of the individual oils, which is why the authors have always recommended using a blend of two or three oils in a treatment.

Quenching

Quenching is an important aspect of synergism, and essential oils display a quenching effect whereby the potential unwanted side effects of one component are nullified by the presence of other component(s). This quenching effect is well known in the perfumery industry, where it is turned to advantage by adding quenching components to its perfumes to prevent skin irritation. This feature can also be made use of when mixing oils. The peel oils from *Citrus paradisi* [grapefruit] or *Citrus sinensis* [sweet orange], when added to *Cymbopogon citratus* in a 50:50 mix, successfully quench the irritant properties of the latter (Witty 1992, personal communication). Comparing two eucalyptus oils, *Eucalyptus globulus* [Tasmanian blue gum] and *E. smithii* [gully gum], each contains around 65% of 1,8-cineole (an oxide which is a skin irritant), yet the former is contraindicated for use on young children and the latter is not (Pénoël 1992/93).

Isolates

Isolates are sometimes used in pharmaceutical preparations but they are not advised for use in aromatherapy. Citral on its own is a severe skin irritant, but *whole* lemon oil, which contains citral, is not, thanks to the presence of (+)-limonene and its synergistic quenching effect. Although citral produces sensitization reactions in humans when applied alone, it produces no such reactions when applied as a mixture with other compounds (Opdyke 1976b).

Phenol is a well known antiseptic which used to be used in hospitals, but the phenol in *Thymus vulgaris* ct. thymol, although it is 20 times more effective and exhibits the mucosal irritating properties of the group far less (Mills 1991 p. 282). Schnaubelt (1998 p. 25) echoes this when he says that pure phenol is toxic, but natural plant phenols, such as thymol, 'have additional side chains that transform them into non-toxic, effective antiseptics'.

Tests carried out with the isolates phenyl acetaldehyde, citral and cinnamic aldehyde – found in *Citrus aurantium* (flos) [neroli bigarade], *Cymbopogon citratus*, *C. flexuosus* [lemongrass] and *Cinnamomum verum* (cort.) [cinnamon bark] oils, respectively – showed them to be skin sensitizers. The whole essential oils in which the aldehydes are present (at up to 85%) were found not to provoke sensitizing reactions. It appeared that some other component (s) of the natural oil inhibited the induction or expression of sensitization (Opdyke 1976b). To test this, several terpenes and alcohols found along with the particular aldehyde in the natural composition were combined with each of the aldehydes in

Table 3.1 Results of quenching tests on mixtures of cinnamic aldehyde with other essential oil components

Second test material	Relative proportions*	Results of sensitization test
Dipropylene glycol	1: 1	+
Phenylethyl alcohol	1: 1	+
Eugenol	1: 1	–
Eugenol	1: 1[†]	–
Eugenol	2.5: 1[†]	+
Cinnamic alcohol	1: 1	+
Benzyl salicylate	1: 1	+
(+)-limonene	1: 1	–

*Ratio (w/w) of cinnamic aldehyde to second test material. Each mixture was tested at an overall concentration of 6% in petrolatum by the maximization procedure (Kligman 1966, Kligman & Epstein 1975).
[†]Duplicate tests.
Reprinted from Opdyke 1979 p. 255, with kind permission from Elsevier Ltd.

question. It appears to be a consistent finding that each of these aldehydes, although producing sensitization reactions when applied alone, produces no sensitization reactions in selected simple mixtures with other compounds (Opdyke 1979) (Table 3.1). The irritant quality of oils with a high citral content (even 70%) can be quenched by adding an oil containing an equal amount of (+)-limonene, a terpene present in some citrus oils to around 80–90%.

These findings point to the difference between using a single compound and the use of a natural synergistic mix with inbuilt quenching action. The above-mentioned tests contrast with two earlier tests carried out by Kligman in 1971 and 1972 on 25 volunteers using cinnamon bark oil at 8% concentration and producing 18 and 20 sensitization reactions, respectively (Kligman & Epstein 1975). Cinnamal is not the only component in *C. verum* (cort.) [cinnamon bark] oil that acts as a sensitizer, so perhaps this may be a case of synergy enhancing the unwanted effect. IFRA recommend that this oil is used at a maximum 1% concentration in a fragrance compound (IFRA 1992), equivalent to 0.2% in an aromatherapy massage oil (i.e. one drop in 25 mL carrier oil), although a lower level of use of 0.1% for the skin has been recommended (Tisserand & Balacs 1995 p. 130).

Interaction takes place between the constituents within a single oil and also between two or more essential oils, hence potentially toxic elements may be altered, enhanced or counteracted by other constituents present.

Safe quantities

Essential oils may be applied to the body in a variety of ways, and these are discussed in Ch. 6, but usually their use involves inhalation, application to the skin or ingestion. Essential oils are powerful, otherwise they would be of no use therapeutically, and inappropriate use in whatever way can bring about undesired effects. Dosage, in terms of both quantity and duration, is all important, as too little may mean little or no result, and too much may either have a beneficial effect or create a serious problem. The majority of essential oils may be considered less toxic than the over-the-counter medicines aspirin and paracetamol. Aromatherapy is safe and there need be no hesitation in introducing these natural aromatic products into a hospital environment. Many substances in common use are toxic in overdose, e.g. carrots are beneficial in moderation but a surfeit will produce illness, and this is true of many everyday foods such as tomatoes, saffron or mustard. Many essential oils contain constituents which when isolated are found to be toxic, but many items normally regarded as quite safe also contain substances which, when isolated, could be shown to be toxic – e.g. tea, almonds, apples, pears, radishes, mustard, sage, hops etc. (Griggs 1977).

Valnet (1980 p. 11) cites headaches and the loss of eyebrows in workers handling vanilla, but vanilla ice-cream is eaten and enjoyed without ill effect. An essential oil may be both safe and toxic depending on the dosage – it all depends on the knowledge, skill and experience of the therapist: for example, lavender is sedative in low dose but a high dose can cause insomnia (amphoteric effect).

Ingestion of essential oils

Only therapeutic essential oils should be employed for internal use, although it is not easy to guarantee the purity of an essential oil. Essential oils are absorbed into the blood stream and are metabolized into water- soluble products, allowing for renal elimination. The ingestion of essential oils should be left in the hands of a competent aromatologist (e.g. a licentiate of the Institute of Aromatic Medicine), or an aromatherapist working under the direction of a doctor. Legal requirements and rules of the hospital management board have to be observed, as well as the ethical considerations of any professional body to which the aromatherapist belongs. Nevertheless, some conditions such as enteritis, irritable bowel syndrome and diverticulitis can scarcely be treated in any other way than by ingestion.

Essential oils should always be correctly diluted for internal use; the best medium, if a dispersant is not readily available, is a fixed oil because the essential oils will dissolve easily and completely in it. Runny honey is also a good diluent, with the addition of a little water. Ingestion of essential oils is not advised for pregnant women and very young children.

Ingestion/overdose

When it comes to testing the toxic effects of swallowing essential oils, all studies have been carried out on animals as testing on humans is considered too hazardous. Occasionally some knowledge is derived from an accident involving a child or a deliberate overdose by an adult. Therefore, many of the opinions offered on this subject in the aromatherapy literature must be regarded as speculative.

The ingestion of a large quantity of neat essential oil is unlikely as it would produce a burning sensation in the mouth and throat, and in some serious cases cause nausea, vomiting and diarrhoea. If the overdose is extreme there may follow lethargy, ataxia and coma, or perhaps irritability and convulsions (e.g. pennyroyal). The pupils may be dilated (e.g. camphor) or constricted (e.g. eucalyptus). Table 3.2 shows the lethal dose (LD_{50} is the dose at which 50% of the test subjects die) of some representative oils for a typical adult and a small child. These figures have been extrapolated from figures derived from animal testing and, as previously stated, metabolization in humans is not always the same as in animals so their accuracy cannot be guaranteed. In the absence of other information we must rely on these data as a guide.

The quantities used in aromatherapy are very small, so there is normally an extremely high safety factor when comparing the lethal dose with the effective dose. The effective dose (ED_{50}) is the term used when some sort of response is being monitored in the experimental animal other than the death of the animal. The median effective dose is the dose

Table 3.2 Lethal dose (LD$_{50}$)

Essential oil			LD$_{50}$ g/kg (animal)	Lethal dose* 15 kg child	Lethal dose* 70 kg adult
Latin name	Common name			(mL)	(mL)
Aniba rosaeodora (lig)	Rosewood		4.3	72	334
Boswellia carteri (resin)	Frankincense		5	83	389
Cananga odorata (flos)	Ylang ylang	More than	5	83	389
Cedrus atlantica (lig)	Atlas cedarwood	More than	5	83	389
Chamaemelum nobile (flos)	Roman chamomile		8.56	143	666
Chamomilla recutita (flos)	German chamomile	More than	5	83	389
Cinnamomum verum (cort)	Cinnamon bark		3.4	57	264
Cinnamomum verum (fol)	Cinnamon leaf		2.65	44	206
Citrus aurantium var. *amara* (flos)	Neroli	More than	5	83	389
Citrus aurantium var. *amara* (fol)	Petitgrain orange	More than	5	83	389
Citrus bergamia (per)	Bergamot	More than	10	167	778
Citrus reticulata (per)	Mandarin	More than	5	83	389
Commiphora myrrha	Myrrh		1.65	28	128
Coriandrum sativum (fruct)	Coriander		4.13	69	321
Cupressus sempervirens (fol)	Cypress	More than	5	83	389
Eucalyptus citriodora (fol)	Eucalyptus	More than	5	83	389
Eucalyptus globulus (fol)	Eucalyptus		4.44	74	345
Foeniculum vulgare var. *dulce* (fruct)	Sweet fennel		3.8	63	296
Hyssopus officinalis	Hyssop		1.4	23	109
Juniperus communis (fruct)	Juniper berry		8	133	622
Lavandula angustifolia	Lavender	More than	5	83	389
Lavandula × *intermedia* 'Super'	Lavandin	More than	5	83	389
Melaleuca alternifolia (fol)	Tea tree		1.9	32	148
Melaleuca leucadendron (fol)	Cajuput		3.87	65	301
Mentha × *piperita*	Peppermint		4.5	75	350
Myristica fragrans (sem)	Nutmeg		2.6	43	202
Ocimum basilicum	Basil		1.4	23	109
Origanum majorana	Marjoram		2.24	37	174
Pelargonium graveolens (fol)	Geranium	More than	5	83	389
Pimpinella anisum (fruct)	Aniseed		2.25	38	175

Continued

Table 3.2 Lethal dose (LD50)—cont'd

Essential oil			LD$_{50}$ g/kg (animal)	Lethal dose* 15 kg child	Lethal dose* 70 kg adult
Latin name	Common name			(mL)	(mL)
Pinus sylvestris (fol)	Pine		6.88	115	535
Piper nigrum (fruct)	Black pepper	More than	5	83	389
Pogostemon patchouli (fol)	Patchouli	More than	5	83	389
Rosa damascena, R. centifolia (flos)	Rose otto	More than	5	83	389
Rosmarinus officinalis	Rosemary		5	83	389
Salvia officinalis	Sage		2.52	42	196
Salvia sclarea	Clary		5.6	93	436
Santalum album (lig)	Sandalwood		5.58	93	434
Satureia hortensis	Savory		1.37	23	107
Syzygium aromaticum (flos)	Clove bud		2.65	44	206
Thymus mastichina	Spanish marjoram	More than	5	83	389
Thymus vulgaris ct. thymol	Thyme		4.7	78	366
Vetiveria zizanioides (rad)	Vetiver	More than	5	83	389
Zingiber officinale (rad)	Ginger		5	83	389
Compound	1, 8-Cineole		2.48	41	193
Compound	Carvacrol		0.81	14	63
Compound	Carvone		1.64	27	128
Compound	Linalool		2.79	47	217
Compound	p-Cymene		4.75	79	369
Compound	Pulegone		0.4	7	31
Compound	Safrole		1.95	33	152
Compound	Terpinen-4-ol		4.3	72	334
Compound	Thymol		0.98	16	76
Compound	Camphor		0.9	15	70
Compound	Borneol		2	33	156

*The human lethal doses are extrapolated from animal test results.

at which 50% of the test subjects achieve the desired benefit.

Toxicity figures given in aromatherapy literature do not always make it clear that these doses are per kilogram of body weight, which could lead to the misunderstanding that the figures given are the effective or lethal doses for a person. They are not: they are dependent on the person's weight. For example, the LD$_{50}$ value for the oil from *Salvia officinalis* [sage] is 2.6 g/kg, which equates to a fatal dose of approximately 170 mL for a 60 kg person; the equivalent figure for *Chamaemelum nobile* [Roman chamomile] is 570 mL for a 60 kg person. The quantities involved are so great that anyone in their right mind would jib at taking them; however, illness may be caused at a much lower dose.

The following should never be administered internally:

- Oils obtained from gums (other than by distillation)
- Resins (because of the solvent residue)
- Absolutes (because of the solvent residue)
- Commercial quality oils (i.e. standardized) used by the perfume, food and pharmaceutical industries.

Ingestion of eucalyptus essential oil

Eucalyptus oil poisoning

There have been many cases of eucalyptus oil poisoning and it is puzzling why eucalyptus oil is so frequently taken by mouth, especially in Australia. A difficulty arises because there are very many kinds of eucalyptus oil of varying composition, and in none of the incidents referred to below is the botanical source specified; this may explain the sometimes conflicting recommendations for treatment given below. Ingesting up to 25 mL of eucalyptus oil led to coma in about 50% of 34 cases examined by Gurr and Scroggie (1965), which lasted from 30 minutes to 8 hours, usually with complete recovery after 24 hours: recovery has been noted even after ingestion of 60 mL. Another case of complete recovery was that of a 3-year-old boy who ingested 10 mL of eucalyptus oil and was soon deeply comatose with shallow, irregular respiration. Gastric lavage was given; he regained consciousness after 5 hours and was normal after 24 hours (Patel & Wiggins 1980). Spoerke et al. (1989) reviewed 14 cases of accidental exposure to eucalyptus oil, of which nine were ingestion. They concluded that small amounts seemed to be comparatively harmless and for larger amounts gastrointestinal symptoms were the most common, followed by central nervous system depression; amounts ingested ranged from 5 to 30 mL and patient age varied from 7 months to 20 plus years. Inhalation and skin exposure produced no or minimal symptoms.

A review of 41 child cases of eucalyptus poisoning in South East Queensland showed that 80% were completely asymptomatic, including four children who had swallowed more than 30 mL (maximum 45 mL). Two children were dizzy or ataxic, four had mildly depressed conscious levels, one child had an itchy rash and another had pruritus. A 4-month-old baby who had ingested 30 mL was the only one to display meiosis, hypertonia and hyperreflexia. The presence and severity of symptoms was not related to the amounts ingested (Webb & Pitt 1993); it was suggested that children should not undergo gastrointestinal decontamination unless symptomatic on arrival at hospital. Tibbals (1995) looked at 109 cases of child eucalyptus oil poisoning and recommended that children should receive medical attention regardless of the amount ingested.

Action to be taken

Traditional treatment in the event of an overdose is quite rigorous, involving gastric lavage or emesis and dilution with milk or fixed oil. Temple et al. (1991) reevaluated this protocol after reviewing five cases of child poisoning following ingestion of citronella essential oil. One of these included a 16-month-old child who had ingested 25 mL of the oil, but in all five cases there was little medical intervention and all patients recovered with no ill effects. They concluded that advice given in standard texts based on cases managed with outmoded techniques should be evaluated, as the risks of evacuative and pharmacological interventions were considered greater than the risk of severe poisoning.

An example not to be followed

A nurse practising aromatherapy in a hospice some years ago was concerned to prove the safety of the oils she was administering to patients and took 5 mL of each of about 40 essential oils by mouth (one per week). In a personal communication she stated that she suffered no ill effects apart from sometimes dreaming more vividly than usual. The 40 oils included some that are potentially hazardous, and this extreme example must not be followed. Individuals vary greatly in their reaction to different substances and such actions may produce a disastrous result. There is a large safety factor when using the oils in normal aromatherapy quantities, i.e. two or three drops compared to approximately 100 drops that a 5 mL teaspoon would hold.

Oils in the eye

Undiluted essential oils are never placed in the ear nor on anogenital mucous surfaces and especially not in the eye, even diluted. If by accident essential oil does get into the eye then the advice given as to what to do varies slightly. One course of action is first to flush the eye under a running tap to expel most of the oil, and then to apply a fixed vegetable oil (Baudoux 2000 p. 35). Zhiri (2002 p. 21) agrees that neat essential oils should never be applied to the eyes, ears and anogenital mucosa, and also adds the nose; in case of accidental instillation or ingestion, either ingest or apply as appropriate a vegetable oil (e.g. olive, sunflower) to dissolve the essential oil, then seek medical aid. The authors have had experience of cases of mal use of essential oils in the eyes and on genital areas and have found the vegetable oil method to be effective, with minimum discomfort; essential oils are immediately soluble in vegetable oils, which give a dissolving/flushing action. For the eyes, the vegetable oil may be flooded in, and for the genital area a piece of cloth soaked in a vegetable oil immediately reduces the painful sensation, and usually there are no after effects.

Health professionals working in hospitals and similar establishments should secure the approval of a consultant or other suitably qualified and responsible person before giving oils by mouth (including gargles) or by the rectal and vaginal routes into the body. It is important to preserve procedural safety: the prescriber, dispenser and administrator should be separate persons to guard against error.

Undesired effects

A synthetic modern drug can have a positive effect on a diseased organ or part of the body but it can also have an adverse effect on a healthy part of the body, resulting in a second drug having to be administered. This in turn can give another adverse side effect, which will call for the administration of yet another drug. This cumulative effect of unwanted effects eventually killed the author's mother, who, at the time of her death, was taking 22 different tablets a day, only one pertaining to her original problem.

In aromatherapy a different mindset is required, as essential oils bring many beneficial effects as well as a very occasional unwanted effect. As can be seen from the list of properties given for lavender oil, most of the side effects of essential oils are desirable. For example, lavender oil may be used as part of a treatment for depression and if, as a result, there are other beneficial results such as the alleviation of insomnia and relief from rheumatic pain, this is to be welcomed.

Undesired side effects occur usually as a result of the misuse of the oils, e.g. in the attempt to produce an abortion, or by accidental overdose – typically a toddler swallowing essential oils from a bottle. If essential oils are sold only in bottles with integral droppers and sensible precautions are taken to prevent access to them by children, this can be considered an extremely low risk therapy.

In normal aromatherapy the dose is usually very low but, as with any form of treatment, idiosyncratic reactions are a rare possibility. Such a case was reported by Vilaplana, Romaguera and Grimalt (1991) of a middle-aged woman who developed itching after using a cologne which was found to contain Bulgarian rose oil and geraniol. This was the first time in 326 cases of dermatitis that a person had tested positive to Bulgarian rose oil, and there were no other reported cases of dermatitis to the damask rose family, which prompts a question about the quality of this particular rose oil.

Hazardous oils

Some oils are rarely or never used in aromatherapy because of possible harmful effects (see Appendix B.4 on the CD-ROM). Some examples are *Juniperus sabina* [savin], *Gaultheria procumbens* [wintergreen], *Peumus boldus* [boldo leaf], *Sassafras officinale* [sassafras] and *Thuja occidentalis* [thuja]. Some other essential oils have a general prohibition on their use but without just cause. *Mentha pulegium* [pennyroyal] is alleged to be an abortifacient, but it may be used on men and those who are not pregnant, albeit with care because of its high content of the ketone pulegone.

Hyssopus officinalis [hyssop] is an excellent oil for respiratory disorders (used regularly over 30 years by the author) but is generally listed as toxic, as are *Pimpinella anisum* [aniseed] and several more. *Salvia officinalis* [sage] contains the ketone thujone (around 50%), and although nothing has been proven against the ketone molecule in sage oil, it is prudent to use it with care. Oils such as these may not be suitable for all health problems and may have contraindications, making their use not suitable for certain people in certain circumstances, but for the well trained therapist it is possible to use effectively the so-called hazardous or 'toxic' oils to the greater advantage of their clients. Confusion is aggravated by some authors and aromatherapy companies giving different warnings for different oils.

Epilepsy

It is widely taught that *Hyssopus officinalis* used on a person will provoke an epileptic fit, and this teaching is supposed to be based on a statement by Valnet (1980 p. 11), but what he actually wrote is 'Even in weak doses the essences of sage, rosemary and hyssop can produce *a tendency to epilepsy under certain conditions and in persons whose resistance is low*' (author's italics). Cases of poisoning by sage and hyssop oils in the south of France have been investigated and the sage culprit has been identified as *Salvia lavandulaefolia*, which is rich in camphor. The epileptogenic effects of these two oils were extrapolated from animal tests, and for humans the sub clinical doses for *Hyssopus officinalis* and sage were found to be up to 0.1 mL/kg and 0.4 mL/kg, whereas lethal doses were more than 1.6 mL/kg and 4.0 mL/kg, respectively; the greatest toxicity was due to a combination of pinocamphone and isopinocamphone (Steinmetz et al. 1980). According to Renzini et al. (1999) *Hyssopus officinalis* begins to exhibit cytotoxicity at a concentration of 100 µg/mL and is due mainly to the component linalool, which is present in many essential oils. Millet et al. (1979) investigated – in animals – the convulsant activity of *Hyssopus officinalis* and *Salvia lavandulaefolia* and found the sub clinical dose for hyssop to be less than 0.08 g/kg; above 0.13 g/kg convulsions appeared and were lethal at 1.25 g/kg; this effect they also found to be due to the presence of pinocamphone and isopinocamphone.

Summary

Although some essential oils do present hazards, which frighten the inadequately trained, the properly trained therapist will recognize the hazard and take account of it to minimize or obviate any risk. This will be done by assessing the situation, applying the training received to the best advantage, and using common sense. These powerful oils should not be available to the general public, who may know nothing about their chemistry and effects.

Power and hazards

3 (Part II)

Len Price

CHAPTER CONTENTS

Specific hazards

Dermal toxicity

This term includes irritation, phototoxicity and sensitization. To minimize risk it is important to bear in mind that essential oils must be properly sourced, of the highest quality, botanically identified, well stored and unadulterated (many cases of dermal toxicity can be traced back to substances that have been added for commercial reasons). Steam distilled essential oils are superior to other extracts such as absolutes, concretes, carbon dioxide extracted etc.; lavender absolute was involved in two cases, one a therapist with a 3-year history of dermatitis extending to the face and neck (Bleasel, Tate & Rademaker 2002).

Skin irritation, sensitization

This is a reaction to a substance that produces inflammation and itchiness. Some essential oils are irritating to the skin, and these are usually (but not exclusively) found to contain high proportions of either aldehydes or phenols. Oils in common use which have been found to be irritant are listed in Appendix B.6 (see CD-ROM). Because there appear to be wide variations in tolerance, a given oil might not cause a reaction in the majority of people yet be irritant to one or two more sensitive individuals; dermal irritation produced by essential oils is usually localized and short lived. Assuming that one oil has a 50% presence of an offending component, this is present in the total mix at only 0.5% when the oil is used in a normal massage mix along with two or three other oils at the standard dilution of 3% essential oils in a carrier.

When spread over a large area of skin the possibility of irritation is remote; the degree of irritation is proportional to the strength of the mixture applied.

The following oils have been recorded as being implicated in irritation:

Tagetes – an aromatherapist presented with acute bilateral hand eczema 24 hours after spraying roses with an insecticide and patch testing gave a strong reaction to *Tagetes patula* [French marigold]; the acute eczema was attributed to a cross-reaction with pyrethroid in the insecticide (Bilsland & Strong 1990). Dermatitis caused by the leaves and flowers of *Tagetes minuta*, *T. patula*, *T. erecta* and *T. glandulifera* is common in South Africa, and the essential oil of *Tagetes glandulifera* is sometimes cited as being a skin irritant, but we have not found this to be the case in practice, although it is a photosensitizer.

Brassica nigra [mustard] and *Armoracia rusticana* [horseradish] – two oils from the Cruciferaceae family which are not normally recommended for aromatherapy use because both consist almost entirely of allylisothiocyanate. These oils applied neat to the skin will provoke severe burning and blistering, but it has been known for them to be recommended at the extremely low concentration of one drop of essential oil in 500 mL of carrier oil for rheumatism.

Melaleuca alternifolia – there are many cases reported of skin irritancy and dermatitis involving tea tree oil (Bhushan & Beck 1997, Southwell, Freeman & Rubel 1997). It should be borne in mind that tea trees are cultivated, grown from seed, and therefore the composition of the oil when distilled is variable. This oil is then adjusted at source to conform to laid down parameters (especially the 1,8-cineole content) and so may not have the natural synergy that may be expected. Tea tree oil has a relatively simple composition (about 30 compounds). Some oils are synthesized in a laboratory and are known as reconstructed oils (RCO); they are not natural products and may have unwanted side effects. Seven people had been applying commercial tea tree oil undiluted on the skin for conditions such as fungal infections, pimples and skin rashes, and all developed eczematous dermatitis, some with vesiculation; a common allergen was (−)-limonene: the application of diluted oil to the skin caused no reaction (Knight & Hausen 1994), showing that use of the commercial oil undiluted was ill advised. Treatment of chronic atopic dermatitis by application of undiluted *Melaleuca alternifolia* was unsuccessful and then oral ingestion of the oil mixed with honey was advised, which led to exacerbation of the dermatitis; 1,8-cineole was the allergen (De Groot & Weyland 1992). The reasoning behind this treatment is hard to understand.

Santalum album [sandalwood] – overdose due to daily application for 8 years of sandalwood paste to the forehead led to a hyperpigmented, erythematous plaque and lesions and fissures on thumb and forefinger; sandalwood paste patch test proved positive (Sharma, Bajaj & Singh 1987). The offending compound was not identified.

Pimpinella anisum [aniseed], *Syzygium aromaticum* flos, fol., caul. [clove, bud, leaf and stem] can irritate the skin if used in high concentration because of their phenolic ether and phenol content, respectively.

Cinnamomum verum cort., fol. [cinnamon bark and leaf] – the bark oil contains cinnamal, which is a known skin sensitizer, but the whole oil proves to be less so. A patch test should always be carried out prior to using this oil.

Of 1500 dermatitis patients who were patch tested, 21 had a reaction to essential oils (which were not botanically specified) of pine needle, dwarf pine, clove and eucalyptus, and it was found that some components of the essential oils – carene, phellandrene and eugenol – were sensitizers (Woeber & Krombach 1969). The regional provenance of the essential oils had no great influence on sensitization potency: good quality and lack of ageing were more important. A therapist with a 3-year history of forearm dermatitis was sensitive to a range of oils containing geraniol but was also sensitive to yarrow, laurel and peppermint oils, which do not contain geraniol (Bleasel, Tate & Rademaker 2002).

More than 95% of users of essential oils in aromatherapy are women, hugely outnumbering men: perhaps it is relevant that a Japanese study showed that the skin of men tends to be more than twice as sensitive as that of women, and that in situations of severe stress, lack of sleep, etc. all skins are rendered more sensitive (Hosokawa & Ogwana 1979).

Mucous membrane irritation

Generally speaking, essential oils with a substantial content of phenols (chiefly thymol, carvacrol and eugenol) can be responsible for irritating a mucous membrane. Oils containing aldehydes may also be implicated. In the past it was believed that the hydrocarbon terpenes caused mucous membrane irritation (Gattefossé 1937 p. 40) but this is now thought not to be the case. Any of the oils listed in Appendix B.6 (see CD-ROM) may cause irritation of the mucous membranes of the alimentary, respiratory and genitourinary tracts. A possible exception is lemon oil, which contains less than 5% aldehyde and consists mainly of hydrocarbon terpenes, principally (+)-limonene, which is known to quench the irritant effect of the aldehyde.

Contact sensitization

There are some oils that do not produce any reaction on first contact with the skin but may do so on a subsequent application; there seems to be no common denominator to those essential oils that are sensitizing. The body's reaction involves the immune system, via the cells in the basal layer of the epidermis. Poor storage of oils containing a significant amount of monoterpenes can lead to the formation of sensitizing hydroperoxides: an infamous example is turpentine, which is responsible for skin allergies in workers in the paint industry. Oils to be wary of in this respect are shown in Appendix B.8 (see CD-ROM).

Cross-sensitization

Once a person is sensitized to one substance, that person is more likely to be susceptible to other similar substances, although the risk is low. This need not cause concern, but any aromatherapist who is sensitive to substances should be aware of the possibility. This is a complex topic, not well understood, but one example is that people can become sensitive to benzoin after sensitization to Peru balsam or turpentine. There is a similar relationship between turpentine and peppermint, and a case of turpentine-induced sensitivity to peppermint oil involved a laboratory technician who suffered swelling of tongue, lips and gums after a dental operation. Tests revealed sensitivity to peppermint oil, an ingredient in dental spray and mouthwash, and this was due to α-pinene, limonene and phellandrene, which are also present in turpentine, from which he had previously developed severe eczema of the hands (Dooms-Goossens et al. 1977): *Cymbopogon martinii* [palmarosa] is implicated in cross-sensitization with lavender, lemongrass and geranium.

An aromatherapist had a 12-month history of hand and forearm dermatitis which improved when away from work. Patch testing revealed positive reactions not only to oils of lavender, geranium and lemongrass, but also to oils to which she had not been previously exposed (palmarosa, frankincense, rose, neroli, myrrh), which implied cross-reactivity (Bleasel, Tate & Rademaker 2002). Dermatitis recurred after eating lemongrass-flavoured food – systemic contact dermatitis.

A man allergic to turpentine breathed in the vapour of tea tree oil in hot water to help his bronchitis and developed acute exudative dermatitis of the face, trunk and arms (De Groot 1996). The origin of the essential oil was not stated. A woman who had been treating her acne for a long time with undiluted *Melaleuca alternifolia* [tea tree] essential oil without reaction presented with dermatitis on her forehead and mouth: patch testing was positive to tea tree and colophony (an oleo resin from which turpentine is distilled): crossreaction between turpentine and colophony had already been established (Selvaag, Erikson & Thune 1994). Palmarosa has been implicated in cross sensitization with lavender, lemongrass and geranium (Dooms-Goossens et al. 1977 p. 73), and galbanum resin has been linked in cross-sensitization with Peru balsam (see also Appendix B on the CD-ROM).

Phototoxicity, photosensitivity

Photosensitization is a process in which reactions to normally ineffective radiation are induced in a system by the introduction of a radiation-absorbing substance – the photosensitizer (Kochevar 1987). Photosensitivity may occur when certain essential oil components, particularly the expressed essences, react with the skin under the influence of ultraviolet rays, yet does not occur on skin protected from natural or artificial sunlight. It may result in erythema, hyperpigmentation and perhaps vesicles, depending on the severity of the reaction. Furanocoumarins (psoralens) appear to be primarily responsible for phytophototoxic reactions in humans (Lovell 1993), so care needs to be taken with the citrus essences, which are expressed from the peel and contain furanocoumarin molecules, particularly bergamot. Other oils exhibiting this characteristic at aromatherapeutic doses are *Angelica archangelica* rad. [angelica root], *Juniperus virginiana* [Virginian cedarwood], *Ruta graveolens* [rue], *Lippia citriodora* [lemon verbena] and *Cuminum cyminum* [cumin] (Opdyke 1974) (see Appendix B.7 on the CD-ROM).

Factors that influence the phototoxic response to psoralens are the presence of a suntan, natural pigmentation (dark skin), site of application, skin hydration, and the interval between application of the psoralen and irradiation (it is worth mentioning that aromatherapy oils are applied mainly to areas not normally exposed to sunlight). A particularly notable culprit is the expressed oil of *Citrus bergamia* [bergamot] (Opdyke 1973), which was studied by Zaynoun, Johnson and Frain-Bell (1977), and its use in aromatherapy needs consideration; tests by Pathak and Fitzpatrick (1959) have shown the time interval between applying psoralens and the maximal phototoxic effect to be 30–45 minutes (tested on guinea pig and human skin), and a later test (Arora and Willis 1976) indicated a time interval of up to 75 minutes.

Tests probably carried out for the benefit of the perfumery trade on bergamot oil in ethyl alcohol showed no phototoxic responses at a concentration of 0.5%, and at 1.0% no phototoxic response after 8 hours; the tests were carried out on five subjects (Zaynoun, Johnson & Frain-Bell 1977 p. 231) and also showed that intervals of 1–2 hours between application and irradiation yielded a maximal phototoxic response. Applying this directly to aromatherapy is questionable, as aromatherapists do not use ethyl alcohol as a medium for application, and the flow of psoralen through the horny layer of the skin is dependent on the carrier used (Kaidbey & Kligman 1974, Kammerau et al. 1976). It is known that the horny layer is a major barrier to the penetration of psoralens; in tests, 70–90% of topically applied 8-methoxypsoralen (8-MOP, xanthotoxin, which is not present in bergamot oil) did not enter the horny layer and was finally lost through sloughing (Kammerau et al. 1976). Bergamot oil itself is resorbed through the skin in 40–60 minutes (Römelt et al. 1974, Valette 1945).

The tests by Zaynoun, Johnson and Frain-Bell (1977 p. 232) also showed that using paraffin molle flavum (PMF) as the carrier resulted in increased speed of penetration through the horny layer and produced a shorter period in which phototoxicity persists than when using ethanol, and it is possible that the effects using a vegetable oil as a carrier more closely resemble the results using PMF than those using alcohol.

The IFRA Committee recommends a level of 5-MOP (bergapten, a naturally occurring analogue of psoralen) of 75 ppm in a (fragrance) compound, and assuming a 5-MOP content of 0.35% this equates to a level of expressed bergamot oil in the compound of 2% (Jouhar 1991), which translates to 0.4% (about eight drops in 100 mL) in an aromatherapy preparation applied to skin. The use of 5-MOP is forbidden in the EU except as a normal component of essential oils.

In practical experience over four decades, there has been no reported problem by thousands of therapists who have followed our training and numerous clients who have followed our advice. On this basis, it is suggested that following the application of bergamot oil using the normal aromatherapy dilution (usually less than 1% in synergistic blends) it is reasonably safe to expose the skin of normal people to sunlight provided that more than 2 hours have elapsed since the application. This advice may be tempered in case of any unusual sensitivity in the individual client. It is interesting to note that some other simple coumarin derivatives, such as umbelliferone, herniarin and aesculetin, have a sunlight filter effect because they absorb ultraviolet light of 280–315 nm (Schilcher 1985 p. 228).

It is necessary to be wary of reported cases now that the fragrance industry relies so heavily on synthetic materials. An example is a middle-aged man who used a sandalwood aftershave lotion for 3 weeks which brought about weeping, lichenified dermatitis of the face which worsened in sunlight, even after discontinuing the aftershave lotion. On analysis the commercial sandalwood was found to be composed of synthetic and natural geranium, synthetic and natural sandalwood, cedarwood oil and patchouli oil; he tested positive to both synthetic and natural geranium.

Other sensitivities and toxicities

Prolonged use

If any one oil is used for a very long period there may be a risk of sensitization even though none exists in normal usage. When eau de Cologne (which contains bergamot and other citrus essences) was much in vogue many people wore it daily over a period of years and developed raised erythematous rough skin where the eau de Cologne had been applied – usually on the neck (berloque dermatitis). This reaction can be semi-permanent, lasting for years after fragrance use has ceased before disappearing (Shirley Price's personal experience). Many perfumes have ingredients in common with eau de Cologne and may produce similar reactions. A 47-year-old woman who sold food that was smoked and spiced with juniper berry oil, had for 25 years had a rash that had become generalized, followed by a dry cough and asthma; skin tests with juniper and pine oils proved positive (Rothe, Heine & Rebohle 1973).

Melaleuca alternifolia [tea tree] oil was identified as a possible cause of relapsing eczema in a 53-year-old woman who had prolonged exposure to the oil (Schaller & Korting 1995). She was also allergic to other essential oils, including lavender, jasmine and rosewood, which may also have resulted from prolonged exposure to the oils, but she was in addition allergic to laurel and eucalyptus, to which she had not been previously exposed. This report emphasizes the importance of treating essential oils with respect, especially when using them for prolonged periods. It is good aromatherapy practice to change the oils used during a treatment of long duration.

A survey of effects on therapists

A survey carried out (Wong 1995) on the personal effects on 120 aromatherapists using essential oils in treatments revealed that they occurred on many levels. A few therapists suffered adverse effects, but it was felt that these were due to reactions to clients rather than to the oils themselves. It is emphasized that this was a survey, not a properly constituted trial. Of the 120 therapists surveyed:

- most felt the effects were beneficial
- only two were men
- most had been in practice for less than 4 years
- most gave fewer than 10 treatments per week
- 40 different oils were mentioned.

Effects on particular systems included the following:

The skin

- 105 therapists experienced insignificant or no effect.
- Several experienced skin irritation, often between the fingers, and sweet almond oil and geranium were mentioned by two therapists as the offenders.
- Two therapists appeared to have developed eczema, and previous dermatitis in one had disappeared.

Emotional and mental state

- Only seven therapists surveyed felt that the oils had had no effect, with a majority feeling a moderate to great effect, usually beneficial, helping to calm, relieve headache and help sleep.
- Sleeplessness was mentioned in connection with geranium, bergamot, lemongrass, peppermint and rosemary.

Female reproductive system

- About 28% of the women surveyed felt some effect on their reproductive system, but most did not know whether this was due to the essential oils or to other factors.
- Some said they felt no effects when using oils on clients, but experienced considerable effects when using oils on themselves.
- Most experienced positive effects such as an improvement in PMS, period pains and menopausal symptoms, and a more regular menstrual cycle. *Salvia sclarea* [clary sage] was mentioned many times in this context.
- Six aromatherapists had been pregnant while practising; some found their sense of smell became more acute and they could not tolerate strong aromas.
- A few therapists felt adverse effects such as tender breasts, irregular or heavy menstruation, a change in menstrual cycle and fluctuating hormone levels, but these are common and may not be linked to essential oil use.

Digestive system

- 109 found a slight or no effect.
- Some found that the calming effect of the essential oils helped digestive problems; a few reported flatulence; others had disturbed bowel movements.

Urinary system

- 106 reported a slight or no effect, with 11 reporting moderate to great effect.

Lymphatic system

- 96 felt no effects.
- Of the 22 who reported effects, about half were positive and half negative regarding fluid retention, congestion and swollen glands (some felt their symptoms were due to standing).

Immune system

- 96 felt a positive effect on their immune system and three felt negative symptoms.

Respiratory system

- Approximately half of those surveyed felt improved symptoms in catarrh, coughs, hay fever, asthma, breathing or chest infections.
- A few thought that their symptoms were made worse.

Circulation, muscles and joints

- Any adverse effects were felt to be due to performing massage rather than to essential oils.
- Some felt their joint and muscle problems had improved.

Note that the quality of the oils used by those surveyed is unknown, and it is known that synthetics added to essential oils have effects of their own. In a general survey such as this other circumstances may well have had an effect, e.g. diet, medication, general state of health, allergies etc.; the performance of the massage itself may be responsible for some of the joint and circulation problems reported.

Unwanted effects are rare and mostly following overdose or overuse. The general safety of essential oils normally used in aromatherapy may be judged by the health of workers who handle and inhale significant quantities in the course of their daily work. Some members of our own staff handled, bottled and breathed a wide range of oils during the whole of their working day for over two decades with no reported bad effects. There are many therapists (including ourselves) who have been working full-time with the oils for over three decades who have experienced nothing but good effects, and it may therefore be inferred that aromatherapy is basically safe. There are one or two therapists who have developed sensitivity to a few oils; unfortunately, if the sensitivity is due to a specific molecule in the oil, then wherever it occurs the person may have a reaction; in some cases a reaction may be due to an adulterant rather than a natural component of the essential oil. Therapists who do not use perfumes run less risk of developing sensitivities to essential oils, as the overall quantity of synthetics employed in perfumes in day-to-day situations plays a large part in the growing number of people developing allergies and substance sensitivities (Bennett 1990).

Mutagenicity and teratogenicity

There is no available evidence that any natural essential oil has ever provoked mutagenicity or teratogenicity in an embryo or developing fetus. No tests have been carried out because the possibility of fragrant materials causing either genetic mutation or malformation is regarded as unlikely.

Carcinogenicity

A few oils have been tested for carcinogenicity on animals and the essential oil components safrole and dihydrosafrole have been implicated in the formation of hepatic tumours in rats; calamus oil containing β-asarone produced duodenal tumours (Taylor et al. 1967). For this reason, sassafras, which contains safrole as an important constituent, is not used in aromatherapy. Safrole is significantly present in Brazilian sassafras oil and in trace amounts in white camphor oil. Wiseman et al. (1987) found that β-asarone produced malignant liver tumours in rodents, but another study failed to confirm the carcinogenicity of β-asarone and calamus oil in rats (Ramos-Ocampo 1988). β-Asarone (found in calamus oil) is restricted in foods and drinks to 0.1–1 mg/kg.

Despite some evidence from animal testing (where the doses used were large), it is thought that there is minimal risk in humans undergoing aromatherapy treatment; Tisserand and Balacs (1995 p. 101) suggest that a safe level for external use in aromatherapy is 0.1% maximum of β-asarone (also estragole, methyl eugenol and safrole).

Neurotoxicity

Special care must be taken with a few essential oils containing significant amounts of a ketone, which can be aggressive to nerve tissue. Not all ketones are neurotoxic (Winter 1999 p. 113), but as a class they must be regarded as hazardous in this respect. Particular care must be exercised when using oils containing apiole (e.g. *Petroselinum sativum* (fruct.) [parsley seed]) and ascaridole (e.g. *Peumus boldus* [boldo]). (For the risks of using neurotoxic oils in pregnancy see Ch. 12.) The molecules in essential oils are lipid soluble and as such can pass the blood–brain barrier and access the central nervous system. The degree of lipid solubility varies from one class of molecule to another: e.g. esters are more fat soluble than are alcohols. Once past this barrier there is a potential for toxicity: an accidental overdose of *Syzygium aromaticum* [clove] (5–10 mL) produced convulsions in a child (Hartnoll et al. 1993). It is thought that the ketone thujone found in *Thuja occidentalis, Tanacetum vulgare, Artemisia vulgaris* and *A. absinthium* is toxic to the central nervous system, as is the ketone asarone (found in *Acorus calamus*) (Wenzel & Ross 1957).

Hepatotoxicity

When using essential oils having appreciable quantities of aldehydes there is a risk of toxicity due to build-up in the liver. People taking fennel essential oil over a long period of time show a colour change in the liver tissue (Franchomme & Pénoël 2001 p. 105). Thujone, thymol and turpentine oil may damage the liver following oral ingestion in high doses (Schilcher 1985 p. 229). Liver toxicity seems to arise when innocuous essential oil components are metabolized to toxic chemicals, as with pulegone, found in many of the mint oils. Also to be treated with caution (based largely on animal testing using very high doses) are methyl chavicol (found in *Artemisia dracunculus* [tarragon]), safrole (in *Sassafras albidum*), myristicin and elemicin (in *Myristica fragrans* [nutmeg]) and apiole (in *Petroselinum sativum* (fruct.) [parsley seed]).

Nephrotoxicity

Some essential oils have an effect on the kidneys which is regarded as stimulating and beneficial in low doses, but which could be classed as toxic if the quantity of oil used is excessive or it is used for too long a time. *Juniperus sabina* [savin] is mentioned by Schilcher (1985 p. 229) as causing damage to the kidneys, even when applied externally. Large quantities of the ester methyl salicylate, found in the oils of *Gaultheria procumbens* [wintergreen] and *Betula lenta* [sweet birch], and of safrole (found in *S. albidum* [sassafras]) are nephrotoxic. Sandalwood and turpentine taken orally in excessive doses can also cause kidney damage (Tukioka 1927).

Respiratory sensitivity

See Ch. 6, section on inhalation.

Powerful oils in pregnancy

There are several essential oils which may have unwanted side effects during the first trimester of pregnancy, e.g. they may be emmenagogic and are therefore best avoided at this time, especially as, once in the body fluids, they may pass through the placenta. It is known that, although the placenta acts as a barrier against both neutral and positively charged molecules, those which are negatively charged can cross it fairly easily (Maickel & Snodgrass 1973); it is also known that small molecules with a molecular weight of less than 1000 are able to pass through the placenta (Baker 1960). Therefore, as many essential oil molecules are negatively charged and all have molecular weights of less than 250, it can be assumed that essential oils do pass through the placenta. Their effects on a newly formed fetus have not yet been studied.

Essential oils may, however, be used correctly and safely later in pregnancy, but the situation is not clear. 'Crossing the placenta does not necessarily mean that there is a risk of toxicity to the foetus; this will depend on the toxicity and the plasma concentration of the compound' (Tisserand & Balacs 1995).

Few authors are able to justify their recommendation of particular aromatherapy oils. This lack of firm information has led many aromatherapists to avoid using any allegedly unsafe oils during the whole gestation period, even though some of the proscribed oils are not necessarily unsafe in relation to pregnancy.

Many lists of oils to be avoided during pregnancy include those containing aldehydes and phenols (such as *Cymbopogon citratus* [lemongrass] and *Syzygium aromaticum* [clove bud], whose toxicity is mainly a potential irritant effect on the skin) and contraindications do not specifically relate to pregnancy (see Appendix B.6 on the CD-ROM). Some oils listed contain coumarins and are therefore photo sensitizers (Appendix B.7 on the CD-ROM), but again this does not affect their use with particular regard to pregnancy. The essential oils listed in Appendices B.6 and B.7 should be treated with caution by everyone, not just those who are pregnant. Balacs (1992) began the clarification of this area by giving reasons for his list of oils to be avoided in pregnancy. This article and *The Aromatherapy Workbook* (Price 2000 p. 131) are intended to be more informative and to put back into perspective the use of powerful and extremely useful essential oils during pregnancy.

Another interesting point to consider is that a woman is often unaware of being pregnant at first – occasionally up to 4 weeks or more – and could be using essential oils regularly during that time. Where this is known to have happened, however, no ill effects have been reported.

To save confusion and misuse, members of the general public (and inadequately qualified aromatherapists) are best advised not to use an essential oil appearing on any restrictive list during pregnancy without having been given advice by a competent aromatherapist; there are a number of essential oils which can be safely used during this time.

Misuse of essential oils

A number of essential oils are labelled as toxic without any evidence of their causing harm to human beings, except by gross misuse. Toxicity of the main component of an essential oil does not always constitute proof that the whole essential oil is toxic to humans, whatever the results of research on rats and mice (which are injected with or made to ingest essential oils – see Part I of this chapter). The results of animal testing cannot be directly extrapolated to humans, and because of the small amounts used in aromatherapy massage the effects of the essential oils would be 100 000 times less hazardous than the amounts used in animal testing (Tisserand & Balacs 1991).

Empirical evidence accumulated over many years illustrates that when used in small doses (and for a restricted period), even the so-called toxic oils on the lists referred to do not normally present a hazard. *Mentha pulegium* [pennyroyal] is reputed to be a strong abortifacient and a much impugned oil so far as pregnancy is concerned. The following selection of the many cases of women who took large doses of pennyroyal deliberately are all recorded in medical journals.

- To induce menstruation, one woman took about 15 mL of pennyroyal and suffered acute gastritis, but recovered fully (Allen 1897).
- Another made herself an infusion with about 15 mL of pennyroyal and 'threepennyworth of rum'. She felt sick after 10 minutes and later became unconscious; she vomited when roused shortly afterwards, but recovered by the next day (Braithwaite 1906).
- To induce abortion, a 22-year-old American woman took approximately 10 mL of pennyroyal and felt dizzy within an hour, recovering the same

day. Tests showed her liver and renal functions to be normal and she was discharged 2 days after admission (Sullivan & Peterson 1979).
- A 24-year-old mother of two, taking an unknown amount of pennyroyal and cohosh herb in two separate doses (evening and the following morning), succeeded in aborting on the second day but was admitted to hospital seriously ill. Towards the end of 10 days her general condition was recorded as being satisfactory – all damaged tissues seemed to have recovered fully, except the kidneys. However, she developed pneumonia and died 3 days later (Vallance 1955). [In this case it is not clear whether the abortion was due to pennyroyal or cohosh, or a combination.]
- An 18-year-old American girl took about 30 mL of pennyroyal, thinking she was pregnant. After severe vomiting and vaginal bleeding, she suffered a cardiopulmonary arrest 4 days after ingestion. She died 2 days later following a second cardiopulmonary arrest (Sullivan & Peterson 1979).

Mentha pulegium can contain varying amounts of the ketone pulegone (see Potential toxicity, below) depending on the country of origin and whether cultivated or wild. Lawrence (1989) quotes the pulegone content found in *M. pulegium* from the following countries: Uruguay (1985): 26.8%, Angola (1976): 42%, Greece (1972): 61.9%, Chile (1986): 92.6%.

The average content in the essential oil is normally around 65%, but it is not known what percentage of pulegone was in the oil / herb /infusion used by the women quoted above. It is difficult therefore to be certain about what dosage level is safe and when the amount poses a danger. What is quite clear is that swallowing large quantities (15–25 mL) of any essential oil, even one considered to be safe, constitutes gross misuse and may cause significant unwanted side effects (see Part I of this chapter). Herbal medicines are promoted as more 'natural' and safer than conventional over-the-counter medicines (Huxtable 1992), but herbal preparations are not subject to the same scrutiny and certification; pennyroyal is one widely available herbal medicine that can be life-threatening after ingestion.

Emmenagogic essential oils

Emmenagogic essential oils are recommended to promote menstrual flow in non-pregnant women suffering from amenorrhoea, or irregular or scanty menstruation. The oils listed below are considered by the majority of writers to be emmenagogic. Such oils should not be used in the first trimester of pregnancy, unless needed in an emergency or for a short period of time. Where there is a history of miscarriage, they should not be used at all.

- *Achillea millefolium* [yarrow] contains little or no thujone, as opposed to sage oil, which may contain 50% (Leung & Foster 1996 p. 458), but the plant has been used as an abortifacient in the past (Chandler, Hooper & Harvey 1982) and so the essential oil must be regarded as emmenagogic until proved otherwise. There is also a taxonomic problem with yarrow: Lawrence (1984) speaks of yarrow being a complex of hardly separable species, which is another reason for caution.
- *Foeniculum vulgare* var. *dulce* – also hormone-like, diuretic and galactagogic; facilitates delivery (average phenolic ether content 60%).
- *Myristica fragrans* [nutmeg] – also facilitates delivery; is hallucinogenic in overdose (average phenolic ether content 6%).
- *Pimpinella anisum* [aniseed] – also hormone-like; facilitates delivery (average phenolic ether content 83%).
- *Salvia officinalis* – also hormone-like; prepares the uterus for labour (average ketone content 35%).

The following essential oils are those that some suggest are emmenagogic and should be used with caution during pregnancy. No evidence has yet been produced to support or refute these suggestions, and under the guidance of a competent aromatherapist it would appear that their use may not be detrimental to the wellbeing of a pregnant woman. However, this does not necessarily mean that all of them should automatically be regarded as safe, because even safe oils can be used wrongly and unsafely.

- *Chamaemelum nobile* [Roman chamomile] (contains around 13% of a ketone). **Indicated for menstrual problems (dysmenorrhoea, amenorrhoea) linked to nervous troubles** Valnet 1980 pp. 104–105).
- *Matricaria recutita* [German chamomile] – hormone-like (Franchomme & Pénoël 2001 p. 396) (contains around 30% oxides).

The above two essential oils are recommended for amenorrhoea, but their emmenagogic properties are generally considered to be very mild.

- *Commiphora myrrha, C. molmol* [myrrh]. Myrrh is thought to be an emmenagogue, perhaps because it is hormonal; in Grieve (1991 p. 572)

it is not made clear whether the plant or the essential oil is responsible for the therapeutic action (see *Levisticum officinale* below). As a result, it appears in many British aromatherapy books as a proven emmenagogue. None of the French books cite it as such, and Balacs (1992) considers it to have 'doubtful toxicity'.

- *Juniperus communis* (fruct. ram. fol.) [juniper berry, twig, leaf] – diuretic. Formacek and Kubeczka (1982) found *J. communis* to contain approximately 87% terpenes, with a small percentage of alcohols and no ketones, yet a *J. communis* cited by Franchomme and Pénoël (2001 p. 389) is given as containing ketones (percentages not given). Valnet (1980) gives it as an emmenagogue, though he does not mention amenorrhoea as an indication – only painful menstruation, and it is not clear whether he means the essential oil or a decoction of the berries; this is crucial, as larger plant molecules can have different effects from the smaller volatile molecules. Franchomme makes no reference whatsoever to the reproductive system, nor do four other French aromatherapy books. The property of *J. communis* fruct. [juniper berry] upon which all are agreed is its diuretic effect.
- *Levisticum officinale* [lovage] – diuretic (contains around 50% phthalides, about which not much is known). The essential oil is distilled from the roots. The leaves were once used as an emmenagogue (Grieve 1991 p. 500), which may be the reason why the essential oil has been assumed to be emmenagogic also.
- *Melaleuca cajuputi* [cajuput] – hormone-like (contains around 30–40% oxides). Franchomme (Franchomme & Pénoël 2001 p. 397) is the only person to advocate prudent use of this essential oil during pregnancy; it is not given as emmenagogic.
- *Mentha x piperita* [peppermint] – hormone-like (contains 20–50% alcohols, 15–40% ketones). Like several essential oils, the main constituents in peppermint essential oil are variable, making decisions regarding its emmenagogic properties difficult. The pulegone content is usually 0.3–0.6%, though that of American peppermint may be just under 3% (Gilly, Garnero & Racine 1986). Peppermint is sometimes distilled after drying the plant, when the ratio of menthone (16–36.1%) to menthol (46.2–30.8%) is radically different (Fehr & Stenzhorn 1979). Valnet (1980 p. 173) lists it as an emmenagogue, though Franchomme & Pénoël

(2001 p. 401–402) list it as a hormone-like oil which regulates the ovaries; they do not contraindicate it for pregnant women. Bardeau (1976 p. 216) states that it calms painful periods.

- *Ocimum basilicum* [European basil]. Because of its phenolic ether content (methyl chavicol), which varies within wide limits depending on the species, the origin and the time of harvesting, basil is often cited as an emmenagogue. Valnet (1980) cites it as such, although Franchomme & Pénoël (2001 p. 408) give no mention of its use for any gynaecological condition and state that regardless of the percentage of methyl chavicol, there are no known contraindications. Most of the basil oils available to aromatherapists contain a high percentage of methyl chavicol, the lowest being around 50% (and often as high as 75–80%).
- *Origanum majorana* [sweet marjoram] (contains around 40% terpenes and 50% alcohols). When this essential oil is contraindicated for pregnancy it is no doubt being confused, owing to the use of the common name, with *Thymus mastichina* [Spanish marjoram]. The latter essential oil is a species of thyme and has totally different constituents, with an oxide content of 55–75%. There is no mention in any of the French aromatherapy literature of any emmenagogic effect or of having to treat *O. majorana* with caution, and no evidence has yet been produced to support the contraindication of *T. mastichina*, despite its high oxide content. Until there is, it may be prudent to use this latter oil with care. 'Marjoram' essential oil should not be purchased without knowing its botanical name.
- *Rosa damascena, R. centifolia* [rose otto] – hormone-like (contains over 60% alcohols). Rose otto is cited several times as being antihaemorrhagic (Bardeau 1976 p. 268, Franchomme & Pénoël 2001 p. 421, Roulier 1990 p. 298), but no sources mention its having any emmenagogic properties. Wabner (1992 personal communication) states that it regulates menstruation because of its hormonal influence, but that it is not emmenagogic.
- *Rosmarinus officinalis* [rosemary] – different chemotypes (ketone content 14–35%, oxide content 18–40%). The chemotype labelled by Franchomme (Franchomme & Pénoël 2001 p. 421) as an emmenagogue is the camphoraceous rosemary. He cites the verbenone chemotype as neurotoxic and abortive (which would indicate care when used with pregnant women), but gives no contraindications regarding the reproductive

system for the cineole chemotype. Roulier (1990 p. 298), on the other hand, gives no contraindications regarding the verbenone chemotype, yet warns against use of both the cineole and the camphoraceous type on pregnant women. He gives neither of them as an emmenagogue. The rosemary quoted in Valnet (1980 p. 177), which is not given as a specific chemotype and does not appear to contain verbenone, is given as an emmenagogue.

- *Salvia sclarea* [clary] – hormone-like (contains 60–70% esters). Clary is cited only for its hormonal properties (Roulier 1990 p. 302) specifically in regard to amenorrhoea, but with no mention of it being emmenagogic. It is considered emmenagogic by Holmes (1993), although no authority is given. According to Culpeper (1983), the juice of the herb (not the essential oil), drunk in beer, accelerates menstruation. This could be due to its hormonal properties, as sclareol (the diterpenol responsible for the hormone-like property of clary) is present in the juice in a much higher quantity than in the essential oil, owing to its molecular weight (see Ch. 1).
- *Vetiveria zizanioides* [vetiver] (average ketone content 22%). Only one source (Franchomme & Pénoël (2001 p. 433) has been found to cite this oil as an emmenagogue.

Safety and training

The purpose of training is to ensure minimum risk and maximum benefit to clients; unfortunately, some training programmes instil fear and insecurity through insufficient, inadequate and often incorrect teaching. Aromatherapy schools and colleges should adopt a sensible approach to the subject of toxicity and not – as many do, perhaps owing to inadequate education of the teachers – sensationalize and exaggerate the possible harmful effects of essential oils. It is up to aromatherapists to have an inquiring mind and make sure that the toxicity information they have been taught is constructive to their work, not destructive. This is not to say that essential oils, even if carefully chosen, can be used carelessly: relevant knowledge and care in use are required.

Aromatherapy in the UK developed from a beauty therapy aspect, where a gentle approach was combined with a high dilution unlikely to have any risk in use. Teaching avoided – and still does – the topics of intensive or internal use, where potential hazards need careful consideration. Today essential oils are rarely used undiluted, but in such high dilution (usually 1–4%) that the only precaution necessary is to be aware of contraindications in circumstances such as epilepsy, pregnancy, skin sensitivity etc. With comprehensive knowledge, applied prudently, these advanced uses are equally as safe as any other method.

The concentration of the oils to be used and duration of treatment depend on the correct assessment of the client's state of health. To attack an infection, a strong dose of a powerful – and possibly so-called 'toxic' oil – is required for a short period; for a chronic problem such as asthma, a much smaller dose of 'safe' oils is effective and can be used for a longer time. These choices can be made only if the therapist has sufficient knowledge of the properties and chemistry of an essential oil and the common sense to know whether or not a 'toxic' oil could be used successfully on a particular client to give beneficial results.

General precautions regarding the use of essential oils

- Keep out of the reach of children.
- Essential oils are not to be ingested without specific professional advice.
- Never remove a dropper insert from a bottle of essential oils in order to prevent accidental ingestion; if this should happen, then

medical assistance must be sought immediately.

- Do not apply neat to the skin unless under the direction of a suitably qualified therapist.
- Idiosyncratic reactions to essential oils are possible; immediate medical assistance must be sought.
- Neat essential oils can be removed from the hands by washing thoroughly with a mild detergent to prevent transference to other parts of the body (e.g. the eyes).
- If essential oil does get into the eye, the eye should be flushed with a good-quality carrier oil, which will dissolve the oil (water does not).
- See also Appendix C on the CD-ROM.

Summary

The need for a dispassionate and scientific attitude towards the possible dangers of essential oils has been demonstrated, as has the need for skill in their selection and prescription. Various potentially hazardous situations have been identified, but no harm should occur if the guidelines for safe administration are followed. Despite this, essential oils must be treated as hazardous substances (see Appendix C on the CD-ROM). In order to comply with regulatory requirements, an assessment of the potential risks associated with their use must be carried out in order to prevent anyone who may come into contact with them from being harmed.

References

Adams, T.B., Taylor, S.V., 2010. Safety evaluation of essential oils: a constituent based approach. Başer, K.H.C., Buchbauer, G. (Eds.), Handbook of essential oils: science, technology and applications. CRC, Boca Raton, p. 194.

Allen, W.T., 1897. Note on a case of supposed poisoning by pennyroyal. Lancet i, 1022–1023.

Arctander, S., 1960. Perfume and flavor materials of natural origin. Published by the author, Elizabeth New Jersey, p. 4.

Arora, S.K., Willis, I., 1976. Factors influencing methoxsalen phototoxicity in vitiliginous skin. Arch. Dermatol. 112, 327.

Baker, J.B.E., 1960. The effects of drugs on the fetus. Pharmacol. Rev. 12, 37–90.

Balacs, M.A., 1992. Safety in pregnancy. Int. J. Aromather. 4 (1), 12–15.

Bardeau, F., 1976. La médecine aromatique. Laffont, Paris.

Baudoux, D., 2000. L'aromathérapie: se soigner par les huiles essentielles. Atlantica, Biarritz.

Bennett, G., 1990. Allergy and substance sensitivity. Course notes. Shirley Price Aromatherapy College, Hinckley.

Bhushan, M., Beck, M.H., 1997. Allergic contact dermatitis from tea tree oil in a wart paint. Contact Dermatitis 36 (2), 117.

Bilsland, D., Strong, A., 1990. Allergic contact dermatitis from the essential oil of French marigold (Tagetes patula) in an aromatherapist. Contact Dermatitis 23, 55–56.

Bleasel, N., Tate, B., Rademaker, M., 2002. Allergic contact dermatitis following exposure to essential oils. Australas. J. Dermatol. 43, 211–213.

Braithwaite, P.F., 1906. A case of poisoning by pennyroyal: recovery. Br. Med. J. 2, 865.

Chandler, R.F., Hooper, S.N., Harvey, M.J., 1982. Ethnobotany and phytochemistry of yarrow, *Achillea millefolium*, Compositae. Econ. Bot. 36 (2), 203.

Culpeper, N., 1983. Culpeper's colour herbal. Foulsham, London, p. 47.

De Groot, A.C., 1996. Airborne allergic contact dermatitis from tea tree oil. Contact Dermatitis 35 (5), 304–305.

De Groot, A., Weyland, W., 1992. Contact allergy to tea tree oil. Contact Dermatitis 26, 309.

Deans, S.G., Noble, R.C., Penzes, L., Imre, S.G., 1993. Promotional effects of plant volatile oils on the polyunsaturated fatty acid status during aging. Age 16, 71–74.

Dooms-Goossens, A., Degreef, H., Holvoet, C., Maertens, M., 1977. Turpentine induced hypersensitivity to peppermint oil. Contact Dermatitis 3 (6), 304–308.

Dürbeck, K., 2003. The procurement of genuine authentic essential oils: professional aromatherapy's challenge. IFPA Conference, 12 October, Bristol.

Fehr, D., Stenzhorn, G., 1979. Untersuchungen zur Lagerstabilität von Pfefferminzblättern, Rosmarinblättern und Thymian. Pharmazeutische Zeitung 124, 2342–2349.

Formacek, K., Kubeczka, K.H., 1982. Essential oils analysis by capillary chromatography and carbon-13 NMR spectroscopy. John Wiley, New York.

Franchomme, P., Pénoël, D., 2001. L'aromathérapie exactement. Jollois, Limoges.

Gattefossé, R.-M., 1937. Aromatherapy (trans 1993). Daniel, Saffron Walden, p. 34.

Gilly, G., Garnero, J., Racine, P., 1986. Menthes poivrées – composition chimique analyse chromatographie. Parfumerie Cosmétiques Aromates 71, 79–86.

Grieve, M., 1991. A modern herbal. Penguin, London.

Griggs, B., 1977. New green pharmacy. Vermilion, London, p. 305.

Gurr, F.W., Scroggie, J.G., 1965. Eucalyptus oil poisoning treated by dialysis and mannitol infusion, with an appendix on the analysis of biological fluids for alcohol and eucalyptol. Australas. Ann. Med. 14 (3), 238–249.

Hall, C., 1904 cited in Valnet J 1980. The practice of aromatherapy. Daniel, Saffron Walden, p. 34.

Hartnoll, G., et al., 1993. Near fatal ingestion of oil of cloves. Arch. Dis. Child. 69, 392–393.

Holmes, P., 1993. Clary sage. Int. J. Aromather. 5 (1), 15–17.

Hosokawa, H., Ogwana, T., 1979. Study of skin irritations caused by perfumery materials. Perfumer and Flavorist 4 (4), 7–8.

Hotchkiss, S., 1994. How thin is your skin? New Sci. (29 January) 141 (1910), 24–27.

Howes, A., Chan, U., Caldwell, J., 1990. Structure specificity of the genotoxicity of some naturally occurring alkenylbenzenes determined by the unscheduled DNA synthesis assay in rat hepatocytes. Food Chem. Toxicol. 28 (8), 537–542.

Huxtable, R.J., 1992. The myth of beneficent nature: the risks of herbal preparations. Ann. Intern. Med. 117 (2), 165–166.

IFRA (International Fragrance Association), 1992. Code of practice. IFRA, Geneva.

Jouhar, A.J. (Ed.), 1991. ninth ed Poucher's perfumes, cosmetics and soaps, vol. 1. Blackie, Glasgow, p. 40.

Kaidbey, K.H., Kligman, A.M., 1974. Photopigmentation with trioxsalen. Arch. Dermatol. 109, 674.

Kammerau, B., Klebe, U., Zesche, A., Schaefer, H., 1976. Penetration, permeation and resorption of 80–methoxypsoralen. Comparative in vitro and in vivo studies after topical application of four standard preparations. Arch. Dermatol. Res. 255, 31.

Kligman, A.M., 1966. The identification of contact allergens by human assay. III. The maximization test, a procedure for screening and rating contact sensitisers. J. Invest. Dermatol. 47, 393.

Kligman, A.M., Epstein, W., 1975. Updating the maximization test for identifying contact allergens. Contact Dermatitis 1, 231.

Knight, T.E., Hausen, B.M., 1994. Melaleuca oil (tea tree oil) dermatitis.

J. Am. Acad. Dermatol. 30 (3), 423–427.

Kochevar, I.E., 1987. Mechanisms of drug photosensitization. Photochem. Photobiol. 45, 891–895.

Lawrence, B.M., 1984. Progress in essential oils: yarrow oil. Perfumer and Flavorist 9 (4), 37.

Lawrence, B.M., 1989. Progress in essential oils: pennyroyal. Perfumer & Flavorist 14 (3), 71.

Leung, A.Y., Foster, S., 1996. Encyclopedia of common natural ingredients used in food, drugs and cosmetics. John Wiley, New York, p. 458.

Lovell, R.C., 1993. Plants and the skin. Blackwell Scientific, London, p. 65.

Low, D., Rawal, B.D., Griffin, W.J., 1974. Antibacterial action of the essential oils of some Australian Myrtaceae with special references to the activity of chromatographic fractions of oil of Eucalyptus citriodora. Planta Med. 26, 184–189.

Maickel, R.P., Snodgrass, W.R., 1973. Physiochemical factors in maternal–fetal distribution of drugs. Toxicol. Appl. Pharmacol. 26, 218–230.

Millet, Y., Tognetti, P., Lavaire-Pierlovisi, M., Steinmetz, M.D., Arditti, J., Jouglard, J., 1979. Experimental study of the toxic convulsant properties of commercial preparations of essences of sage and hyssop. Rev E. E. G. Neurophysiology 9 (1), 12–18.

Mills, S., 1991. The essential book of herbal medicine. Penguin Books, London, p. 282.

Nunes, D.S., et al., 2010. Psychopharmacology of essential oils. Başer, K.H.C., Buchbauer, G. (Eds.), Handbook of essential oils: science, technology and applications. CRC Press, Boca Raton, p. 300.

Opdyke, D.L.J., 1973. Bergamot oil expressed. Food Cosmet. Toxicol. 11, 1031–1033.

Opdyke, D.L.J., 1974. Monographs on fragrance raw materials: cumin oil. Pergamon, Oxford, p. 274.

Opdyke, D.L.J., 1976b. Inhibition of sensitisation reactions induced by certain aldehydes. Food Cosmet. Toxicol. 14 (3), 197–198.

Opdyke, D.L.J., 1979. Fragrance raw materials monographs. Food Chem. Toxicol. 17 (3), 253–258.

Opdyke, D.L.J., 1992. Monographs on fragrance raw materials. Food Chem. Toxicol. 30 (special issue viii), 137s.

Orafidiyia, L.O., 1993. The effect of autoxidation of lemongrass oil on its bacterial activity. Phytother. Res. 7, 269–271.

Patel, S., Wiggins, J., 1980. Eucalyptus oil poisoning. Arch. Dis. Child. 55 (5), 405–406.

Pathak, M.A., Fitzpatrick, T.B., 1959. Relationship of molecular configuration to the activity of furocoumarins which increase the cutaneous responses following long wave ultraviolet radiation. J. Invest. Dermatol. 32, 255.

Pénoël, D., 1992. Winter shield. Int. J. Aromather. 4 (4), 11.

Price, L., 1990b. Lecture notes: theory and philosophy of aromatherapy. Shirley Price International College of Aromatherapy, Hinckley.

Price, S., 2000. The aromatherapy workbook. Thorsons, London, p. 131.

Ramos-Ocampo, V.E., 1988. Mutagenicity and DNA damaging activity of calamus oil, asarone isomers and dimethoxypropenylbenzene analogues. Philippine Entomologist 7 (3), 275–291.

Raynor, L., 1999. The genus Echinacea. Herbs 24 (2), 5.

Renzini, G., Scazzocchio, F., Lu, M., Mazzanti, G., Salvatore, G., 1999. Antibacterial and cytotoxic activity of Hyssopus officinalis L. oils. *Journal of Essential Oil Research* 11, 649–654.

Römelt, H., Zuber, A., Dirnagl, K., Drexel, H., 1974. Münchner Medizinische Wochenschrift 116: 537 cited in Schilcher H 1985 Effects and side effects of essential oils. Baerheim Svendsen, A., Scheffer, J.J.C. (Eds.), Essential oils and aromatic plants. Martinus Nijhof/Junk, Dordrecht, p. 228.

Rothe, A., Heine, A., Rebohle, E., 1973. Oil from juniper berries as an occupational allergen for the skin and respiratory tract. Berufsdermatosen 21 (1), 11–16.

Roulier, G., 1990. Les huiles essentielles pour votre santé. Dangles, St-Jean-de-Braye.

Schaller, M.S., Korting, H.C., 1995. Allergic airborne contact dermatitis from essential oils used in aromatherapy. Clin. Exp. Dermatol. 20 (2), 143–145.

Schilcher, H., 1985. Effects and side effects of essential oils. Baerheim Svendsen, A., Scheffer, J.J.C. (Eds.), Essential oils and aromatic plants. Martinus Nijhof/Junk, Dordrecht, p. 229.

Schnaubelt, K., 1998. Advanced aromatherapy. Healing Arts Press, Vermont.

Schroeder, J., 1689. Pharmacopoeia medico-chymica, thesaurus pharmacologus. (Ulm 1641, 1649, 1655, 1662, 1705) (Frankfurt 1640, 1669, 1677) (Lyons 1649, 1656, 1665, 1681) (Leyden 1672) (Geneva 1689) (Nürnberg 1746).

Selvaag, E., Erikson, B., Thune, P., 1994. Contact allergy due to tea tree oil and cross sensitisation to colophony. Contact Dermatitis 31, 124–125.

Sharma, R., Bajaj, A.K., Singh, K.G., 1987. Sandalwood dermatitis. Int. J. Dermatol. 26 (9), 597.

Simpson, E., 1994. Essential oils and the ageing process. Aroma 93: harmony from within. Conference Proceedings. Aromatherapy Publications, Brighton, pp. 107–110.

Smith, R.L., Cohen, S.M., Doull, J., Feron, V.J., Goodman, J.I., Marnett, L.J., et al., 2005. Criteria for the safety evaluation of flavouring substances – The Expert Panel of the Flavor and Extract Manufacturers Association. Food Chem. Toxicol. 43, 1141–1177.

Southwell, I.A., Freeman, S., Rubel, D., 1997. Skin irritancy of tea tree oil. Journal of Essential Oil Research 9, 47–52.

Spoerke, D.G., Vandenburg, S.A., Smolinske, S.C., Kulig, K., Rumack, B.H., 1989. Eucalyptus oil: 14 cases of exposure. Vet. Hum. Toxicol. 31 (2), 166–168.

Steinmetz, M.D., Tognetti, P., Mourgue, M., Jouglard, J., Millet, Y., 1980. Concerning the toxicity of certain commercial essential oils – essences of hyssop and sage. Plantes Med. Phytother. 14 (1), 34–45.

Stewart, D., 2004. The chemistry of essential oils made simple. Care Publications, Missouri.

Sullivan, J.B., Peterson, R.G., 1979. Pennyroyal poisoning and hepatoxicity. J. Am. Med. Assoc. 242 (26), 2873–2874.

Taylor, J.M., Jones, W.I., Hagan, E.C., Gross, M.A., Davis, D.A., Cook, E.L., 1967. Toxicity of oil of calamus (Jammu variety). Toxicol. Appl. Pharmacol. 10, 405.

Temple, W.A., Smith, N.A., Beasley, M., 1991. Management of oil of citronella poisoning. J. Toxicol. Clin. Toxicol. 29 (2), 257–262, Discussion 263.

Tibbals, J., 1995. Clinical effects and management of eucalyptus oil ingestion in infants and young children. Med. J. Aust. 163 (4), 177–180.

Tisserand, R., Balacs, M.A., 1991. Research reports. Int. J. Aromather. 3 (1), 6.

Tisserand, R., Balacs, M.A., 1995. Essential oil safety. Churchill Livingstone, New York, p. 105.

Tukioka, M., 1927. Proceedings. Imperial Academy Tokyo 3, 624.

Tyman, J.H.P., 1990. Essential Oils Trade Association Symposium. Brunel University, June.

Valette, C., 1945. Société de Biologie Comptes Rendus 13 October cited in: Katz A E 1947 Pénétration transcutanée des essences. Parfumerie Modern 39, 64–66.

Vallance, W.B., 1955. Pennyroyal poisoning: a fatal case. Lancet ii, 850–851.

Valnet, J., 1980. The practice of aromatherapy. Daniel, Saffron Walden.

Vilaplana, R.C., Grimalt, F., 1991. Contact dermatitis from geraniol in Bulgarian rose oil. Contact Dermatitis 24, 301.

Webb, N.J.A., Pitt, W.R., 1993. Eucalyptus oil poisoning in childhood: 41 cases in south east Queensland. J. Paediatr. Child Health 29, 368–371.

Wenzel, D.G., Ross, C.R., 1957. J. Am. Pharm. Assoc. 46, 77.

Winter, R., 1999. A consumer's dictionary of cosmetic ingredients. Three Rivers, New York, p. 113.

Wiseman, R.W., et al., 1987. Structure–activity studies of hepatocarcinogenicities of alkenylbenzenes derivatives related to estragole and safrole on administration to preweanling male C57BL/6J × C3H/HeJF1 mice. Cancer Res. 47, 2275–2283.

Woeber, K., Krombach, M., 1969. Sensitisation from volatile oils. Berufsdermatosen 17 (6), 320–326.

Wong, M., 1995. The healing touch: survey results. Aromatherapy Quarterly 46, 26–29.

Zaynoun, S.T., Johnson, B.E., Frain-Bell, W., 1977. A study of bergamot and its importance as a phototoxic agent. II. Factors which affect the phototoxic reaction induced by bergamot oil and psoralen derivatives. Contact Dermatitis 3, 225–239.

Zhiri, A., 2002. Huiles essentielles chémotypées et leurs synergies. Amyris, Bruxelles.

Sources

AOC, 1997. Report from research and scientific sub-committee for Executive and Council meetings. 27 November.

British Pharmacopoeia, 1993. HMSO, London, p. 273.

Guba, R., 2000. Toxicity myths – the actual risks of essential oil use. Int. J. Aromather. 10 (1–2), 37–49.

Lamy, J., 1985. De la culture à la distillerie: quelques facteurs influant sur la composition des huiles essentielles. Chambre d'Agriculture de la Drôme, Valence, p. 5.

Skoula, M., Harborne, J.B., 2000. The taxonomy and chemistry of Origanum. In: Kintzios, S.E. (Ed.), Oregano – the genera Origanum and Lippia. Taylor and Francis, London, pp. 67–108.

Traditional use, modern research

4
(Part I)

Len Price

CHAPTER CONTENTS

Introduction

Different approaches to the healing of people have always existed and today they are generally viewed as being complementary and supplementary to each other rather than alternative or antagonistic. The use of essential oils as part of traditional plant-based medicine has led to the accumulation of a large body of empirical knowledge about their effectiveness in different conditions. This chapter looks at their therapeutic properties, and shows where modern science confirms traditional usage.

Different approaches

The predominant contemporary approach is that of allopathic medicine, where illness is regarded as being due to an outside agent. Throughout the ages this concept has been looked upon in various ways and illness attributed to 'evil spirits', 'ill will' or 'microbes', and nowadays to 'bacteria' and 'viruses'. The aim has always been to target and exterminate this outside agent, freeing the body from attack.

This focusing on the causative agent has brought about an enormous increase in the knowledge of the separate bodily systems, resulting in specialization, and it is left to the general practitioner to preserve an overview of the whole person.

For many decades now medicine and pharmacy have focused on analysis and simplification, as evidenced in the production of medicines, mostly composed of a single well-defined molecule whose structure and therapeutic action are well understood. This style of analysis and simplification is the heritage of Descartes, who said that to know the body better it was necessary to divide it into its constituent parts.

The holistic approach

An aromatherapist looks at the whole person to ascertain the cause of the illness, and the treatment that follows aims to strengthen the body's natural defence system to cope with attacks by pathogens. The weakness is then considered in relation to the body as a whole and studied in the context of the living environment, then the aromatherapist chooses the essential oils for healing.

> I had seen the miracles of modern medicine in Intensive Care; in daily practice it was not the same. Sick people fell ill again; sick people suffered side effects; new sicknesses appeared when I treated them with chemical medicines. But what struck me most of all was the complete absence of the human dimension.
>
> Dr Jean-Claude Lapraz, quoted in Griggs (1997)

Fall and rise of plant-based medicine

A century ago many medicines were based on plants and plant extracts because of their easy availability: in a rural environment people could gather plants and process their own medicines – necessary because money was scarce, there was little state assistance and private health insurance was practically unknown. Dr Jean-Claude Lapraz made this observation (quoted in Griggs 1997).

When I was a boy my grandfather had a farm in the country, and I noticed that everybody used plants: they drank them in infusions, they made an oil to treat burns – Oh yes, plants worked, I saw that clearly. But later, in all the years I spent in medical school, nobody ever mentioned plants. Not a single one.

After the Second World War, orthodox medicine took advantage of developments in science and technology, resulting in a shift from natural medicines to rapidly acting drugs. At this time state medicine was introduced in some Western European countries (including the UK), to the great benefit of individuals and society. This wonderful step forward struck a near-mortal blow to folk/plant medicine because, with the availability of free treatment, the knowledge of centuries was discarded, or at best put to one side. People were no longer content with plants which were slow both to prepare and to heal. They had great expectations of the new synthetic drugs, which appeared then to produce immediate and startling results without any real effort on the part of the sufferer.

In the 1960s and 1970s there was a resurgence of caring for the ecological balance of nature, the use of natural as opposed to synthetic products, and the eating of organically grown foods. This new outlook also encompassed the field of medicine, and as a result many alternative (as they were viewed then) approaches to healing took root and flourished. These are now known as parallel or complementary approaches, where much attention is paid to a holistic style of treatment.

Plant remedies are popular for small problems (such as headaches) which are too insignificant to warrant visiting a doctor, as well as for chronic complaints, which by definition are not susceptible to orthodox treatment. People are prepared to try alternative procedures at their own expense for 'must learn to live with it' conditions. The most popular and successful aromatherapy treatments are, in the editors' experience, for stress and chronic conditions such as arthritis and rheumatism.

Acceptance of aromatherapy

Studies suggest that about half of the adult population in industrialized countries use complementary/alternative treatments to ward off or treat a wide variety of health problems. Should doctors bother with this strange aromatherapy? It is understandable that 'unproven' complementary treatments and medicaments are viewed with a certain amount of caution. The editors hope that this book will convince doubters that there is something of substance to be looked into, something which can be used alongside orthodox treatments. The attitude of health professionals to alternative and complementary therapies is changing for the better, and over the years the intrinsically safe practice of aromatherapy has grown and is finding acceptance in many hospital departments today, as shown by the surveys quoted below.

1986 Although most general practitioners knew little about the techniques of complementary medicine (CAM), a majority found that they had been useful to their patients. Most had referred patients for this type of treatment during the previous year even though they felt that complementary practitioners needed statutory regulation (Wharton & Lewith 1986).

1987 Most general practitioners discussed CAM with their patients and over half of them referred patients to alternative practitioners (Anderson & Anderson 1987).

1994 A survey of Israeli doctors found that 60% of all physicians had made referrals to CAM practitioners at least once (Borkan et al. 1994). A survey of UK doctors revealed that 93% of all general practitioners (GPs) and 70% of hospital doctors had suggested a referral to alternative treatment at least once; 20% of GPs and 12% of house doctors practised an alternative therapy (Perkin, Pearcy & Fraser 1994), and Fisher & Ward (1994) reported that harmonization of training and regulation in Europe was an urgent requirement for the immediate future.

1995 A review of 12 surveys of doctors found that 46% considered CAM to be effective, but noted that young doctors were significantly more in favour than were older doctors (Ernst, Resch & White 1995) [the experience of the editors also]. In Canada 73% of doctors surveyed wanted to know more about the major CAM; they believed that these therapies were most needed for chronic conditions and musculo-skeletal disorders (Verhoef & Sutherland 1995b). Many GPs believed that alternative medicine had ideas and methods from which conventional medicine could benefit (Verhoef & Sutherland 1995a), and in a questionnaire 73% of physicians felt that they should have some knowledge of the most important alternative treatments (Verhoef & Sutherland 1995b). In a survey of USA doctors over 70% indicated that they would like to learn more about CAM (Berman et al. 1995).

1998 A comprehensive review suggested that large numbers of physicians either refer to or practise some of the well-known forms of CAM, and that many believed the therapies to be both useful and efficacious (Astin et al. 1998).

1999 The situation in Japan lags behind Europe and North America: the majority of Japanese doctors practise kampo (Chinese herbal medicine) but only 8% practise other forms of CAM, among which is aromatherapy (Imanishi et al. 1999).

2002–2004 In New Zealand a study showed that 25% of adults had visited a CAM practitioner during the previous 12 months.

2003 An increasing number of GPs were practising CAM to treat their NHS patients. Analysis revealed that GP therapists identified positive clinical gains associated with their direct integrative practice, e.g. successfully treating conditions for which conventional medicine proved ineffective, and providing safer techniques in medical cases where the practitioner suspected or anticipated potential side effects from conventional treatments. The positive gains experienced should not be ignored by those considering the future provision and practice of CAM within the general practice environment (Adams 2003).

2005 More than 70% of the developing world population still depended on the CAM systems of medicine. Evidence-based CAM therapies have shown remarkable success in healing acute as well as chronic diseases. Alternative therapies have been used by people in Pakistan as the first choice for many problems, and Shaikh and Hatcher (2005) concluded that a positive interaction between CAM and the orthodox systems had to be harnessed to work for the common goal of improving the health of the people.

2006 In New Zealand 300 general practitioners completed a questionnaire which revealed that 20% practised a form of CAM (most commonly acupuncture), 95% referred patients to CAM (most commonly chiropractic), 32% had had formal training, 29% were self-educated in one or more CAM therapies, and 67% felt that an overview of CAM should be included in conventional medical education. Some CAM therapies are on the border of acceptance by the medical profession, whereas others that have little evidence behind them are still viewed with much scepticism (Poynton et al. 2006).

2007 Although there has been a marked increase in the use of CAM in the UK in recent years, many doctors believe that CAM lacks scientific evidence, and such perceptions may remain a significant barrier to greater integration of CAM within the NHS (Maha & Shaw 2007). In France, medical doctors prescribe essential oils for internal use in capsules, diluted in alcohol or in suppositories and pessaries, as well as externally in dressings, inhalations, ointments and in foot, hand or whole body baths; massage is not used, although topical application in low dilution (40% or more) is used occasionally. The original concept of aromatherapy in England was to use the essential oils highly diluted (0.5–2%) in a fixed vegetable oil in massage only; this unfortunately led to the belief that that is all there is to it, and the editors have been active in trying to correct this image. UK training now includes inhalation, baths, compresses, and in some schools intensive and internal use (including pessaries, suppositories, gargles, capsules) is taught on aromatology courses. Essential oil therapy has now been introduced into many hospitals, hospices and clinics, and many GPs respect their patients' decision to use CAM while encouraging them to continue with standard treatment; in most cases the doctor–patient relationship is not affected. Health professionals need to take a greater interest in essential oils and use their skills with these active agents to their fullest capabilities. The editors have tried to address the question of proof with regard to aromatherapy, although it is still as much tradition as science.

Orthodox drugs

These are predominantly synthetic (but may include isolated natural components) and are used mostly symptomatically. Unwanted side effects (iatrogenic disease) are always present to some degree, which may necessitate further medication. Antidepressants (e.g. fluoxetine) can cause side effects including nausea, vomiting and diarrhoea, and this may be the reason for the continued use of tricyclic drugs (e.g. dothiepin hydrochloride) despite the risks shown by research. The clinical testing of drugs is rigorous but carried out over a comparatively short timescale compared with traditional plant usage, and are usually available only on prescription; less powerful drugs and tablets are available over the counter.

Side effects not only come from the drug itself but are due also to additives such as colouring. Pollock et al. (1989) carried out a survey of 2204 orthodox drugs and found 419 different additives present in 930 formulations; these additives may cause a variety of reactions in some people, e.g. nettle rash, watery eyes and nose, blurred vision, oedema, bronchoconstriction (Bowker undated), hypersensitivity reactions and photo allergy (Lawrence 1987). Nothing is added to essential oils.

Essential oils

These are natural plant products extracted by steam distillation; those used in aromatherapy are obtained from a single, specified botanical source.

Aromatherapists have to depend on honest suppliers who can guarantee not only the exact source of their oils, but also that they are not the 'commercial' products used by the perfume and food industries. Any essential oil conforming to a BP formula will have been modified to fit a specification and may not be properly identified.

Essential oil research studies

'Essential oils are products of complex composition, comprising the volatile principles contained in the plants and more or less modified during the preparation process' (Bruneton 1995). These complex mixtures are comprised of single compounds and the number can vary from about 30 to 1200, each constituent contributing to the beneficial or adverse effects of the oils. The intimate knowledge of essential oil composition allows for a better and specially directed application, and such detailed knowledge can only be obtained by means of carefully performed capillary-gas chromatography experiments (Buchbauer 2000). There is a real need for a simple, reliable and reproducible method to study the bioactivity of essential oils and their constituents which can detect a broad spectrum of action or specific pharmacological activities in aromatic plants. Standardization of some of

these methods is therefore desirable to permit more comprehensive evaluation of plant oils, and greater comparability of the results obtained by different investigators (Lahlou 2004).

Many papers on the biological activity of essential oils have been published, the data showing much variation between the same oils. The reasons for these differences can be understood by taking account of factors influencing the chemical composition of the oils – climatic, seasonal and geographic conditions, time of harvest, distillation equipment and technique (Panizzi et al. 1993). The effect of plant maturity at the time of oil production and the existence of chemotypic differences also affect this composition (Lahlou & Berrada 2003). These variations are of distinct importance in the study of their biological and pharmacological activities, as the value of an essential oil in aromatherapy must be related to its chemical composition (Lawrence 2000). Generally, essential oils are poorly soluble in water, which causes problems when studying their biological and pharmacological properties.

Research

Past research is not necessarily negated by more recent research, and the quality of the information should not be judged solely on the date of publication: a later date does not necessarily guarantee better-quality information. Something that is proven remains so until challenged by new evidence. Sometimes recently published research is merely a repetition of extant research and does not advance useful knowledge. In the past some papers on essential oils have been published where:

1. the oil being tested is not properly identified
2. only the common name has been used (more than 60 plant species are commercially available under the name oregano (Skoula & Harborne 2002))
3. no analysis has been undertaken of the oil under test
4. the oil batch was analysed but oil from another batch was used for the investigation
5. oils intended for the perfume or food industries (which probably are not the same as therapeutic oils) have been used in tests.

Franz and Novak (2010) write that repeatability of results is not given, owing to weak experimental design, incorrect description of the plant material used or inappropriate sampling. The observation by Janssen et al. (1987) is still worthy of note that 'most papers do not often cite the geographic origin and the exact composition of the essential oil studied, which somewhat detracts from the findings'.

Essential oil interaction with drugs

Essential oils are known to be active: they gain access to cells by virtue of being fat soluble and are metabolized by the body. As active agents they may react with other drugs present in the body, although there has been no evidence so far that would imply any significant adverse reaction, and essential oils have been used together with allopathic drugs successfully in hospitals (Barker 1994 personal communication). In a study on rats, eucalyptol administered subcutaneously or by aerosol was found to increase the in vitro liver metabolism of aminopyrine, p-nitro-anisol and aniline, and in vivo the metabolism of pentobarbital (Jori, Bianchetti & Prestini 1969).

Nevertheless, this is a cloudy area and, until laboratory investigations into possible reactions between essential oils and other drugs have been carried out, it is possible only to surmise what may happen. If sedative pills to help sleep are being prescribed then it is unwise with our current level of knowledge to use an essential oil such as rosemary, which keeps the mind alert: better to select oils such as *Lavandula angustifolia* [lavender], *Vetiveria zizanioides* [vetiver] and *Valeriana officinalis* [valerian], which are known to aid relaxation and sleep. It has been suggested that when a person is on medication the drugs involved could possibly affect the metabolization of essential oil molecules. In some cases metabolism may be increased, e.g. clofibrate (a blood lipid level reducer), steroids and phenobarbitones (antiepileptic); in other cases the drugs involved may reduce the metabolism of essential oil molecules, e.g. imidazole (antifungal) and plant drugs caffeic acid, myristicin and tannic acid. The study by Buchbauer et al. (1993) indicates an area of possible future study in that some essential oils or their components may interact with caffeine, e.g. neroli, methyl salicylate, isoeugenol.

Some essences have been found to complement the action of antibiotics. Laboratory tests have shown that niaouli (*Melaleuca viridiflora*) will increase the activity of streptomycin, cocaine and, more especially, of penicillin (Quevauviller & Parousse Perrin 1952a,b). Results obtained when using turpentine derivatives in conjunction with antibiotics have shown, from tests in vitro and on mice, that the action of the antibiotics is considerably augmented by being administered in a solution of oxygenated turpentine derivatives. On the other hand, some constituents of essential oils (aldehydes, ketones and some alcohols) inactivate antibiotics and so limit their use in ointment form (Valnet 1980 p. 39).

In vitro tests investigating the inhibitory effect of *Matricaria recutita* and its major constituents (chamazulene, *cis*-spiroether, *trans*-spiroether, α-bisabolol) on human cytochrome P450 enzymes (CYP1A2, CYP2C9, CYP2D6 and CYP3A4) indicated inhibition of each of these human drug metabolizing enzymes, therefore interactions with drugs whose route of elimination is mainly via cytochromes (especially CYP1A2) are possible (Ganzera et al. 2006).

The aroma of jasmine has been shown to shorten pentobarbital-induced sleeping time in mice; *cis*- and *trans*-phytol were considered the stimulant-like compounds in solvent extracted oil (Kikuchi et al. 1989), and *Cymbopogon citratus* injected peritoneally in rats was found to be analgesic, to prolong phenobarbitone-induced sleeping time and to potentiate the effects of morphine (Seth, Kokate & Varma 1976).

There are no human studies with whole therapeutic-grade oils that have ever demonstrated a negative reaction that should be a cause for concern (Stewart 2005 p. 397).

The therapeutic properties of essential oils

4 (Part II)

CHAPTER CONTENTS

There are many reasons why essential oils need to be included in the armoury of the fight against disease. They have many positive properties and effects which are desirable and have few drawbacks. They are capable of being anti-inflammatory, antiseptic, appetite stimulating, carminative, choleretic, circulation stimulating, deodorizing, expectorant, granulation stimulating, hyperaemic, insecticidal, insect repelling and sedative (Schilcher 1985 p. 217). They are natural antimicrobial agents able to act on bacteria, viruses and fungi, and many trials have been performed in this field (see below).

Essential oils are applied to the skin, ingested or inhaled, and all are harmless unless used incorrectly. They are much used in products for the home (obvious examples are lemon and lavender) and are well accepted, and the aroma can have beneficial effects on the person using them (see Ch. 7).

The aromatherapist determines the therapeutic materials to be used so that the treatment is tailored to the individual patient. Generally speaking there is an absence of unwanted side effects from the use of essential oils (see Synergism in Ch. 3 Part I); also, plant extracts are ecologically sound, causing no pollution, unlike antibiotics, which are flushed down the drain and pollute the land (Verdet 1989).

Antiseptic, antibacterial

Essential oils have multiple actions and effects, e.g. when used for a respiratory infection an oil may be not only antiseptic but also mucolytic and anti-inflammatory (Duraffourd 1987 p. 17). In the digestive system, the oils are antiseptic in action but do not act unfavourably on flora and the digestive secretions, in contrast to some unwelcome effects of antibiotics. The molecules of essential oils are not inimical to the human body: they support the immune system and can be considered as *pro-* and *eu*biotic as opposed to synthetic *antibiotics*.

Essential oils are especially valuable as antiseptics because their aggression towards microbial germs is matched by their total harmlessness to tissue; one of the chief drawbacks of some antiseptics used today is that they are likely to be as harmful to the cells of the organism as to the cause of the disease. It is very important to remember that antiseptics can destroy not only the microorganisms but also the surrounding cells (Valnet 1980 p. 44).

The use of essential oils is a sure way of avoiding the phenomenon of developed resistance in microbes as experienced with antibiotics, because the aromatic essences are able to destroy even resistant strains

Case 4.1

Antibacterial, antiinfectious, cicatrizant (A deep, open wound)

Mary Zorzou – Aromatherapist

Assessment

Mrs M came to the clinic with a deep wound, approximately 1 cm in width, from a caesarean operation that had become infected with *Staphylococcus*.

Treatment was as follows:

Thymus vulgaris (population) hydrolat (antibacterial, antiseptic, cicatrizant) was sprayed constantly on the wound

A blend was made with a base of 5 mL each of aloe vera gel and hypericum oil and the following essential oils:

2 drops *Pelargonium graveolens* [geranium] – antibacterial, antiinfectious, anti-inflammatory, cicatrizant

2 drops *Lavandula angustifolia* – antibacterial, anti-inflammatory, cicatrizant

2 drops *Melaleuca alternifolia* [tea tree] – antibacterial, anti-infectious

This blend was applied directly onto the wound 2 or 3 times a day and 1-2 drops of hypericum hydrolat and hypericum oil were also put into the wound 3 times a day. Hypericum oil was placed on bread and eaten with half a glass of hypericum hydrolat (diluted 50/50).

Outcome

The wound began to shrink within a week.

The antibacterial and cicatrizant essential oils of *Boswellia carteri* [frankincense], *Pelargonium graveolens* [geranium] and *Pogostemon patchouli* [patchouli] were put into aloe vera gel and applied twice a day to help minimise the scar. The skin was almost perfectly recovered after six weeks.

selectively (Pellecuer, Allegrini & De Buochberg 1974). Germs resistant to synthetic antibiotics are susceptible in certain cases to some essences in high dilution, e.g. 1 in 16,000 for *Satureia montana* (Belaiche 1979 p. 31) (Table 4.1).

Acquired resistance on the part of a germ can be avoided by prescribing three or four essential oils in combination. The editors strongly advise using a synergistic mix of oils in any treatment: it is unlikely that bacteria will be resistant to all oils in the mix.

Testing for antiseptic and antibacterial activity

Tests have been carried out on the antiseptic and antibacterial properties of essential oils for more than a century, and now there is a reasonably good knowledge base on this aspect of the effects of essential oils – Koch's 1881 investigation of turpentine with respect to the anthrax bacillus and Chamberland's 1887 investigation into the activity of cinnamon oils, angelica and geranium. Since then the antiseptic and bactericidal powers of many essential oils have been tested many times in laboratories across the world using the aromatogram technique, a recognized standard test; the results obtained are repeatable and universally accepted: it is virtually the same as the antibiogram test.

Antibiogram and aromatogram

An antibiogram can test the validity of an antibiotic agent for the treatment of, say, a chest infection. A sample of sputum is taken and a culture grown in a dish. The antibiotic is introduced into the centre of the culture and its activity against the offending microorganism measured by the diameter of a clear 'killing zone', which indicates the power of the antibiotic: the greater the diameter, the greater the effectiveness of the antibiotic agent. An aromatogram is carried out in exactly the same way except that essential oil is used instead of an antibiotic. Both methods are subject to the proviso that in vitro activity is not always echoed in vivo, which is modified by absorption, metabolism, bioavailability etc. Finding the most effective essential oil to counteract a specific germ can be a lengthy undertaking: if there were no previous experience to draw on it would be necessary to test all the oils available to the therapist. This testing procedure has confirmed the antiseptic

Table 4.1 Antibacterial spectrum of *Satureia montana* on some species and strains resistant to antibiotics (after Pellecuer et al. 1976)

Bacteria tested	Origin of bacteria	Type of resistance	Active dose in mg/ml
Staphylococcus aureus	IP 6454	Penicillin	0.250
Staphylococcus aureus	IP 6455	Penicillin Streptomycin Tetracycline	0.250
Staphylococcus aureus	IP 52149	Penicillin Streptomycin Tetracycline	0.250
Staphylococcus aureus Sarcina lutea	Ip 52150 Natural	Streptomycin 100γ of tetracycline	0.250 0.062
Bacillus subtilis	Natural	Streptomycin	0.250
Escherichia coli	Natural	Ampicillin Colomycin	0.250
Staphylococcus pathogen	Natural no. 1	Resistant to 500γ of virginiamycin	0.062
Staphylococcus pathogen	Natural no. 2		0.062
Staphylococcus pathogen	Natural no. 3		0.062
Staphylococcus pathogen	Natural no. 5		0.125
Staphylococcus pathogen	Natural no. 8		0.250
Staphylococcus pathogen	Natural no. 10		0.125

powers of many oils and at the same time has revealed previously unsuspected antiseptic powers in other oils. *Foeniculum vulgare* var. *dulce* [fennel] was known only for being an appetite stimulant, *Myristica fragrans* [nutmeg] as a stomachic and *Artemisia dracunculus* [tarragon] as an antispasmodic, but now the antiseptic qualities of these oils are also recognized. A huge number of aromatogram results have now been published, making it possible to list the major essential oils by their antimicrobial properties (Table 4.2).

Essential oils provide a very pleasant and effective means of disinfecting the air in an enclosed area (Kellner & Kober 1954, 1955, 1956) and are therefore ideal for use in sick rooms, burns units, reception areas, waiting rooms etc. A test describing the use of a blend of pine, thyme, peppermint, lavender, rosemary, clove and cinnamon essential oils for the bacteriological purification of the air concluded that 'the atmospheric dispersion of the prepared liquid brought about a very marked disinfection of the air, as demonstrated by the considerable reduction in the number of pre-existing micro-organisms, some types being destroyed completely' (Valnet 1980 pp. 36–38).

Methicillin resistant *Staphylococcus aureus* (MRSA)

Hospital-acquired infections and antibiotic-resistant bacteria continue to be major health concerns worldwide. Particularly problematic is MRSA and its ability to cause severe soft tissue, bone or implant infections, but recent experience has indicated that essential oils have an important part to play in dealing with this resistant bacterium. At a presentation to the Royal Society of Medicine, Michael Smith, pathologist, stated that several essential oils (including *Ormenis multicaulis, Origanum vulgare, Thymus vulgaris* ct. thymol, *Lavandula intermedia* 'Super', *Cupressus sempervirens, Mentha* x *piperita, Ravensara aromatica, Juniperus communis* (unspecified), *Citrus limon, Cymbopogon martinii, Eucalyptus globulus* and *Eucalyptus smithii*) were effective against MRSA (cited in Buckle 1997 p. 125). Sherry et al. (2001) successfully used a blend of phytochemicals (*Eucalyptus globulus, Melaleuca alternifolia, Thymus* sp., *Syzygium aromaticum*, citrus extracts and bioethanol) to treat two cases of MRSA infection with no reported recurrence. More recently several

Table 4.2   Antibacterial effects of essential oils

Latin name	Common name	Bacillus megaterium	Bacillus mycoides	Bacillus pumilis	Bacillus subtilis	Bacterioides fragilis	Clostridium perfringens	Clostridium sporogenes	Corynebacterium diphtheriae	Diplococcus pneumoniae	Enterobacter aerogenes	Enterobacter cloaceae	Enterococci	Escherichia coli	Helicobacter pylori	Klebsiella species	Klebsiella ozonae	Klebsiella pneumoniae	Lactobacillus plantarum	Mycobacterium phlei
Abies balsamea	balsam fir needle													X						
Artemisia dracunculus	tarragon									X			X	X		X				
Boswellia carteri	frankincense				xx											X				X
Carum carvi	caraway										xx			X		X				
Chamaemelum nobile	Roman chamomile																			
Cinnamomum verum (cort.)	cinnamon bark									xxx			xxx	xxx		xxx				
Cistus ladaniferus	labdanum												X							
Citrus aurantium var. amara (flos)	neroli												X	X		X				
Citrus aurantium var. amara (fol.)	petitgrain									X		X	X			X				
Citrus bergamia (per.)	bergamot										X					X				
Citrus limon (per.)	lemon									X			X	X						
Coriandrum sativum (fruct.)	coriander								X	X				X		xx				
Citrus paradisi	grapefruit																			
Cupressus sempervirens	cypress													X						
Cymbopogon citratus	lemongrass																			
Cymbopogon martini	palmarosa																			
Eucalyptus citriodora	lemon scented gum	X												xx						
Eucalyptus dives	broad leaved peppermint													xx						
Eucalyptus globulus	Tasmanian blue gum									xxx			X	xx		xx				
Eucalyptus radiata	narrow leaved peppermint													xx						
Eucalyptus smithii	gully gum																			
Eucarya spicata	Australian sandalwood																			
Foeniculum vulgare var. dulce (fruct.)	fennel									X				X						
Helichrysum angustifolium	everlasting											X		X				X		
Hyssopus officinalis	hyssop								xx											
Kunzea ericoides	kanuka																			
Laurus nobilis	bay																			
Lavandula angustifolia	lavender								X	xx	xx		xx	xx		xx				
Lavandula latifolia	spike lavender																			
Leptospermum scoparium	manuka																			
Matricaria recutita	German chamomile																			
Melaleuca alternifolia	tea tree					X	xx	xx	xx	xx	X			xx	X					
Melaleuca leucadendron	cajuput									xxx			xx	xx		xxx				
Melaleuca viridiflora	niaouli												X	X						

Mycobacterium tuberculosis	Moraxella species	MRSA	Neisseira catarrhalis	Neisseria gonorrhoeae	Neisseria meningitidis	Proteus species	Propionibacterium acnes	Pseudomonas aeruginosa	Salmonella species	Salmonella pullorum	Salmonella typhi	Salmonella typhimurium	Sarcina species	Shigella sonnet	Staphylococcus species	Staphylococcus albus	Staphylococcus aureus	Staphylococcus epidermidis	Staphylococcus faecalis	Streptococcus species	Streptococcus faecalis	Streptococcus beta-haemolytic	Vibrio cholerae	Vibrio parahaemolyticus	Yersinia enterocolitica
															x										
								X		X						x	x					x			x
													x				x	x							
						xx				x							xx								
																	x								
		X				xxx			xx	xxx						xxx	xxx			xx		xxx			xx
																	x								
						x																x			
																x	xx					x			
									x								x				xx				
x	X				x												x		X						
						x				x							x								xx
																				x					
x	X																x					x			
	X																			x				x	
	X															x									
																xx									
																xx									
		X				xx				x						xx	xx			x		?			
								x									x								
		X																							
																	xxx								
						x				x							x								
								x									x	x							
xxx																x	x		x			x			
																					x				
											x						x							x	
	x	X				x				x						x	xx			x	xx	xxx			x
																	x	x							
																	x								
		X	x			x	x	xx			xxx					x	xx	x		x					
						xx										xx	xx					x			
x						x											xx					x	x		

Continued

Table 4.2 Antibacterial effects of essential oils—cont'd

Latin name	Common name	Bacillus megaterium	Bacillus mycoides	Bacillus pumilis	Bacillus subtilis	Bacterioides fragilis	Clostridium perfringens	Clostridium sporogenes	Corynebacterium diphtheriae	Diplococcus pneumoniae	Enterobacter aerogenes	Enterobacter cloaceae	Enterococci	Escherichia coli	Helicobacter pylori	Klebsiella species	Klebsiella ozonae	Klebsiella pneumoniae	Lactobacillus plantarum	Mycobacterium phlei
Mentha arvensis	cormint				x															
Mentha × piperita	peppermint				xx					x				xx		xx				
Myristica fragrans (sem.)	nutmeg										x			xx		xx				
Myrtus communis	myrtle													x						
Ocimum basilicum var. album	basil									x	x			x						
Origanum majorana	marjoram								xx	x	xx			xx		xx				
Origanum vulgare, O. heracleoticum	oregano				xx									xx						
Ormenis mixta	Moroccan chamomile													xx						
Pelargonium graveolens P. × asperum	geranium									xx	xx		x			x				
Pimpinella anisum	aniseed																			
Pinus sylvestris	pine									xx		xx		xx		xx				
Piper nigrum	black pepper													x					x	
Ravensara aromatica	ravensara																			
Rosa damascena	rose otto														x					
Rosmarinus officinalis	rosemary						xx	x		x	xx			x		xx				
Rosmarinus officinalis ct. verbenone	rosemary verbenone																			
Salvia officinalis	sage				x					x				xx				x		
Satureia hortensis	summer savory									xxx			xx	xx		xx				
Satureia montana	winter savory									xxx			xx	xx		xx				
Syzygium aromaticum (flos)	clove bud							xx		xxx	xx		xxx	xx		xx				
Tagetes patula, Tagetes minuta	taget, French marigold	x	x	x										x						
Thymus capitatus	Spanish oregano									xxx			xxx	xxx		xxx				
Thymus serpyllum	wild thyme									x			x	x		x				
Thymus mastichina	Spanish marjoram																			
Thymus vulgaris ct. thymol	thyme									xxx	xxx			xxx		xxx				

Not all the oils in this table have been tested for all the bacteria shown. Other oils mentioned as antibacterial but unspecified are:

Illicium verum   star anise

Inula helenium   elecampane

Melissa officinalis   lemon balm

Mentha arvensis   cornmint

Terebinth   turpentine

Pogostemon patchouli   patchouli

Mycobacterium tuberculosis	Moraxella species	MRSA	Neisseira catarrhalis	Neisseria gonorrhoeae	Neisseria meningitidis	Proteus species	Propionibacterium acnes	Pseudomonas aeruginosa	Salmonella species	Salmonella pullorum	Salmonella typhi	Salmonella typhimurium	Sarcina species	Shigella sonnet	Staphylococcus species	Staphylococcus albus	Staphylococcus aureus	Staphylococcus epidermidis	Staphylococcus faecalis	Streptococcus species	Streptococcus faecalis	Streptococcus beta–haemolytic	Vibrio cholerae	Vibrio parahaemolyticus	Yersinia enterocolitica
																				X					
XX		X				XX		XX		XX							XX		X	X	X	X			XX
				X						X															X
								X																	
								X	X								X				X				X
						XX		X		XX							XX								XX
		X						XX			XX						XX								
		X																							
						X		X		XX					XX	X						XX			XX
													X		X	X		X					X		
						XX									XX	XX						XX			
										X									X						X
		XX																							X
						X				X					X	X				XX	X	X			
														X					X						
		X				X		X	X	X				X	XX				X	X	X				
X						X		XX		XX					XXX	XXX					X	XXX			XX
X						X		XX		XX					XXX	XXX				XXX	XXX				XX
XX		X				XX		XX		XX					XXX	XX				X	X	XX			XX
								X							X	X									
						XXX									XXX	XXX						XX			
						X										X						XX			
XX																									
		X				XXX		X		XXX		XX	XXX		XXX	XXX					X	XXX	XXX		

common and hospital-acquired bacterial and yeast isolates (six *Staphylococcus* strains including MRSA, four *Streptococcus* strains and three *Candida* strains, including *Candida krusei*) were tested by Warnke et al. (2009) for their susceptibility to eucalyptus, tea tree, white thyme, lavender, lemon, lemongrass, cinnamon, grapefruit, clove bud, sandalwood, peppermint, kunzea and sage oil with the agar diffusion test. Large zones of inhibition were observed for white thyme, lemon, lemongrass and cinnamon oil, and other oils also showed considerable efficacy. Almost all the tested oils demonstrated efficacy against hospital-acquired isolates and reference strains.

Analgesic

Many essential oils have analgesic properties and there seems to be no single reason. It is thought that the effect is partly due to the anti-inflammatory, circulatory and detoxifying effects of some oils and to the anaesthetic effect of others. The phenol eugenol found in the oil of clove is well known for its use in calming dental pain, wintergreen oil (containing methyl salicylate, an ester) has traditionally been used in rubs for muscle pain, and menthol has been used specifically for headaches. On the skin, oils rich in terpenes have an analgesic effect, especially those containing *p*-cymene (Franchomme & Pénoël 2001 p. 99); many aromatherapists report that the oil of *Melaleuca alternifolia* [tea tree] has this effect, as have azulene and chamazulene (found in the chamomiles). Some essential oils have a universal sedative or soporific action leading to an easing of pain, e.g. *Chamaemelum nobile, Cananga odorata, Citrus reticulata* (fol.) (Rossi et al. 1988), *Citrus bergamia* per., fol. (Franchomme & Pénoël 2001 p. 99). According to Roulier (1990), the analgesic and antalgic essential oils are white birch, chamomile, frankincense, wintergreen, clove, lavender and mint (common names only given).

At Monklands Hospital in Scotland more than 75% of patients suffering from chronic complaints (e.g. back or shoulder pain, long-term problems, premenstrual tension, depression, anxiety or mood swings) referred by local GPs found that complementary therapies helped to provide short-term relief of their symptoms. The patients were treated with essential oils, reflexology or acupuncture during an 8-week trial (Anderson 1998) (see Appendix B.9 on the CD-ROM for a list of effective oils).

Antifungal

Many essential oils have been reported as having an antifungal effect (Table 4.3) and many investigations have taken place, some more than half a century ago (Schmidt 1936), showing the fungicidal and fungistatic effects of cinnamon, clove, fennel and thyme; these were active against *Candida albicans, Sporotrichon* and *Trichophyton* species (Gildemeister & Hoffmann 1956 p. 140). The fungicidal activity of the oil of *Chamomilla recutita* and its components, including chamazulene and (–)-α-bisabolol, has been well investigated and shown to

Case 4.2

Analgesic (headache)

Nic Gerard – Aromatherapist

Assessment

N was prone to headaches, which occasionally turned into migraine.

Normally she used lavender hydrolat as a compress on his forehead, which cleared headaches but not a migraine.

Intervention

She had just attended an Open Day at PPA and had bought a bottle of Len Price's special hydrolat blend (an experiment when he had some plants left in his field but not enough of each one to fill the still).

Two days later she had a severe headache, which felt like the beginning of a migraine, and because she saw

there were two types of lavender as well as peppermint in the special blend, she thought she 'would give it a try' (along with a little sweet marjoram massaged into the back of her neck).

She felt the headache lifting within moments and eventually it eased considerably. She had also been taking it in water throughout the day since the weekend, and had not had a headache since.

Outcome

'I have to say I really love it – please tell your Dad and ask him to make some more!'

Case 4.3

Antifungal (*Candida albicans*)

Alan Barker – Aromatologist

Assessment

Mrs F (aged 40) was suffering from a continuous urinary tract infection (with inflammation, incontinence and pain) which antibiotics failed to control. She was given intermittent self-catheterization (ISC) and by April 1992 major surgery (removal of the bladder) was considered. She also developed a vaginal inflammation – thrush, being eventually unable to perform the ISC and complaining of constant pain and swelling of the abdomen (caused by having to have residual catheterization using microcatheters).

It was suggested to the consultant that aromatherapy be tried. Mrs F's vagina was the consistency of 'raw liver' and she suffered frequent discharges, thus intercourse was impossible. Her husband attended with her and was checked over, as this side of the partnership, although important, is often overlooked – Mrs F had had this recurrent form of *candida* for several years and the relationship was beginning to suffer.

Intervention

The couple's normal diet plan for an average week was looked at and gradual changes over a period of time were arranged.

A colonic massage with essential oils was decided upon for Mrs F, to benefit the swelling, pain and infection. Equal quantities of the following oils were used in a 15 min massage and at 50% dilution with grapeseed oil:

- *Citrus bergamia* (per.) [bergamot]
- *Eucalyptus globulus* [blue gum]
- *Melaleuca alternifolia* [tea tree]
- *Melaleuca viridiflora* [niaouli]

Mr F was taught how to perform a simple, clockwise abdominal massage, to be carried out once daily to aid Mrs F's constipation. This was a good morale booster for him, as he had previously felt helpless – he now became part of her recovery process. The 3% mix for him to use contained the following essential oils:

- *Zingiber officinale* (antispasmodic and laxative)
- *Foeniculum vulgare* var. *dulce* (appetite stimulant, laxative and circulation stimulant)
- *Mentha x piperita* (analgesic, antiinflammatory and stomachic).

Treatment with live yogurt and essential oils was also given; the client's vagina was too swollen to use a tampon soaked in this mix, so the yogurt mixture was poured into the vagina (the client was propped up with raised legs to allow the mix to penetrate). Although messy and difficult, the swelling had reduced enough after several days to insert a tampon, changing it morning and night.

Treatment at home involved:

- tea made with marigold flowers plus 1 drop bergamot 3 times a day for 3 weeks
- 6 acidopholus tablets daily
- essential oils for the bath
- abdomen massage oil – using the mix above
- 10 ml yogurt with 5 drops tea tree – used as above.

Outcome

By the end of a month Mrs F was already feeling benefits from the treatment and the yogurt treatment was changed to oral yogurt tablets.

A few months later the abdominal swelling was going down and the urinary tract was almost clear. Mrs F was on only 3 acidopholus tablets daily, the marigold tea and yogurt with tea tree internally occasionally. Abdomen massage by her husband continued once or twice a week only and with a reduced concentration of oils to 1.5%.

The couple's relationship is now close once more, partially due to Mr F's eagerness to help.

---

be effective against *Trichophyton rubrum*, *T. mentagrophytes*, *T. tonsurans*, *T. quinckeanum* and *Microsporum canis* in concentrations of 200 mg/mL (Janssen et al. 1984, 1986, Szalontai, Verzar-Petri & Florian 1976, 1977, Szalontai et al. 1975a,b). *Satureia montana* has been found to be active against *Candida* sp. (Pellecuer et al. 1975). A general review of some essential oils with antifungal properties was carried out by Pellecuer et al. (1976) and in other trials a number of compounds found in essential oils, especially the aldehydes and esters, were effective against various fungi, including candida infection (Larrondo & Calvo 1991, Maruzella 1961, Thompson & Cannon 1986). *Melaleuca alternifolia* has been investigated in vaginal infection with candida and found to be effective (Belaiche 1985, Pena 1962, Shemesh & Mayo 1991). Rosemary, savory and thyme also have antifungal properties (Pellecuer, Roussel & Andary 1973) and *Ocimum basilicum* has both antifungal and insect-repellant properties (Dube, Upadhyay & Tripath 1989).

Anti-inflammatory

The oils of *Lavandula angustifolia* [lavender] and *Chamomilla recutita* [German chamomile] are widely used to soothe minor inflammations such as

Table 4.3   Antifungal effects of essential oils

Latin name	Common name	General antifungal properties*	Acinetobacter calcoacetica	Aspergillus species	Aspergillus flavus	Aspergillus fumigatus	Aspergillus nidulans	Aspergillus niger	Aspergillus ochraceous	Aspergillus parasiticus	Candida species	Candida albicans	Candida glabrata	Chaetomium species	Clamidia sporogenes	Clostridium perfringens	Colletotrichum gloeosporioides	Cryptococcus neoformans	Epidermophyton species	Fusarium species	Fusarium oxysporum	Fusarium moniliforme	Listeria monocytogenes
Artemisia dracunculus	Tarragon											X											
Cinnamomum verum (cort)	Cinnamon bark				X			X	X	X		XX	X					X					
Cinnamomum verum (fol.)	Cinnamon leaf				X			X				X	X										
Cistus ladaniferus	Labdanum											X											
Citrus aurantifolia (per.)	Lime			X																	X		
Citrus aurantium var. amara (fol.)	Petitgrain bigarade	X										XXX											
Citrus aurantium var. amara (flos)	Neroli	X																					
Citrus aurantium var. amara (per.)	Bitter orange			X																	X		
Citrus aurantium var. sinensis (per.)	Sweet orange			X	X			X		X													
Coriandrum sativum	Coriander										X												
Cuminum cyminum (fruct.)	Cumin				X			X		X													
Cymbopogon martinii	Palmarosa			X							X												
Cymbopogon citratus	Lemongrass			X							X												
Ellettaria cardamomum	Cardamom				X				X	X													
Eucalyptus citriodora	Lemon scented gum	X						X				X											
Eucalyptus dives	Broad leaved peppermint							X				X											
Eucalyptus globulus	Tasmanian blue gum										X	X											
Eucalyptus radiata	Narrow leaved peppermint							X				X											
Eucaria spicata	Australian sandalwood											XXX											
Foeniculum vulgare var. dulce	Fennel											X											
Hyssopus officinalis	Hyssop					X																	
Illicium verum	Star anise	X																					
Inula helenium	Elecampane	X																		X			
Kunzea ericoides	Kanuka										X									X			
Lavandula angustifolia	Lavender										X	XX						XX					
Lavandula × intermedia 'Super'	Lavandin																						
Lavandula latifolia	Spike lavender											X											
Leptospermum scoparium	Manuka											X											
Matricaria recutita	German chamomile																						
Melaleuca alternifolia	Tea tree	X						XX			X	XX						X					
Melaleuca leucadendron	Cajuput	X										XX											
Melaleuca viridiflora	Niaouli											X											
Melissa officinalis	Lemon balm	X																					

Malassezia furfur	Moraxella species	Mycobacterium fortuitum	Mycobacterium smegmatis	Microsporum audounii	Microsporum canis	Microsporum cookei	Microsporum gypseum	Mucor species	Nigrospora oryzae	Penicillium species	Penicillium chrysogenum	Pityosporum ovale	Rhizopus species	Saccharomyces cereviciae	Sclerotium rolfsii	Sporotrichium species	Tinea capitis	Tinea pedis	Trichoderma viride	Trichophyton species	Trichophyton beigelii	Trichophyton mentagrophytes	Trichophyton quinckeanum	Trichophyton rubrum	Trichophyton souclanense	Trychophyton tonsurans	Trichophyton violaceum	Trichothecium roseum	Zygorrhynchus species
					x											x				x		x		x					
					x																	x		x					
													X																
													X																
								X																X			X		
								X																X			X		
									X																				
		x												X								X							X
																X			X										
				x																X		X					X		
																							X						
												X																	
												X																	
																	X												
																X	X												
					x																	X	X	X		X			
	x											X				X	X												

Continued

Table 4.3   Antifungal effects of essential oils—cont'd

Latin name	Common name	General antifungal properties*	Acinetobacter calcoacetica	Aspergillus species	Aspergillus flavus	Aspergillus fumigatus	Aspergillus nidulans	Aspergillus niger	Aspergillus ochraceous	Aspergillus parasiticus	Candida species	Candida albicans	Candida glabrata	Chaetomium species	Clamidia sporogenes	Clostridium perfringens	Colletotrichum gloeosporioides	Cryptococcus neoformans	Epidermophyton species	Fusarium species	Fusarium oxysporum	Fusarium moniliforme	Listeria monocytogenes
Mentha arvensis	Cornmint	x		x																			
Mentha x piperita	Peppermint										x	x											
Mentha spicata	Spearmint																						
Myrtus communis	Myrtle	x						x			x	x											
Nardostachys jatamansi	Spikenard	x			x		x	x													x	x	
Nepeta cataria	Catnep							xx				xx											
Ocimum basilicum	Basil	x			x		x	x		x				x							x	x	
Origanum heracleoticum	Greek oregano	x						xx				xx											
Origanum majorana	Sweet marjoram	x																					
Pelargonium graveolens	Geranium											?			x								
Pelargonium asperum	Geranium											x											
Pinus sylvestris	Pine											xx											
Pogostemon patchouli	Patchouli	x																	x				
Rosmarinus officinalis	Rosemary									x		x											x
Rosmarinus officinalis ct. verbenone	Rosemary verbenone											x											
Salvia officinalis	Sage		x								x	x			x			x					
Satureia montana, S. hortensis	Winter savory	x										x											
Syzygium aromaticum (flos)	Clove bud							xx	xx	xx	x	xx											
Tagetes glandulifera, T. patula	Marigold							x															
Thymus capitatus	Spanish oregano											xxx											
Thymus mastichina	Spanish marjoram											x											
Thymus serpyllum	Wild thyme											x											
Thymus vulgaris (pop.)	Thyme	x									x	x											
Thymus vulgaris ct. linalool, geraniol	Sweet thyme											x											
Thymus vulgaris ct. thymol, carvacrol	Thyme	x								x	x	xxx									x		
Santalum spicatum	Australian sandalwood							x			x												

Malassezia furfur	Moraxella species	Mycobacterium fortuitum	Mycobacterium smegmatis	Microsporum audounii	Microsporum canis	Microsporum cookei	Microsporum gypseum	Mucor species	Nigrospora oryzae	Penicillium species	Penicillium chrysogenum	Pityosporum ovale	Rhizopus species	Saccharomyces cereviciae	Sclerotium rolfsii	Sporotrichium species	Tinea capitis	Tinea pedis	Trichoderma viride	Trichophyton species	Trichophyton beigelii	Trichophyton mentagrophytes	Trichophyton quinckeanum	Trichophyton rubrum	Trichophyton souclanense	Trychophyton tonsurans	Trichophyton violaceum	Trichothecium roseum	Zygorrhynchus species
																									x				
x																				X			X						
																		X											
										X		X																	
											X				X														
xx																				XX		XX							
					x		x												X		X		X	X			X		
																							X						
		x																											
	x																												
																X				X									
																		X	X										
																X				X									
xx																X				X									

sunburn, small burns and insect bites, and plenty of people can testify to their effectiveness in this respect. Jakovlev, Isaac and Flaskamp (1983) showed the anti-inflammatory effect of yarrow, chamomile and turpentine. Although chamazulene and (–)-α-bisabolol found in chamomile oils are anti-inflammatory agents (Weiss 1988 p. 24), other azulenes that may be added to anti-inflammatory preparations are not so effective, e.g. guaiazulene (manufactured from guaiol) and elemazulene (from elemol). Also (+)-α-bisabolol and synthetic (–)-α-bisabolol are not as effective as the natural form.

Otitis media is an infectious and inflammatory disease which may lead to impairment of hearing; over a 2-year period Kang Mok Yoo, an otolaryngologist in South Korea, used aromatherapy to treat 200 patients suffering from chronic mucoid otitis media with effusion and found that the success rate was 90% achieved in just 13 days on average (personal communication) (Table 4.4 and Appendix B Table B1 on the CD-ROM).

Antipruritic

Lavender and tea tree oils (both unspecified) were diluted in jojoba wax and sweet almond oil used in massage in a study to determine the effects of aromatherapy on pruritus and *Stratum corneum* hydration pruritus in patients undergoing haemodialysis: the results showed pruritus to be significantly decreased and skin hydration greatly enhanced (Ro et al. 2002).

Antitoxic

Chamomile oil has been found to be capable of inactivating toxins produced by bacteria. The amount of oil obtained by distilling 0.1 g of chamomile is sufficient to destroy, within 2 hours, three times that amount of staphylococcal toxins – the highest concentration of toxin so far found in the human organism; streptococcal toxins proved even more sensitive (Weiss 1988 p. 26).

Case 4.4

Anti-inflammatory (gangrene)

L. Cooke – Aromatherapist

Client assessment

Mr A developed gangrene on the toes of his left foot and the whole area was inflamed. There was also a large patch on his shin and a smaller area below his knee. As the gangrene was in its acute stage, Mr A wanted to see an aromatherapist that he knew, to try anything she might suggest, before it reached the stage of needing amputation. The consultant was in agreement, as there was nothing the hospital could do except amputate.

Intervention

To reduce the inflammation, the following oils were applied in a cold compress to each area and left for 60 minutes:
- 8 drops *Eucalyptus globulus* [blue gum] – anti-inflammatory, bactericidal, rubifacient
- 8 drops *Lavandula angustifolia* [lavender] – analgesic, antibacterial, anti-inflammatory, cicatrizant
- 150 mL cold water.

The three pieces of cotton – the size of the areas to be treated – were first wetted (and squeezed well) in cold water, before being immersed in this well-stirred blend, making sure all the liquid was absorbed. Each was squeezed lightly to remove excess liquid before being applied to the areas concerned.

The foot and leg were then massaged using the following blend:

- 16 drops *Juniperus communis* fruct. [juniper berry] – analgesic, depurative
- 16 drops *Pelargonium graveolens* [geranium] – analgesic, antibacterial, anti-infectious, anti-inflammatory, cicatrizant, haemostatic
- 16 drops *Eucalyptus globulus* – as above
- 75 mL carrier lotion
- 25 mL hypericum.

Mr A was given the rest of the blend to apply at home twice a day.

Outcome

The inflammation died down quickly and after several days the dark patches on his leg formed a hard scaly skin, which subsequently flaked off.

The recovery was put down to the fact that the gangrene had been treated in its acute stage.

Two and a half years later Mr A had an accident and the patches reappeared on the same three areas as before. He refused to go into hospital, sending instead for the aromatherapist, who repeated the treatment above. In between visits, the district nurse was given permission to apply the lotion on every visit.

The leg made a complete recovery once again.

Antiviral

Most people practising aromatherapy have reported success in the control of viruses causing *herpes simplex* type I, but there is no consistency in the choice of oils used (as can be seen from Table 4.5). Speaking from personal experience, the editors have found the oils *Melissa officinalis, Pelargonium graveolens* and *Eucalyptus smithii* to be helpful for *herpes simplex I* (cold sore). The use of melissa agrees with tests showing this plant to be antiviral (Cohen, Kucera &

Herrman 1964, Herrman & Kucera 1967, Kucera & Herrman 1967). For *herpes zoster* (shingles) the oil of *Pelargonium graveolens* [geranium] is specifically recommended; it is best applied at the first sign of an attack to prevent virus replication. Used early it prevents blisters from forming and damps down the pain. For *herpes simplex II* (genital herpes) the many oils suggested include *Melaleuca alternifolia* [tea tree] and *M. viridiflora* [niaouli] (Franchomme & Pénoël 2001 pp. 397, 398), but little success has been reported. Despite the lack of

Case 4.5

Antiviral

Dr D. Pénoël – Aromatologist

Client assessment

Clément was suffering from Molluscum contagiosum, a serious viral infection, which had developed while the family were on holiday in Corsica. His whole body (including his genitals) was covered with boils; he was feverish and screaming with pain day and night.

His parents firmly believed in natural medicine and did not wish to send Clément to the hospital, knowing that no allopathic cure existed for viral diseases. The boy was also prone to eczema and allergic reactions. Not only was the medical condition of the child assessed, but the family were asked to undertake the therapeutic programme prescribed.

Intervention

A toxin-free diet was established for Clément to help the detoxification process that accompanies any infectious disease.

Because of the extreme cutaneous condition, the hydrolat of *Melissa officinalis* [melissa] (undiluted) – antiviral, anti-inflammatory, calming – was selected first and sprayed around the little boy, who felt relief for the first time in many days of intense suffering.

The following essential oils were then chosen and blended:
- *Chamaemelum nobile* [Roman chamomile] – anti-inflammatory, calming, vulnerary
- *Matricaria recutita* [German chamomile] – cicatrizant, antiallergic, anti-inflammatory
- *Melaleuca alternifolia* [tea tree] – analgesic, antiinfectious, anti-inflammatory, antiviral, immunostimulant
- *Thymus vulgaris* ct. linalol [sweet thyme] – antiinfectious, anti-inflammatory, antiseptic, antiviral, immunostimulant
- *Juniperus communis* fruct. [juniper berry] – analgesic, antiseptic, antiviral, depurative

These were made up in three ways:
- A 5% concentration with a 95% blend of vegetable carrier oils, also active in the healing process: macerated oils of calendula (60%) and St John's Wort (25%) and oil of *Calophyllum inophyllum* (5%). The parents were asked to apply this blend to each boil, using a fine paintbrush.
- A blend of the essential oils above was given to the parents to be used internally – 1 drop blended in honey six times per day.
- 3 drops, diluted in vegetable oil, were put into capsules, to use as suppositories.

A second blend of essential oil was made with equal quantities of:
- *Melaleuca cajuputi* (cajuput)
- *Melaleuca alternifolia*
- *Myrtus communis* (red myrtle)

This was to be applied without dilution to the sole of the each foot six times a day.

After the first treatment at the clinic, the blends and suppositories were given to the parents to continue treatment at home; the spraying equipment was lent to them for the period of intensive care.

The parents were asked to telephone every day to report Clément's progress and to return to the clinic after 9 days.

Outcome

After three days the problem had improved enormously. The treatment was continued, but reducing the number of applications per day.

Nine days later the family returned to see me. Clément's skin was almost perfect and he had regained his vitality. This remarkable and speedy result was helped not only by the determination of the parents, but also by the high-quality aromatic and vegetable oils.

Table 4.4 Anti-inflammatory effects of essential oils

Latin name	Common name	Unspecified	Acne	Boils	Arteritis	Arthritis	Blepharitis	Bronchitis	Bursitis	Cellulitis	Colitis	Coronaritis	Cystitis	Dermatitis	Eczema	Emphysema
Achillea millefolium	Yarrow															
Acorus calamus	Sweet flag							x					x			
Aloysia triphylla	Verbena												x			
Boswellia carteri	Frankincense															
Cinnamomum verum (fol.)	Cinnamon leaf															
Cistus ladaniferus	Labdanum					x							x			
Citrus aurantium var. *amara* (fol.)	Petitgrain		x													
Citrus aurantium var. *amara* (per.)	Orange bitter	x														
Citrus limon (per.)	Lemon			x												
Commiphora myrrha, C. molmol	Myrrh	x														
Coriandrum sativum	Coriander															
Cuminum cyminum	Cumin					x										
Cymbopogon citratus, C. flexuosus	Lemongrass					x				x						
Elettaria cardamomum	Cardamum	x														
Eucalyptus citriodora	Lemon-scented gum					x						x	x			
Eucalyptus globulus	Tasmanian blue gum							x					x			
Eucalyptus radiate	Narrow-leaved peppermint		x					x								
Eucalyptus staigeriana	Lemon-scented ironbark	x														
Foeniculum vulgare var. *dulce*	Fennel												x			
Helichrysum angustifolium	Everlasting					x					x			x		
Hyssopus officinalis	Hyssop							x					x			x
'*Inula helenium, I. graveolens*'	Elecampane							x					x	x		
Juniperus communis (ram)	Juniper twig	x														
Lavandula angustifolia	Lavender		x										x		x	
Litsea cubeba	May chang												x			
Matricaria recutita	German chamomile												x	x		
Melaleuca alternifolia	Tea tree															
Melaleuca viridiflora	Niaouli						X	X				X				
Melissa officinalis	Melissa x	X														
Mentha x *piperita*	Peppermint							x			x		x		XX	
Mentha spicata	Spearmint												x			
Myrtus communis	Myrtle															
Nepeta cataria	Catnep					X										
Ormenis mixta (flos)	Moroccan chamomile											x	x	x	x	
Pelargonium graveolens	Geranium					x					x					
Picea mariana	Black spruce															
Pinus mugo var. *pumilio*	Dwarf pine	X														
Pinus sylvestris	Pine							X								
'*Pogostemon cablin, P. patchouli*'	Patchouli		X											X	X	
Ravensara aromatica	Ravensara															
'*Rosa centifolia, R. damascena*'	Rose													x		
Rosmarinus officinalis	Rosemary												x			
Syzygium aromaticum (flos)	Clove bud					X			X	X						
Thymus satureioides	Moroccan thyme					XX							x			
Thymus vulgaris ct. *geraniol*	Sweet thyme					X										
Thymus vulgaris ct. *linalool*	Sweet thyme							x					x		X	
Thymus vulgaris ct. *thujanol-4*	Thujanol thyme				X										X	
'*Valeriana officinalis, V. walachii*'	Valerian	X														
Zingiber cassumunar	Plai, phrai					X			X		X					

Fol(ium) = leaf
Flos = flower
Caul(is) = stem
Cort(ex) = bark
Sem(en) = seed
Rad(ix) = root
Ram(unculus) = twig
Per(icarpium)
Lig(num) = wood
Rhiz(oma) = rhizome

Enterocolitis	Gall bladder inflammation	Gastritis	Gingivitis	Gout	Hepatitis	Insect bites, stings	Laryngitis	Neuritis	Orchitis	Otitis	Pericarditis	Phlebitis	Pleurisy	Prostatitis	Rheumatism	Rheumatoid arthritis	Rhinitis rhinopharyngitis	Salpingitis	Sinusitis	Stomatitis	Tendonitis	Tonsillitis	Tracheitis	Urethritis	Vaginitis
								X						X	X										
		X		X																					
															X										
															X										
																		X		X					
																X									
				X		X									X										
															X										
X					X				X						X										
											X														X
							X						X						X						
										X							X								X
				X																					
		X															X		X						
															X		X		X						
							X																X		X
						X				X		X							X						
		X													X										
										X									X						
														X			X		X					X	X
X		X			X		X												X						
														X											
															X										
				X		X																			
															X										
															X							X			
														X	X										
	X			X											X										
															X										
			X																						
	X			X			X								X										
																	X	X							
																				X					
										X				X	X									X	
										X				X	X									X	
																							X		

Table 4.5 Antiviral effects of essential oils

Latin name	Common name	Unspecified	Adenovirus	Childhood infections	Herpes genitalis	Glandular fever	Herpes simplex	Herpes varicella
Aniba rosaeodora	Rosewood							
Cinnamomum verum (fol.)	Cinnamon leaf	x						
Cinnamomum verum (cort.)	Cinnamon bark							
Cistus ladaniferus	Labdanum			x				
Citrus aurantifolia (per.)	Lime							
Citrus aurantium var. *bergamia* (per.)	Bergamot						x	
Citrus limon (per.)	Lemon						x	
Commiphora molmol	Myrrh							
Cuminum cyminum	Cumin	x						
Cupressus sempervirens	Cypress							
Cymbopogon martinii	Palmarosa							
Eucalyptus dives	Broad-leaved peppermint	x						
Eucalyptus globulus	Tasmanian blue gum						x	
Eucalyptus radiata	Narrow-leaved peppermint							
Eucalyptus smithii	Gully gum							
Helichrysum angustifolium (flos)	Everlasting							
Hyssopus officinalis	Hyssop						x	
Inula helenium	Elecampane							
Laurus nobilis (fol.)	Bay leaf							
Lavandula × *intermedia* 'Super'	Lavandin Super							
Lavandula latifolia	Spike lavender							
Litsea cubeba	May chang							
Melaleuca alternifolia	Tea tree						x	
Melaleuca leucadendron	Cajuput							
Melaleuca viridiflora	Niaouli				xx		x	
Melissa officinalis	Melissa						x	
Mentha × *piperita*	Peppermint							
Nepeta cataria	Catnep						xx	
Ocimum basilicum	Basil							
Origanum majorana	Sweet marjoram						x	
Pelargonium graveolens P. × *asperum*	Geranium						x	
Pimenta dioica (fol.)	Pimento							
Pimenta racemosa (fruct.)	West Indian bay							
Piper nigrum	Pepper		x					
Ravensara aromatica	Ravensara							x
Rosmarinus officinalis	Rosemary						x	
Rosmarinus officinalis ct. *verbenone*	Rosemary verbenone							
Satureia montana	Winter savory							
Salvia officinalis	Sage				x	x		
Satureia hortensis	Summer savory							
Satureia montana	Winter savory							
Syzygium aromaticum (flos)	Clove bud						xx	
Thymus serpyllum	Wild thyme							
Thymus vulgaris ct. *phenol*	Thyme					X		
Thymus vulgaris ct. *geraniol*	Sweet thyme							
Thymus vulgaris ct. *linalool*	Sweet thyme							
Thymus vulgaris ct. *thujanol-4*	Sweet thyme	x						

Influenza	Viral enteritis	Viial enterocolitis	Viral hepatitis	Viral infections	Viral meningitis	Viral neuritis	Warts	Veruccae	Zoster	Viremia virus	Multiple sclerosis	Poliomyelitis
X												
				X			X	X				
X							X	X				
X							X	X				
			X									
X												
										X		
X												
X												
X												
X												
	X											
	X					X						
		X										
						X						
	X	X										
						X						
X	X		XX									
									X			
			X			X			X			
			X			X						
									X			
		X	X			X			X		X	X
X				X								
X	X		X									
X	X		X						XX			
			X									
	XX		X									
		X										
X	X				X	X			X			
				X								
				X								
X	XX	X	X									
X												
X												
	XX			X				X				
	XX			X				X	X			

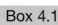

Box 4.1

Antiviral (avian and swine flu prevention)

The following blend was formulated by the editors' daughter and son-in-law for their flight to China (they wanted to ensure that they had some protection in that incubator of viruses!) for use by inhalation and in the bath; it was in a 10 mL bottle, so that it would not be a problem at the security checks:

- 4 mL *Ravensara aromatica* – antibacterial, antiinfectious, antiviral
- 2 mL *Eucalyptus radiata* – antiinfectious, strong antiseptic, antiviral
- 2 mL *Melaleuca viridiflora* – antibacterial, antiinfectious, antiviral, immunostimulant

- 2 mL *Syzygium aromaticum* – antibacterial, antiinfectious, antiviral, immunostimulant.

It was used by inhalation on Dr Stephen's moustache, although a paper tissue had to serve for Penny; a face-mask would work well also for those without the necessary equipment. Did it work? They travelled for 2 weeks on seven flights and in contact with a great many people without any evidence of viral infection, despite a punishing schedule and becoming extremely exhausted. The regime of baths and inhalation continued for 14 days after their return, as a precaution.

---

scientific support, many aromatherapists find that *herpes simplex* type II and other viral infections such as glandular fever and influenza do respond to essential oil treatment, and there is research to support the use of *Piper nigrum* [black pepper] (Lembke & Deininger 1988). *Cymbopogon flexuosus* [lemongrass], *Mentha arvensis* [cornmint] and *Vetiveria zizanioides* [vetiver] (Pandey et al. 1988), and *Eucalyptus viminalis*, *E. macarthurii* [woolly-butt] and *E. dalrympleana* appear to be effective both in vitro and in ovo on two strains of influenza virus (Vichkanova, Dzhanashiya & Goryunova 1973). There have been other papers published on this topic in India, Russia and China, and a Swiss patent was filed in 1979 for an antiviral preparation using essential oils.

Table 4.5 shows the essential oils that have been recommended for antiviral use. The information has been culled from many sources, which often use only the plant's common name. Many other oils have been mentioned anecdotally as having antiviral properties, but without specific indications.

Several constituents found naturally in a wide range of essential oils (anethole, β-caryophyllene, carvone, cinnamic aldehyde, citral, citronellol, eugenol, limonene, linalool, linalyl acetate, α-sabinene, γ-terpinene) were found to be active against *herpes simplex* (Lembke & Deininger 1985, 1988). If the oils are effective it could well be because of some property common to all of them – perhaps lipid solubility. The in vitro studies conducted so far indicate that many essential oils have antiviral properties but that they affect only enveloped viruses and only when they are in a free state, before the virus has entered or is attached to the host cell (e.g. Schnitzler et al. 2008). This is in contrast to the majority of synthetic agents, which either stop complete penetration of viral particles into the host cell or interfere with replication once the virus is inside the cell (Harris 2010 p. 319).

Balancing

Aromatherapists are aware of the remarkable balancing powers of essential oils, which can be puzzling because of the apparently contradictory effects. Essential oils are complex mixtures of natural constituents, some stimulating and others sedative, so a single oil may demonstrate an arousing effect on one occasion and a sedative effect on another: this is known as the adaptogenic effect.

Hyssop essential oil contains the ketone pinocamphone and is said to be toxic in high doses, causing epileptic attacks in those so predisposed (Valnet 1980), yet this oil is used in Case study 4.6 and has been used by the editors in an epilepsy case with beneficial effects, reducing the number of attacks from three per week to less than one. *Rosmarinus officinalis* [rosemary] in low dose is a hypotensor and in high dose a hypertensor; similar properties are often ascribed to *Cananga odorata* [ylang ylang] but are not proven.

Case 4.6

Balancing (epilepsy)

A. Barker – Aromatologist

Patient assessment

Seven-year-old M was hyperactive and epileptic, going in a few seconds from daydreaming to petit mal convulsions.

He was on a high dose of Epanutin, which his mother was not very happy about.

The following essential oils were used in high concentration as recommended by Valnet (1980):

- 15 drops *Hyssopus officinalis* [hyssop]
- 20 drops *Salvia officinalis* [sage]
- 25 drops *Ocimum basilicum* [sweet basil]

These were used in 30 mL of carrier oil (10% dilution) only on the kidney area of M's back, and so the quantity of essential oils being applied was in reality quite small.

Outcome

The convulsions ceased within a week, and M is now on a minimum dose of Epanutin. The massage oil concentration was reduced to 1.5% and treatments to one a month. M's mother is now looking at withdrawing conventional drug therapy.

Deodorant

Bad odours arise sometimes from the disease process and sweet-smelling oils act to prevent degradation, replace the odours and tackle the bacteria causing these effects. The use of familiar essential oils is more acceptable to the client (who may be in a weakened state) than is the imposition of synthetics, and they are helpful in a healing situation where malodours are generated, for example in some severe burn injuries. Valnet (1980 p. 44) wrote that 'the odour of essential oils does not cover up the bad smells of infected gangrenous or cancerous wounds; it suppresses them by physicochemical action'.

For a number of years the editors supplied an essential oil blend for this purpose to a burns unit at the request of the consultant surgeon: the nurses found it particularly useful when bathing patients with burns. Essential oils find a similar use in incontinence cases, making life more pleasant for all concerned.

The deodorizing effect of some fragrant materials is made use of in underarm and foot deodorants. Compounds and oils recommended as effective against body odour are eugenol, linalool and essential oil *Pogostemon patchouli* [patchouli] (Decazes 1993). Elsewhere,

chamomile preparations, *Cymbopogon citratus* [lemongrass], *Lavandula x intermedia* [lavandin] and *Myristica fragrans* [nutmeg], *Salvia sclarea* [clary sage] and *Zingiber officinale* [ginger] are mentioned in this respect.

The use of essential oils to treat malodorous wounds in cancer patients is becoming widespread in many palliative care units, although no formal clinical trials have so far been conducted (Harris 2010 p. 323). Bad-smelling wounds can be deodorized by the use of hypericum oil, thyme and citrus oils (Schilcher 1985 p. 222). Warnke et al. (2004) reported smell reduction in 25 malodorous patients with inoperable squamous cell carcinoma of the head and neck: Megabac, a commercial product containing grapefruit, eucalyptus and tea tree essential oils, was applied topically to the wounds daily and the smell disappeared completely in 2–3 days, and signs of superinfection and pus secretion were reduced in the necrotic areas. *Lavandula angustifolia* [lavender], *Melaleuca alternifolia* [tea tree] and *Pogostemon cablin* [patchouli] essential oils, used alone or in blends at 2.5–5% concentration in a cream base, successfully reduced the smell of fungating wounds (Mercier & Knevitt 2005).

Digestive

Carminative. Essential oils have strong effects on the digestive system (Table 4.6) and are used in appetite-stimulating and digestive drinks; apart from the strong carminative effect offered by many essential oils there are other benefits, such as increased secretory activity of the stomach and gallbladder, plus antiseptic and spasmolytic effects. The essential oils concerned are mainly from the botanical family Apiaceae – *Carum carvi*, *Coriandrum sativum*, *Foeniculum vulgare* var. *dulce*, *Pimpinella anisum* and also *Mentha x piperita*, *Ocimum basilicum* and the chamomiles (Schilcher 1985 p. 224). *Thymus serpyllum* [creeping thyme] has been shown to stimulate bile production (Chabrol et al. 1932), and essential oils containing the alcohols menthol and thujanol-4 seem to be beneficial to liver function (Gershbein 1977, Zara 1966).

The combination of peppermint and caraway essential oils acts locally in the gut as an antispasmodic (Micklefield et al. 2000, 2003) and has a relaxing effect on the gallbladder (Goerg & Spilker 2003) and caraway oil inhibits gallbladder contractions, increasing gallbladder volume by 90% (Georg & Spilker 1996). *Rosmarinus officinalis* has always been associated with improving the liver function. In animals an intravenous infusion of rosemary doubled the volume

Table 4.6 Essential oils and the digestive system. Sources same as for Appendix A

		Properties							
Latin name	**Common name**	Antispasmodic	Aperitive	Astringent	Carminative	Choleretic	Hepatic stimulant	Litholytic U=urinary K=kidney G=gall
Achillea millefolium	Yarrow						x	K
Angelica archangelica (rad)	Angelica root	x			x			
Carum carvi	Caraway	x			x	x		
Chamaemelum nobile (flos)	Roman chamomile		x		x			
Citrus aurantium var. *amara* (flos)	Neroli						x	
Citrus aurantium var. *amara* (fol.)	Petitgrain							
Citrus aurantium var. *amara* (per.)	Orange bitter						x	
Citrus bergamia (per.)	Bergamot	x	x		x			
Citrus limon (per.)	Lemon	x	x	x	x			G,U
Citrus reticulata (per.)	Mandarin				x		x	
Commiphora myrrha	Myrrh							
Coriandrum sativum	Coriander	x			x			
Cupressus sempervirens	Cypress	x		x				
Eucalyptus smithii	Gully gum							
Foeniculum vulgare var. *dulce* (fruct.)	Fennel				x	x		U
Hyssopus officinalis	Hyssop							U
Juniperus communis (fruct.)	Juniper berry		x	x	x		x	U,K
Matricaria recutita (flos)	German chamomile	?						
Melaleuca alternifolia	Tea tree							
Melaleuca leucadendron	Cajuput	x						
Melaleuca viridiflora	Niaouli				x		x	G
Melissa officinalis	Melissa	x				x	x	
Mentha arvensis	Cornmint							
Mentha × *piperita*	Peppermint	x		x	x		x	
Myristica fragrans (sem.)	Nutmeg	x			x			
Nepeta cataria	Catnep							G
Ocimum basilicum var. *album*	Basil	x			x		x	
Origanum majorana	Marjoram				x			
Pelargonium graveolens	Geranium			x			x	
Pimpinella anisum	Aniseed	x	x		x			
Pinus sylvestris	Scots pine							G
Piper nigrum	Pepper						x	
Rosmarinus officinalis	Rosemary				x	x	x	G
Salvia officinalis	Sage		x	?		x		
Santalum album	Sandalwood			x				
Satureia montana, S. hortensis	Winter and summer savory	x			x	x		
Syzygium aromaticum (flos)	Clove bud	x						
Thymus serpyllum	Wild thyme							
Thymus vulgaris 'Population'	Thyme				x			
Zinziber officinale	Ginger				x			

	Indications										
Pancreatic stimulant	Colic	Colitis, gastroenteritis	Constipation	Diarrhoea	Digestion painful	Digestive stimulant	Diverticulitis	Enteritis, gastritis	Indigestion	Nausea	Ulcers (gastric and duodenal)
						X					
	X								X		
	X								X		
		X		X					X		
X											
									X		
	X		X						X		
	X					X			X		
X	X			X	X	X			X	X	
			X						X		
							X				
		X				X					
				X							
						X					
		X				X			X		
	X					X			X		
X	X	X					X				
						X	X			X	X
			X								
		X		X			X	X			X
	X						X		X	X	
			X						X	X	X
	X	X		X	X	X	X		X	X	
						X					
	X		X			X			X		
	X	X	?	X		X		X	X		X
X		X		X			X				
	X					X	X		X		
			X			X					
	X		X	X	X	X		X	X		
	X					X			X		
		X									
	X		X	X	X	X					
	X										
						X					
	?		X	X	X	X				X	

95

Case 4.7

Digestive (flatulence – twin babies)

L. Cantele – Nurse aromatherapist

Client assessment

The clients, 5-week-old twin babies, were suffering from severe flatulence and constipation. They were in pain and constantly crying. Neither of the children was sleeping well due to the stomach pain and inconsolable crying fits.

Intervention

The following massage oil was prepared for the mother to use at home every evening:

- 5 drops *Rosmarinus officinalis* [rosemary] – analgesic, digestive (sluggish and painful digestion)
- 3 drops *Chamaemelum nobilis* [Roman chamomile] – calming, digestive
- 4 drops *Origanum majorana* [sweet marjoram] – analgesic, digestive (flatulence)
- 50 mL sweet almond oil

After a treatment by the therapist, the mother was shown how to give her babies a simple abdominal massage herself. She was also asked to apply a little of the blend to the soles of the babies' feet.

Outcome

After 2 days, the mother called to say that the results were so encouraging after the initial treatment and her massage the following night that she was going to continue over the next few days.

After a week, the babies were sleeping better – they were no longer waking up during the night with flatulence and pain.

The babies are now 7 months old. From time to time they become constipated, but the mother simply applies the essential oil mix twice during the day – abdomen and feet – and before they go to bed, which solves the problem straightaway.

of bile secreted (Valnet 1980 p. 177); it is given as a carminative and cholagogue (Lautié & Passebecq 1984 p. 74) and to stimulate hepatobiliary secretions (Duraffourd 1982 p. 107).

Citrus oils generally have a favourable effect on the digestive system, being mildly appetite stimulating and digestive. *Citrus aurantium* var. *amara* (per.) is given as a treatment for constipation as it encourages intestinal peristalsis and also acts as a cholagogue (Duraffourd 1982 p. 95); this oil is also mentioned for dyspepsia, flatulence and gastric spasm (Franchomme & Pénoël 2001 p. 365).

A significant reduction in irritable bowel symptoms was noted in tests using Mintoil enteric-coated capsules (containing peppermint oil) against placebo,

showing a reduction of >50% in bloating, discomfort, diarrhoea, passage of gas and incomplete or urgent defecation (Cappello et al. 2007). Pittler and Ernst (1998) reviewed five double-blind placebo-controlled trials and found that there was a significant difference between peppermint oil and placebo in three cases but not in the other two. They concluded that peppermint had a beneficial role in treatment, but that its role was not established.

Diuretic

Juniperus communis fruct. [juniper berry] is associated with the kidneys. At normal dosage it is a beneficial stimulant, although it has a toxic effect on inflamed kidneys. It has a diuretic effect (Duraffourd 1982, p. 67, Franchomme & Pénoël 2001 p. 389, Lautié & Passebecq 1984 p. 51, Viaud 1983, Gattefossé 1937 p. 71) although this is denied

Case 4.8

Diuretic (water retention)

S. Price – Aromatologist

Client assessment

Mrs L was suffering from oedema in her legs and ankles, which had been controlled by diuretic tablets from her doctor. She had come off these of her own accord, as she was unable to support the frequency of toilet visits they caused – at most awkward moments.

She had heard of aromatherapy and asked if anything could help her swollen legs. As she said she had stopped taking her diuretic tablets, it was ethically possible to treat her with essential oils.

Intervention

The essential oils chosen for Mrs L were those with diuretic properties: *Citrus limon* [lemon], *Cupressus sempervirens* [cypress], *Foeniculum vulgare* [fennel] and *Juniperus communis* [juniper].

10 drops of each were put into 50 mL grapeseed oil and Mrs L was shown how to apply it firmly in an upward direction only. This she had to do every night, and report back in 2–3 weeks.

Outcome

When Mrs L returned, she was delighted with the reduction of swelling in her legs, with no over-frequent visits to the toilet. A few days earlier she had paid her regular visit to the doctor, who had looked at her legs and said 'Ah, Mrs L, I see you have gone back onto your tablets!', whereupon she explained that that was not the case – and that she had visited an aromatherapist. 'H'm!' was the reply!

by Schilcher (1985 p. 226). Terpene-free oil containing mainly terpinen-4-ol has marked diuretic effects (Schneider 1975); the level of this alcohol may be only 2–5% in juniper oils (which consist of more than 90% hydrocarbon monoterpenes).

Cicatrizant, granulation promoting

Lavandula angustifolia [lavender] oil is well known for its healing property, yielding positive and rapid results on minor burns (Gattefossé 1937). Hypericum and chamomile oils have been used traditionally for wound healing, and in the case of chamomile the validity of this has been borne out (Glowania, Raulin & Swoboda 1987, Thiemer, Stadler & Isaac 1973). St John's wort (*Hypericum perforatum*) flowers are macerated in a fixed oil (usually olive or sunflower), producing a red oil containing the essential oil and hypericin, which was much used in the past for the external treatment of wounds and burns (Weiss 1988 p. 296); the editors have found that *Pelargonium graveolens* [geranium] together with *Lavandula angustifolia* [lavender] and *Boswellia carteri* [frankincense] is effective.

Hormone-like activity

Some essential oils seem to normalize hormonal secretions and it is thought that this action may be either direct or effected via the hypophysis (Franchomme & Pénoël 2001). No work has so far been done to establish how the oil molecules could do this, but treatment is easy and pleasant for the client with no unwanted side effects. The hormone-like action of some plant extracts has been widely noted. Extracts of fennel seed have a slight oestrogenic effect in animal experimental models (Foster 1993) and fennel has been used for thousands of years as a menstrual cycle regulator and for premenstrual syndrome (Stewart 2005 p. 411); fennel oil promotes milk in nursing mothers. Bernadet (1983) and others advise the use of essential oils for such disorders as dysmenorrhoea and amenorrhoea.

There are compounds in some volatile oils that have a structural similarity to natural human hormones, and these promote efficient endocrine gland activity by natural means. Sclareol (Fig. 2.7), viridiflorol (Fig. 2.6A) and *trans*-anethole (Fig. 4.1A) are examples of compounds that have structures similar to folliculin or analogous to oestrogen. The sclareol

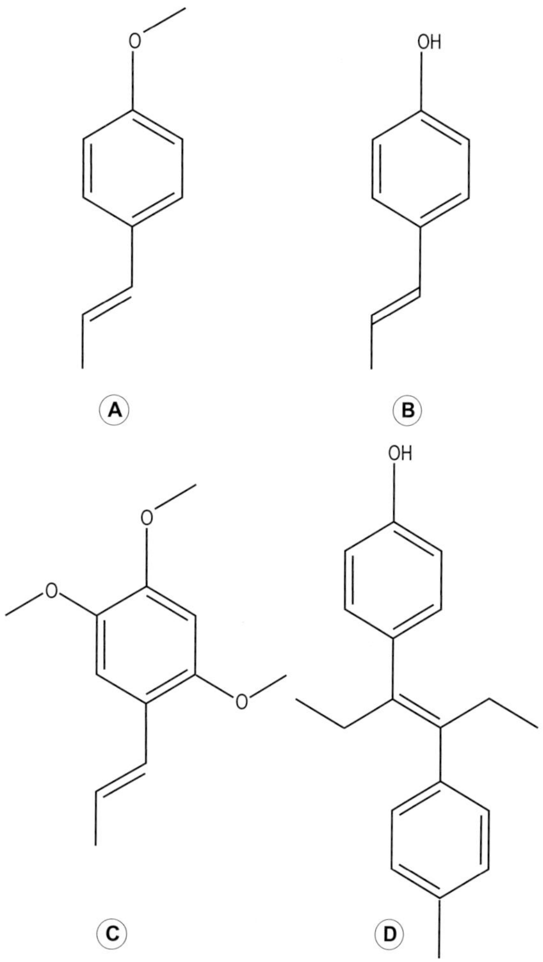

Figure 4.1 • (A) *trans*-Anethole; (B) *p*-anol; (C) β-asarone; (D) diethyl stilbestrol.

containing *Salvia sclarea* [clary] oil is useful for PMS and menopausal symptoms. Other compounds, found in *Pinus sylvestris* [pine needle], are similar to cortisone (Franchomme & Pénoël 2001 p. 417). The essential oil of *Vitex agnuscastus* balances progesterone levels and moderates excess oestrogen by direct action on the pituitary (Lucks 2003 p. 15), and cypress contains a chemical structure which is a homologue of the ovarian hormone (Valnet 1980 p. 71).

The essential oils of pine (needles), borneol, geranium, basil, sage, savory and rosemary are said to stimulate the cortex of the suprarenal gland, and anise excites the anterior pituitary body, as does mint (Valnet 1980 p. 70). Monoterpenes, in particular α-pinene and β-pinene and δ3-carene, which are found in many essential oils, mimic the action of cortisone in so far as they have a modulating effect on the activity of the adrenal cortex. They cause release of the adrenocortical hormone cortisol, which additionally alleviates pain, inflammation and, to some extent, allergic reactions (von Braunschweig 1999 p. 17).

The following plant volatile molecules are said to be hormone-like: anethole (*para*-anol methyl ether), citral, eugenol, carvacrol, thymol, gingerol, lachnophyllum methyl ester, matricaria methyl ester, viridiflorol and sclareol.

Anethole, *p*-anol methyl ether

This molecule (Fig. 4.1A) is generally believed to have oestrogen-like properties, being emmenagogic and lactogenic; it is found in *Foeniculum vulgare* var. *dulce* [fennel] oil 52–86%. Anethole, fennel oil and aniseed oil have been shown to have oestrogenic activity in rats (Zondec et al. 1938). The structure of the molecule has a similarity to a derivative of stilben, viz. diethyl stilbestrol (Fig. 4.1C), to which its mode of action may be compared. Essential oils containing this molecule, e.g. *Pimpinella anisum* [aniseed], may be used in the menstrual cycle before ovulation (Franchomme & Pénoël 2001 p. 189, 193). *trans*-Anethole has weak oestrogen-like properties (Zondec et al. 1938). Albert-Puleo (1980 2:337) suggests that polymers of anethole such as dianethole and photoanethole are active oestrogenic compounds. NB: Essential oils rich in anethole are to be used orally with caution in people with oestrogen-dependent cancers, in endometriosis, pregnancy and breastfeeding (Tisserand & Balacs 1995 p. 75).

> Anethole has structural similarity to the catecholamines adrenaline, noradrenaline and dopamine: this may account for some of the sympathomimetic effects of fennel and anise (which also contain large quantities of anethole) such as ephedrine like bronchodilator action and amphetamine like facilitation of weight loss. The traditional lactogenic effect may be due to competitive inhibition of dopamine inhibition of prolactin secretion as much as to any direct hormonal activity. The relationship of anethole to psychoactive chemicals like mescaline, asarone and myristicin from nutmeg has been noted and may account for a psychoactive and aphrodisiac tradition for fennel and anise.
>
> Mills (1991 p. 425)

Some plant materials have long been regarded as psychotropic agents, and this property may arise from myristicin and elemicin compounds: these have a structural similarity to amphetamines, which exert hallucinogenic effects (Fig. 4.2). Apiole, found in

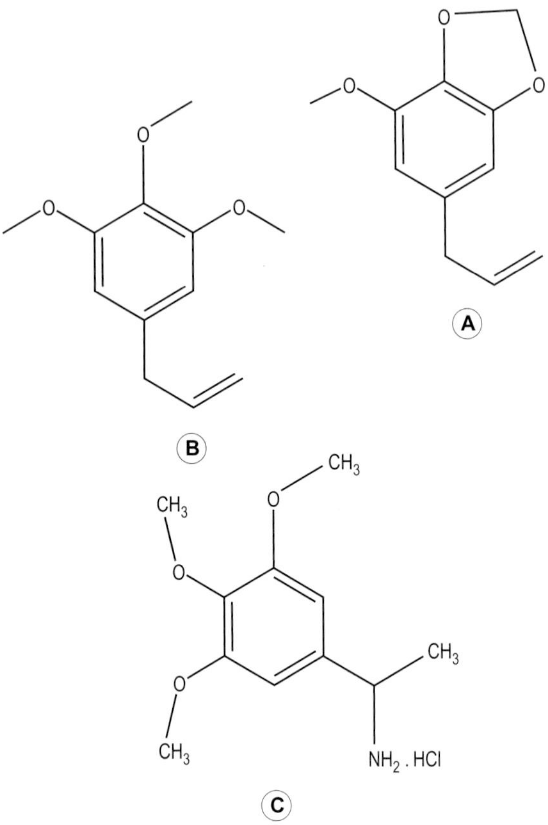

Figure 4.2 • (A) Myristicin; (B) elemicin; (C) amphetamine corresponding to elemicin.

parsley, and dillapiole also bear a relationship to these compounds (Trease & Evans 1983 p. 691).

Citral (Figs 2.11A, 2.11C)

This molecule was shown to have an oestrogenic effect, causing prostatic hyperplasia in rats (Abramovici et al. 1985, Geldof et al. 1992). Tisserand and Balacs (1995 p. 146), referring to *Cymbopogon flexuosus* [lemongrass], say that a mild hormone-like (oestrogenic) action may be assumed from the citral content, but that as used in aromatherapy it is not known whether the effect will be oestrogenic or androgenic.

Eugenol, carvacrol (Fig. 2.9C), thymol (Fig. 2.8B), gingerol

Hormones play a part in the mechanisms of prostaglandins and these molecules, found in the essential oils of *Syzygium aromaticum*, *Thymus vulgaris* and *Zingiber officinale*, have an influence on prostaglandin E (Bennett & Stamford 1988, Wagner et al. 1986).

Lachnophyllum methyl ester, matricaria methyl ester

Esters as a rule are not hormone like, but these two esters are exceptions: and are used in the treatment of delayed puberty (Franchomme & Pénoël 2001 p. 207). Cis- and trans- forms of *Lachnophyllum* methyl ester occur at 40–60% in the essential oil of *Coniza bonariensis* (Asteraceae); this essential oil has no known contraindications.

Viridiflorol (Fig. 2.6A)

This is a sesquiterpenol that occurs up to 15% in the essential oil of *Melaleuca quinquenervia* [niaouli] and has an oestrogen-like influence in ovaries and testicles (Franchomme & Pénoël 2001 p. 398).

Sclareol (Fig. 2.7)

This is a diol that occurs up to 7% in the essential oil of *Salvia sclarea* [clary] (Lamiaceae) and has a similarity to the oestrogens; allegedly aphrodisiac according to Franchomme & Pénoël (2001 p. 424).

Essential oils affecting the thyroid gland

Allium sativum [garlic] – thyroid stimulant (Franchomme & Pénoël 2001 p. 349).
Onion (*N*-propyl disulphide) and garlic (methyl disulphide, allyl disulphide) – inhibit iodine metabolism in rats (Cowan et al. 1967, Salji et al. 1971).
Daucus carota [carrot seed] – helps the pituitary gland to regulate the production of thyroxin.
Commiphora myrrha [myrrh] – balances the production of thyroxin. Rose (1992 p. 118) advises that myrrh be used in inhalation in the early morning to stimulate and regulate the thyroid.
Pinus sylvestris [pine] – thyroid stimulant.
Cymbopogon martinii [palmarosa] – considered to have a normalizing effect on the thyroid gland (Rose 1992 p. 122).
Picea mariana [black spruce] – said to be cortisone like and useful in cases of hyperthyroidism.
Sassafras albidum [sassafras] – oral administration of safrole or sassafras oil in rats

Case 4.9

Hormonal (PMS)

C. O'Malley – Aromatherapist

Assessment

Kay worked in an office with several other girls – and the therapist. She was a chatty, happy person, well liked. However, when her period was due she became a different person – snapping people's heads off and generally reacting with bad temper at the slightest challenge. She realized after a while that her behaviour was affecting the others in the office. The therapist suggested she try aromatherapy and Kay accepted.

Intervention

The essential oils chosen were those which are hormone-like, alleviating PMS:

- 2 drops *Chamomilla recutita* [German chamomile]
- 5 drops *Pimpinella anisum* [aniseed]
- 8 drops *Salvia sclarea* [clary]
- A few drops of *Lavandula angustifolia* were added – to her liking, as she was not too keen on the aroma without it
- 30 mL grapeseed carrier oil

Kay was asked to apply this blend to her abdomen every night and morning immediately after she finished menstruating each month, until the next period commenced.

She was also given a pure blend of the oils (in the same proportions) to use in the bath which she took twice a week.

Outcome

After the first month, the girls felt that Kay was marginally easier to live with.

By the second month there was a noticeable difference, and by the third month Kay herself felt much more relaxed and able to cope. She continued the two treatments for 6 months, then decided she was so much better – and happier – that she would stop the night and morning applications.

The therapist suggested she stop only the morning application first, continuing to apply it at night for 2 months, before stopping altogether. This she did, but never gave up the bath blend, as she loved the aroma while bathing. Kay was with the firm for a further 3 years before getting married and moving away, and in all that time she was her original happy and efficient self – her PMS was non-existent.

gives rise to cellular changes in the adrenal, pituitary and thyroid glands; also in the testes or ovaries (Abbot et al. 1961).

Not referenced: many essential oils are said to have a tendency to normalize hormonal secretions by encouraging the endocrine glands naturally to work more efficiently. The author's searches found these mentioned – artemisia, basil, cinnamon, clary sage, cumin, cypress, lavender, melissa, myrtle, peppermint, pine, thyme, valerian. Both *Pimenta dioica* [allspice] and eugenol are said to enhance trypsin activity and have larvicidal properties (Harkiss personal communication) (Table 4.7).

Hyperaemic

Essential oils promote local peripheral circulation owing to a primary irritation of the skin, and the effects of this are twofold:

- The freeing of mediators (e.g. bradykinin) which cause vasodilatation.
- Humoral reactions resulting in the anti-inflammatory effect.

On the skin there is a sensation of warmth, comfort and pain relief following the use of rubefacients such as *Eucalyptus globulus* [Tasmanian blue gum], *Rosmarinus officinalis* [rosemary] and *Juniperus communis* ram. [juniper twig], which cause increased local blood circulation. Local skin irritation may also have some effect on internal organs (e.g. cardiac ointment used in angina). Some essential oils are vesicants, e.g. *Brassica nigra* [mustard] and *Armoracia lapathifolia* [horseradish] as the principal constituent is allylisothiocyanate. Croton oil also is a vesicant, and its use is proscribed by the Medicines Act 1968.

Immunostimulant

Melaleuca viridiflora has been reported to have an immunostimulant effect by increasing the level of immunoglobulins (Pénoël 1981), and other oils have been mentioned by various writers as strengthening the immune system, but with no common agreement. This may be so because many oils possess a range of properties (antifungal, antiseptic, antiviral, etc.) which are beneficial to the immune system (see Appendix B.9 on the CD-ROM for a list of effective oils.)

Case 4.10

Immunostimulant (headaches and insomnia)

Muriel Raynes – Aromatherapist

Client assessment

Norman (mid-60s) was referred for aromatherapy by his doctor as he wasn't sleeping and suffered from severe headaches, both thought to be a result of full-time caring for his wife, who had Parkinson's disease.

The doctor felt that his immune system was low and that aromatherapy would help relieve his stress and headaches, possibly enabling a sounder sleep. Norman was physically and mentally tired, saying his head 'felt solid'. Emotionally he was low – and tearful as he expressed his frustration at his condition. His arms and legs had patches of psoriasis and he complained of coldness and aching in his knees.

Intervention

The main aim was to ease anxiety and depression, promote sleep and relieve his headaches.

Norman was given six massage sessions over 2 weeks, with emphasis on his shoulders, which ached. The carriers and essential oils chosen were:

- 10 mL grapeseed oil

- 2 drops *Boswellia carteri* [frankincense] – analgesic, antidepressant, energizing, immunostimulant
- 2 drops *Lavandula angustifolia* – analgesic, balancing, calming (aids insomnia), tonic
- 1 drop *Origanum majorana* (sweet marjoram) – analgesic, calming (aids insomnia), neurotonic

For use in between treatments, Norman was given a 50 mL lotion containing five drops of frankincense and two drops each of lavender and *Marjoram nobile* [Roman chamomile] – anti-inflammatory, calming and sedative, stimulant. This was to be applied twice daily to his shoulders.

Outcome

After the first session Norman was more relaxed. He appreciated the treatments, which he said made him feel less stressed.

By the third treatment his shoulders were much less tense and he said he felt more able to cope.

After his last session the headaches had ceased and he felt less tense in his shoulders. Emotionally, he was better able to relax at home and felt more positive about the future.

Insecticidal and repellent

Plant volatile oils may be used over a long period without promoting resistance – some plants use essential oils to repel attacking insects, and they are still effective after thousands of years. Citronella is universally used as an insect repellent, and tests show other oils to have this property too, e.g. *Ocimum basilicum* [sweet basil] (Dube, Upadhyay & Tripath 1989). Of a number of essential oils and some of their components investigated for insecticidal activity, only a few demonstrated this attribute: *Cinnamomum camphora* [camphor], *C. verum* [cinnamon], *Cymbopogon nardus* [citronella], *Syzygium aromaticum* flos [clove bud] and eucalyptus oils, plus two aldehydes and a ketone (cinnamal, citral and carvone) (Gildemeister & Hoffmann 1956). The editors' experience indicates that *Thymus vulgaris* ct. thymol [thyme] and *Melaleuca alternifolia* [tea tree] are effective parasiticides (head and pubic lice), and tests in which the editors were involved tend to confirm this. *Mentha arvensis* [cornmint] is effective as a house fly repellent (Table 4.8 and Appendix A on the CD-ROM).

Mucolytic and expectorant

Accumulated secretions in the mucous linings can hold germs and it is necessary to break down the mucus in order to kill them. Many oils are mucolytic thanks to their content of powerful ketones (carvone, menthone, thujone, pinocamphone etc.) and in some cases lactones. The expectorant effect is due to the breaking down of secretions and to cilial activity; several oils have in the past been tested to determine expectorant properties (Boyd & Pearson 1946, Gordonoff 1938, Schilcher 1985 p. 223). Besides *Eucalyptus globulus* and other essential oils containing the oxide 1,8-cineole, *Pimpinella anisum*, *Foeniculum vulgare* var. *dulce*, *Pinus sylvestris* and *P. mugo* var. *pumilio*, *Thymus vulgaris* ct. phenol and *T. serpyllum* are also expectorants. These oils, whether used by external application or by inhalation, reach the bronchi and are eliminated from the lungs in the exhaled air. Russian research endorsed this property of some essential oils when inhaled (Eremenko et al. 1987): all 96 patients suffering from chronic bronchitis showed a significant increase in the permeability of the respiratory tracts and clearing of the airway as well as a decrease in immunoglobulin E, indicating reduced infection levels. The study shows that the vapour of some essential oils (camphor, eucalyptus, peppermint and menthol) can improve the function of the lungs and bronchials, relieve mucous congestion, chest infections, colds and influenza. Kehrl et al. (2004) used 1,8-cineole on 152 patients with acute rhinosinusitis and concluded that this compound was a safe and effective treatment for acute non-purulent rhinosinusitis before antibiotics are indicated.

 Case 4.11

Mucolytic and expectorant (Bronchial inflammation)

Client assessment

Tim had suffered with bronchial inflammation and accumulation of mucus in his lungs for 5 years, since undergoing treatment for cancer in the throat/pharyngeal area and radiotherapy to the thorax. The resultant scarring and fibrosis reduced his lung capacity. His dependency on antibiotics increased as chest infections increased also. He was experiencing difficulty in expectorating accumulated mucus, which was usually dark brown, thick and tenacious. In addition, he was often very tired.

An intensive application of the following essential oils was used:

- 25 mL *Eucalyptus smithii*
- 10 mL *Abies balsama* [Canadian balsam]
- 5 mL *Eucalyptus radiata*
- 5 mL *Lavandula spica* [spike lavender]
- 5 mL *Melaleuca alternifolia* [tea tree]
- 5 mL *Cymbopogon citratus* [lemongrass]
- 5 mL *Thymus vulgaris* ct. geraniol [sweet thyme]

4 mL of the blend was applied twice a day to the soles of his feet, having first warmed them with a heater

Outcome

Within 10 minutes of applying the blend some sputum was expectorated, with very little effort or coughing, continuing to be produced for about an hour. Almost at the same time his nose began to run, accompanied by short bursts of sneezing. Within 1 week the mucus was coming up more easily, was a lighter colour and less thick.

After 3 weeks the sputum was whitish-clear and Tim was not coughing at all during the night. He felt brighter, more alert and relaxed.

Table 4.7   The influence of essential oils on the hormonal system

Latin name	Common name	Adrenal (cortex)	Adrenal (medulla)	Amenorrhoea	Antidiabetic	Choleretic cholagogic	Cortisone-like	Dysmenorrhoea	Emmenagogic	Hypophys/gonads	Hypophysis
Achillea millefolium	Yarrow			X		X		X			
Aloysia triphylla	Verbena				X						
Anethum graveolens	Dill seed					X					
Angelica archangelica (rad.)	Angelica root								X		
Cananga odorata	Ylang ylang				X						
Carum carvi	Caraway								X		
Chamaemelum nobile	Roman chamomile			X				X	X		
Cinnamomum verum (cort.)	Cinnamon bark								X		
Citrus aurantium var. amara (per.)	Orange bitter						X				X
Citrus limon (per.)	Lemon										X
Commiphora myrrha	Myrrh								?		
Cupressus sempervirens (fol. strob.)	Cypress										
Cymbopogon citratus C. flexuosus	Lemongrass										
Foeniculum vulgare var. dulce (fruct.)	Fennel			X				X	X		
Hyssopus officinalis	Hyssop							X	X		
Illicium verum	Star anise										
Laurus nobilis	Bay leaf								X		
Lavandula angustifolia	Lavender								X		
Matricaria recutita	German chamomile			X							
Melaleuca leucadendron	Cajuput								?		
Melaleuca viridiflora	Niaouli			X				X	X	X	
Melissa officinalis	Lemon balm					XX					
Mentha × piperita	Peppermint							X			
Mentha spicata	Spearmint					X					
Myristica fragrans	Nutmeg								X		
Myrtus communis	Myrtle			X				X			
Nardostachys jatamansi	Spikenard										
Origanum majorana	Sweet marjoram										
Pelargonium graveolens P. × asperum	Geranium				X						
Picea mariana	Black spruce						X				
Pimenta racemosa	West Indian bay							X	X		
Pimpinella anisum	Aniseed			X					X		
Pinus sylvestris	Pine	X						X		X	
Piper nigrum	Black pepper										
Rosa centifolia, R. damascena	Rose otto								?		
Rosmarinus officinalis	Rosemary	X		X	X				X		
Rosmarinus officinalis ct. verbenone	Rosemary verbenone										
Salvia officinalis	Sage		X	X	X			X	X		
Salvia sclarea	Clary			XX				X	?		
Santalum album	Sandalwood										
Syzygium aromaticum (flos)	Clove bud										
Tagetes patula, T. glandulifera	French marigold			X					X		
Thymus vulgaris ct. linaloot	Sweet thyme										
Thymus vulgaris ct. thujanol	Thyme					X					
Thymus vulgaris ct. thymol	Thyme	X									
Vetiveria zizanioides	Vetiver			X					X		
Zingiber officinale	Ginger										

Hypothalamus	Impotence/frigidity	Lactogenic	Menopause	Oestrogen-like	Oligomenorrhoea	Ovaries	Pancreas (diabetes)	Pituitary (anterior)	Pituitary (posterior)	PMS	Sex hormones (testes)	Thymus	Thyroid	Thyroid	Uterotonic (facilitates delivery)
					X										
								X							
			X												
					X										
X								X							
X							X		X						
													X		
						X									
												X			
		X	X	X	X	X				X					X
					X										
			X	X	X										
					X										
					X										
										X					
				X		X									
						X									X
	X					X									X
													X		
						X									
														X	
							X							X	
		X	X	X	X						X				X
	X					X						X	X		
X															
X					X										
X				X		X						X			
			X	X	X									X	
			X	X	X										
X												X			
X													X		X
															X
				X		X									
	X														

Table 4.8 Insecticidal, larvicidal and repellent properties of essential oils

Latin name	Common name	Clothes moths	Fleas	Cockroaches	Gnats	Houseflies	Insects (unspecified)	Lice	Mosquitoes (unspecified)	Mosquito larvae	Aedes aegypti	Allocophora foveicollis	Anopheles funestus	Anopheles gambiae	Anopheles stephensi	Culex quinquefasciatus	Culicoides variipennis	Dermatophagoides pteronyssinus (house dust mites)	Pediculosus capitis (head louse)	Pediculosus pubis (pubic louse)
Acorus calamus (rad.)	Calamus					RS	S													
Cymbopogon nardus	Citronella				R				R											
Eucalyptus globulus	Tasmanian blue gum								R											
Laurus nobilis	Bay leaf			R																
Melaleuca alternifolia	Tea tree																			I
Melaleuca leucadendron	Cajuput		R					R										I		
Mentha arvensis	Cornmint																			
Myrtus communis	Myrtle					R		R											IL	
Mentha × piperita	Peppermint		R		R	RI	RI		RI	L										
Ocimum basilicum	Sweet basil					RI	RI	I	RI		I									
Pelargonium graveolens	Geranium				R		I		R			R		I		I				
Syzygium aromaticum (flos)	Clove bud	R					I		R											
Thymus vulgaris (population)	Thyme						I	I	L											
	I = insecticidal																			
	L = larvicidal																			
	R = repellent																			
	S = renders sterile																			
Compound																				
	Carvone (unspecified)																			
	Cinnamal																			
	Citral															R				
found in eucalyptus oil	p-Menthane-3, 8-diol											R	R							
	p-Menthane-3, 8-diol + Isopulegol + Citronellol											R	R			R				
found in Tagetes patula	(Z, E)-Ocimenone									L										
	I = insecticidal																			
	R = repellent																			
	L = larvicidal																			
	S = makes sterile																			

Compiled from information in Appendix A (see CD-ROMq.v.)

Sedative

In the past there has been little apart from anecdotal evidence for the sedative properties of essential oils, but now several oils have been investigated and found to be effective. They include *Melissa officinalis*, which is calming to the central nervous system because of its citronellal and other monoterpene content (Becker & Förster 1984, Mills 1991), and the valerian oils, which contain small amounts of valepotriates (Becker 1983, Becker & Reichling 1981, Boeters 1969, Schmiedeberg 1913). *Valeriana officinalis* contains only about 1.5% of these, but this figure can rise to

12% in other species. Recently other tests have been carried out which prove for the first time the sedative, calming effects of other oils, such as *Citrus aurantium* var. *amara* (flos) [neroli] and *Passiflora incarnata* [passion flower] (Buchbauer 1993, Buchbauer, Jirovetz & Jäger 1992, Buchbauer et al. 1993) (Table 4.9). The aromatic water collected during the distillation of orange flowers also has sedative properties, and more effective still is the essential oil of C. *aurantium* var. *amara* (fol.) [petitgrain] (Duraffourd 1982 p. 97). Lavender is recognized as a calming oil (Guillemain, Rousseau & Delaveau 1989) and is now used in many hospital wards to aid sleep. It is thought that the

Table 4.9   Effects of fragrance compounds and essentials oils on the motility of mice after a 1-hour inhalation period

Compound	Effect on motility %[a]	Effect on motility after caffeine %[b]
Anethole	−10.81	−1.26
Anthranilic acid methyl ester	+17.70	+38.22
Balm leaves oil (Austria)	−5.21	+16.29
Benzaldehyde	−43.69	−34.28
Benzyl alcohol	−11.21	−23.68
Borneol	−3.05	−1.88
Bornyl acetate	−7.79	+2.27
Bornyl salicylate	−17.29	−2.99
Carvone	−2.46	−47.51
Citral	−1.43	+17.24
Citronellal	−49.82	−37.40
Citronellol	−3.56	−13.71
Coumarin	−15.00	−13.75
Dimethyl vinyl carbinol	+5.36	−2.11
Ethylmaltol	+9.73	+2.09
Eugenol	+2.10	−38.73
Farnesol	+5.76	+36.34
Farnesyl acetate	+4.62	−30.71
Furfural	+3.04	−4.51
Geraniol	+20.56	+1.20
Geranyl acetate	−29.18	−7.46

Continued

Table 4.9 Effects of fragrance compounds and essentials oils on the motility of mice after a 1-hour inhalation period—cont'd

Compound	Effect on motility %[a]	Effect on motility after caffeine %[b]
Isoborneol	+46.90	−11.23
Isobornyl acetate	+3.16	−22.35
Isoeugenol	+30.05	−74.34
β-Ionone	+14.20	−27.97
Lavender oil (Mont Blanc)	−78.40	−91.67
Lime blossom oil (France)	−34.34	+30.41
Linalool	−73.00	−56.67
Linalyl acetate	−69.10	−46.67
Maltol	+13.74	−50.04
Methyl salicylate	+16.64	−49.88
Nerol	+12.93	+29.31
Nerol oil	−65.27	+1.87
Orange flower oil (Spain)	−4.64	−14.62
Orange terpenes	+35.25	−33.19
Passion flower oil (USA)	+8.15	−27.93
2-phenyl ethanol	+2.67	−30.61
2-phenyllethyl acetate	−45.04	+12.42
α-Pinene	+13.77	+4.73
Rose oil (Bulgaria)	−9.50	+4.31
Sandalwood oil (East India)	−40.00	−20.70
α-Terpineol	−45.00	−12.50
Thymol	+33.02	+19.05
Valerian root oil (China)	−2.70	−12.01

[a]motility of untreated control animals = 100%
[b]motility of control animals after pretreatment with 0.1% caffeine solution (0.5 mL, ip) = 100%
(from Buchbauer et al. 1993 p. 661)

sedative effect of *Lavandula angustifolia* is due in part to the presence of coumarins in the oil, even though the content is low at 0.25%. *Cymbopogon citratus* essential oil was shown in rats to have a marked depressive effect on the central nervous system, producing an effect comparable to that of chlorpromazine hydrochloride (Seth, Kokate & Varma 1976).

Spasmolytic

Some essential oils have been found to relieve smooth muscle spasm (Debelmas & Rochat 1964, 1967a,b, Taddei et al. 1988), hence their usefulness for some problems of the digestive tract. The oils with this property are chamomile oils containing (−)-α-bisabolol

Case 4.12

Spasmolytic (Chronic leg cramp)

S. Price – Aromatologist

Client assessment

Mrs P had suffered with cramp in her calves and feet for several years, occurring most of the time during the night. Her doctor had not taken much interest, telling her to rub them when it occurred and this would ease it. Having heard of aromatherapy, she decided to see whether it could help her.

Intervention

Mrs P was asked first if she would be prepared to apply an oil blend to her legs every night before retiring. Having been assured that Mrs P would do anything to help, the therapist made up the following prescription:

- 16 drops *Ocimum basilicum* [European basil] – analgesic, antispasmodic
- 16 drops *Origanum majorana* [sweet marjoram] – analgesic, antispasmodic
- 100 mL grapeseed carrier oil

Mrs P was asked to telephone if there was no improvement after a week, and to make another appointment for a month's time.

Outcome

There was no phone call and Mrs P arrived after a month to say that she had had no cramp at all for a week. Because of this, the frequency of use of her essential oil mix was reduced to once every 2 nights, and an appointment made for another 4 weeks' time.

At her next appointment, Mrs P reported that she had still had no cramp at night, so her frequency of use was reduced to twice a week.

At the next visit, Mrs P reported having cramp during the last week, but she had forgotten to apply her oil the night before. This showed that twice a week was the minimum number of applications to achieve good results.

When Mrs P went to Australia to live with her daughter, she took with her a 5 L can of the blended oils – she didn't want to risk being without them!

(Achterrath-Tuckerman et al. 1980, Melegari et al. 1988), *Carum carvi, Cinnamomum verum* (cort.), *Citrus aurantium* var. *amara* (per.), *Foeniculum vulgare* var. *dulce, Melissa officinalis* and *Mentha x piperita* (Schilcher 1985 p. 225).

In successful practical experience essential oils have been used to ease spasm in skeletal muscle also. The editors have used *Ocimum basilicum* [sweet basil] and *Origanum majorana* [marjoram] successfully over the years, and a fuller list has been published (Price 2000 pp. 266–287). *Cupressus sempervirens* [cypress] is also credited with this property (Franchomme & Pénoël 2001 p. 373).

Molecular structure

A relationship between the molecular structure of the essential oil components and their therapeutic effect has been studied and published (Franchomme & Pénoël 2001). This is an interesting piece of work and, although not proven rigorously, is nevertheless very useful to therapists when studying and selecting oils; the principles involved are to be found in Price (2000 pp. 52–54). Balacs (1991) comments that it is based on the presence of key chemical groups in the oil molecules. If this approach is valid, it may well be that essential oil molecules are interacting with the same receptors on nerve cells and in other tissues which respond to drugs (see also Hormone-like, above).

Summary

The numerous therapeutic properties of essential oils have been examined and scientific confirmation of traditional wisdom given where possible. Financial backing is lacking for clinical trials on essential oil therapy unless they form part of a commercial formulation. Nevertheless, it is hoped that in the future more controlled trials will take place, and that the importance of the effects of a whole essential oil will be given precedence over the activity of isolated components.

References

Abbot, D.D., et al., 1961. Chronic oral toxicity of oil of sassafras and safrole. Pharmacologist 3 (73), 62.

Abramovici, A., et al., 1985. Benign hyperplasia of ventral prostate in rats induced by a monoterpene (preliminary report). Prostate 7, 389–394.

Achterrath-Tuckerman, U., Kunde, R., Flaskamp, O., Theimer, I., Theimer, K., 1980. Pharmacological investigations with compounds of chamomile. V. Investigations on the spasmolytic effect of compounds of chamomile. Planta Med. Stuttgart 39, 38–50.

Adams, J., 2003. The positive gains of integration: a qualitative study of GPs' perceptions of their complementary practice. Primary Health Care Research and Development 4 (2), 155–162. Cambridge University Press.

Albert-Puleo, M., 1980. Fennel and anise as oestrogenic agents. J. Ethnopharmacol. 2, 337–344.

Anderson, E., Anderson, P., 1987. General practitioners and alternative medicine. Journal of Royal College of General Practitioners 37 (295), 52–55.

Anderson, M., 1998. Sweet smell of success for Monklands hospital. Scottish Nurse 2 (8), 7.

Astin, J.A., et al., 1998. A review of the incorporation of complementary and alternative medicine by mainstream physicians. Arch. Intern. Med. 158, 2303–2310.

Balacs, T., 1991. Essential issues. Int. J. Aromather. 3 (4), 24.

Becker, H., 1983. Dtsch. Apoth. Ztg. 123, 2470.

Becker, H., Förster, W., 1984. Biologie, Chemie und Pharmakologie pflanzlicher Sedativa. Zeitschrift Phytotherapie Stuttgart 5, 817–823.

Becker, H., Reichling, J., 1981. Dtsch. Apoth. Ztg. 121, 1185.

Belaiche, P., 1979. Traité de phytothérapie et d'aromathérapie. vol. 3. Maloine, Paris.

Belaiche, P., 1985. L'huile essentielle de Melaleuca alternifolia (Cheel) dans les infections vaginales à Candida albicans. Phytothérapie 15 (September), 13–14.

Bennett, A., Stamford, F., 1988. The biological activity of eugenol, a major constituent of nutmeg, on prostaglandins, the intestine and other tissues. Phytother. Res. 2, 124–129.

Berman, B.M., Singh, B.K., Lao, L., Singh, B.B., Ferentz, K.S., Hartnol, S. M., 1995. Physicians' attitudes towards complementary or alternative medicine: a regional survey. J. Am. Board Fam. Pract. 8 (5), 361–366.

Bernadet, M., 1983. La phyto-aromathérapie pratique. Dangles, St-Jean-de-Braye.

Boeters, M., 1969. Behandlung vegetativer Regulationsstörungen mit Valepotriaten (Valmane). Münchner Medizin Wochenschrift 11, 1873–1876.

Borkan, J., Neher, J.O., Anson, O., Smoker, B., 1994. Referrals for alternative therapies. Journal of Family Practitioners 39 (6), 545–550.

Bowker (undated). Food additives and the patients they affect. CBA and Associates Ltd, London (leaflet).

Boyd, E.M., Pearson, G.L., 1946. The expectorant action of volatile oils. Am. J. Med. Sci. 211, 602–610.

Bruneton, J., 1995. Pharmacognosy, Phytochemistry, Medicinal Plants. Intercept, Hampshire.

Buchbauer, G., 1993. Biological effects of fragrances and essential oils. Perfumer & Flavorist 18 (January/February), 19–24.

Buchbauer, G., 2000. The detailed analysis of essential oils leads to the understanding of their properties. Perfumer & Flavorist 25, 64–67.

Buchbauer, G., Jirovetz, L., Jäger, W., 1992. Passiflora and lime blossoms: motility effects after inhalation of the essential oil and of some of the main constituents in animal experiment. Archiva Pharmaceutica (Weinheim) 325, 247–248.

Buchbauer, G., Jirovetz, L., Jäger, W., Plank, C., Dietrich, H., 1993. Fragrance compounds and essential oils with sedative effects upon inhalation. J. Pharm. Sci. 82 (6), 660–664.

Buckle, J., 1997. Clinical aromatherapy in nursing. Arnold, London, p. 125.

Cappello, G., Spezzaferro, M., Grossi, L., Manzoli, L., Marzio, L., 2007. Peppermint oil (Mintol®) in the treatment of irritable bowel syndrome: a prospective double blind placebo controlled randomized trial. Dig. Liver Dis. 39, 530–536.

Chabrol, E., Charonnat, R., Maximum, M., Busson, A., 1932. Le serpolet: cholagogue. Comptes Rendus Société Biologie 109, 275–276.

Chamberland, M., 1887. Les essences au point de vue de leurs propriétés antiseptiques. Annales Institut Pasteur 1, 153–154.

Cohen, R.A., Kucera, L.S., Herrman, E. C., 1964. Antiviral activity of Melissa officinalis extract. Proc. Soc. Exp. Biol. Med. 117, 431–434.

Cowan, J.W., et al., 1967. Antithyroid activity of onion volatiles. Aust. J. Biol. Sci. 20, 683–685.

Debelmas, A.M., Rochat, J., 1964. Etude comparée sur la fibre lisse des solutions aqueuses saturées d'essence de thym, de thymol et de carvacrol. Bulletin des Travaux. Société de Pharmacie de Lyon 4, 163–172.

Debelmas, A.M., Rochat, J., 1967a. Action des eaux saturées d'huiles essentielles sur la musculature lisse. 25th International Congress of Pharmaceutical Science. In: Butterworth, London, pp. 601–607.

Debelmas, A.M., Rochat, J., 1967b. Activité antispasmodique étudiée sur une cinquantaine d'échantillons différents. Plantes Médicinales et Phytothérapie 1, 23–27.

Decazes, J.-M., 1993. The masking effect of perfume ingredients. Symposium at Stoke-on-Trent: Fragrance – more than just a pleasant smell? Society of Cosmetic Chemists .

Dube, S., Upadhyay, P.D., Tripath, S.C., 1989. Antifungal, physiochemical, and insect-repelling activity of the essential oil of Ocimum basilicum. Can. J. Bot. 67 (7), 2085–2087.

Duraffourd, P., 1982. En forme tous les jours. In: La Vie Claire, Périgny, p. 107.

Duraffourd, P., 1987. Les huiles essentielles et la santé. La Maison du Bien-Etre, Montreuil-sous-Bois.

Eremenko, A.E., Nikolaevskii, V.V., Kostin, N.F., Meshkov, V.V., 1987. Letuchie fraktsii fitontsidov na osnove efirnykh masel v sostav lechebno-reabilitatsionnykh kompleksov pri khronicheskikh bronkhitakh. Volatile fractions of essential oil based phytoncides as a component of therapeutic-rehabilitative complexes in chronic bronchitis (in Russian). Tikhomirov AA Ter. Arkh. 59 (3), 126–130.

Ernst, E., Resch, K.L., White, A.R., 1995. Complementary medicine. What physicians think of it: a meta analysis. Arch. Intern. Med. 155 (22), 2405–2408.

Fisher, P., Ward, A., 1994. Complementary medicine in Europe. Br. Med. J. 309 (6947), 107–111.

Foster, S., 1993. Herbal renaissance. In: Gibbs Smith, Layton, Utah, p. 93.

Franchomme, P., Pénoël, D., 2001. L'aromathérapie exactement. Jollois, Limoges.

Franz, C., Novak, J., 2010. Sources of essential oils. In: Baser, K.H.C., Buchbauer, G. (Eds.), Handbook of essential oils: science, technology and application. CRC Press, Boca Raton, p. 73.

Ganzera, M., Schneider, P., Stuppner, H., 2006. Inhibitory effects of the essential oil of chamomile (*Matricaria recutita* L.) and its major constituents on human cytochrome P450 enzymes. Life Sci. 78 (8), 856–861.

Gattefossé, R.M., 1937. Aromatherapy (transl 1993). In: Daniel, Saffron Walden, p. 87.

Geldof, A.A., et al., 1992. Oestrogenic action of commonly used fragrance agent citral induces prostatic hyperplasia. Urol. Res. 20, 139–144.

Gershbein, L.E., 1977. Regeneration of rat liver in the presence of essential oils and their components. Food Cosmet. Toxicol. 15, 173–181.

Gildemeister, E., Hoffmann, F., 1956. Die ätherischen Öle. vol. 1. In: Akadamie Verlag, Berlin, p. 119.

Glowania, H.J., Raulin, C., Swoboda, M., 1987. Effect of chamomile on wound healing – a clinical double-blind study. Z. Hautkr. (Berlin) 62 (17), 1262, 1267–1271.

Goerg, K.J., Spilker, T., 1996. Simultane sonographische Messung der Magen und Gallenblasenentleerungmit gleichzeitiger Bestimmung der orozökalen Transizeit mittels H2-Atemtest. In: Low, D., Rietbrock, N. (Eds.), Phytopharmaka II. Forschung und klinische Anwendung. Steinkopff, Damstadt.

Goerg, K.J., Spilker, T., 2003. Effect of peppermint oil and caraway oil on gastrointestinal motility in healthy volunteers: a pharmacodynamic study using simultaneous determination of gastric and gall bladder emptying and orocaecal transit time. Aliment. Pharmacol. Ther. 17, 445–451.

Gordonoff, T., 1938. Ergebnisse der Physiologie, biologischen Chemie und experimentallen. Pharmakologie 40, 53.

Griggs, B., 1997. New green pharmacy. In: Vermilion, London, p. 293.

Guillemain, J., Rousseau, A., Delaveau, P., 1989. Neurodepressive effects of the essential oil of Lavandula angustifolia Mill. Ann. Pharm. Fr. 47 (6), 337–343.

Harris, B., 2010. Phytotherapeutic uses of essential oils. In: Başer, K.H.C., Buchbauer, G. (Eds.), Handbook of essential oils: science, technology and applications. CRC Press, Boca Raton.

Herrman Jr., E.C., Kucera, L.S., 1967. Antiviral substances in plants of the mint family (Labiatae). II. Nontannin polyphenol of *Melissa officinalis*. Proc. Soc. Exp. Biol. Med. 117, 369–374.

Imanishi, I., Watanabe, S., Satoh, M., Ozasa, K., 1999. Japanese doctors' attitudes to complementary medicine. Lancet 354 (9191), 1735–1736.

Jakovlev, V., Isaac, O., Flaskamp, E., 1983. Pharmacological investigations with compounds of chamomile. VI. Investigations on the antiphlogistic effects of chamazulene and matricin. Planta Med. 49, 67–73.

Janssen, A.M., Chin, N.L.J., Scheffer, J.J. C., Baerheim Svendsen, A., 1986. Screening for antimicrobial activity of some essential oils by the agar overlay techniques. Pharmazeutisch Weekblad (scientific edn) 8, 289–292.

Janssen, A.M., Scheffer, J.J.C., Baerheim Svendsen, A., Aynehchi, Y., 1984. Pharmazeutisch Weekblad (scientific edn) 6, 157.

Janssen, A.M., Scheffer, J.J., Baerheim Svendsen, A., 1987. Antimicrobial activity of essential oils: a 1976–1986 literature review. Aspects of the test methods. Planta Med. 53, 395–398.

Jori, A., Bianchetti, A., Prestini, P.E., 1969. Effect of essential oils on drug metabolism. Biochem. Pharmacol. 18, 2081–2085.

Kellner, W., Kober, W., 1954. Möglichkeiten der Wewendung ätherischer Öle zur Raumdesinfektion. I. Mitteilung: Die Wirkung gebrèuchlicher ätherischer Öle auf Testkeime. Arzneimittelforschung [Drug Research] 4 (5), 319.

Kellner, W., Kober, W., 1955. Möglichkeiten der Werwendung ätherischer Öle zur Raumdesinfektion. II. Arzneimittelforschung [Drug Research] 5 (4), 224.

Kellner, W., Kober, W., 1956. Möglichkeiten der Werwendung ètherischer Öle zur Raumdesinfektion. III. Arzneimittelforschung [Drug Research] 6 (12), 768.

Kehrl, W., Sonneman, U., Dethlefson, U., 2004. Therapy for acute nonpurulent rhinosinusitis with cineole: results of a double blind, randomised, placebo controlled trial. Laryngoscope 114, 738–742.

Kikuchi, A., Tsuchiya, T., Tanida, M., Uenoyama, S., Nakayama, Y., 1989. Stimulant like ingredients in absolute jasmine. Chem. Senses 14 (2), 304.

Kucera, L.S., Herrman Jr., J.C., 1967. Antiviral substances in plants in the mint family (Labiatae). 1. Tannin of Melissa officinalis. Proc. Soc. Exp. Biol. Med. 124, 865.

Lahlou, M., Berrada, R., 2003. Composition and niticidal activity of essential oils of three chemotypes of Rosmarinus officinalis L. acclimatised in Morocco. Flavor & Fragrance Journal 18, 124–127.

Lahlou, M., 2004. Methods to study the phytochemistry and bioactivity of essential oils. Phytother. Res. 18, 435–448. Published online in Wiley InterScience. DOI: 10.1002/ptr.1465. www.interscience.wiley.com.

Larrondo, J.V., Calvo, M.A., 1991. Effect of essential oils on *Candida albicans*: a scanning electron microscope study. Biomedical Letters 46 (184), 269–272.

Lautié, R., Passebecq, A., 1984. Aromatherapy. In: Thorsons, Wellingborough, p. 74.

Lawrence, B.M., 2000. Essential oils: from agriculture to chemistry. Int. J. Aromather. 10, 82–98.

Lawrence, F. (Ed.), 1987. Additives – your complete survival guide. Century, London.

Lembke, A., Deininger, R., 1985. Preparation and method for stimulating the immune system. German Patent 3508875 A 1 21 November 1985.

Lembke, A., Deininger, R., 1988. Virus inactivating pharmaceutical containing formates and black pepper oil. European Patent (EP) 259617 A 2 16 March 1988.

Lucks, B.C., 2003. Essential oils in holistic menopause management. In: Essence, Winter (2) (3).

Maha, N., Shaw, A., 2007. Academic doctors' views of complementary and alternative medicine (CAM) and its role within the NHS: an exploratory qualitative study. BMC Complement Altern. Med. 7, 17 doi: 10.1186/1472-6882-7-17.

Maruzella, J.C., 1961. Antifungal properties of perfume oils. J. Am. Pharm. Assoc. 50, 655.

Medicines Act, 1968. HMSO, London.

Melegari, M., Albasini, A., Pecorari, P., Vampa, G., Rinaldi, M., Rossi, T., et al., 1988. Chemical characteristics and pharmacological properties of the essential oil of Anthemis nobilis. Fitoterapia 59 (6), 449–455.

Mercier, D., Knevitt, A., 2005. Using topical aromatherapy for the management of fungating wounds in a palliative care unit. J. Wound Care 14, 497–501.

Micklefield, G., Greving, I., May, B., 2000. Effects of peppermint oil and caraway oil on gastroduodenal motility. Phytother. Res. 14, 20–23.

Micklefield, G., Jung, O., Greving, I., May, B., 2003. Effects of intraduodenal application of peppermint oil and caraway oil on gastrointestinal motility in healthy volunteers. Phytother. Res. 17, 135–140.

Mills, S.Y., 1991. Essential book of herbal medicine. In: Penguin, London, p. 452.

Pandey, M.P., Prasad, J., Awasthi, L.P., Kaushik, P., 1988. Antiviral effect of the essential oils from lemongrass (Cymbopogon flexuosus), mint (Mentha arvensis) and vetiver (Vetiveria zizanioides). Indigenous medicinal plants including microbes and fungi. National seminar on conservation and ethnobotanical aspects. In: Today and Tomorrows Printers and Publishers, New Delhi, pp. 47–49.

Panizzi, L., Flamini, G., Cioni, P.L., Morelli, I., 1993. Composition and antimicrobial properties of essential oils of four Mediterranean Lamiaceae. J. Ethnopharmacol. 39, 167–170.

Pellecuer, J., Roussel, J.L., Andary, C., 1973. Propriétés antifongiques comparatives des essences des trois Labiées méditerranéennes: romarin, sarriete et thym. Travaux de la Société de Pharmacie de Montpelier 33 (4), 587.

Pellecuer, J., Allegrini, J., De Buochberg, S., 1974. Etude in vitro de l'activité anti-bactérienne et antifongique de l'essence de Satureia montana L. Labiées. J. Pharm. Belg. 29 (2), 137–144.

Pellecuer, J., Allegrini, J., De Buochberg, S., Passat, J., 1975. Place de l'essence de Satureia montana L. Labiées dans l'arsenal thérapeutique. Plantes Médicinales et Phytothérapie 9 (2), 99–106.

Pellecuer, J., Allegrini, J., Seimeon, M., De Buochberg, S., 1976. Huiles essentielles bactéricides et fongicides. Revue de l'Institut de Lyon 1 (2), 135–159.

Pena, E.F., 1962. Melaleuca alternifolia oil – its use for trichomonal vaginitis and other vaginal infections. J. Obstet. Gynaecol. (June), 793–795.

Pénoël, D., 1981. Phytomédecine. CIMP, La Courtête 1/2, 63.

Perkin, M.R., Pearcy, R.M., Fraser, J.S., 1994. A comparison of the attitudes shown by general practitioners, hospital doctors and medical students towards alternative medicine. J. R. Soc. Med. 87 (9), 523–525.

Pittler, M.H., Ernst, E., 1998. Peppermint oil for irritable bowel syndrome: a critical review and meta-analysis. Am. J. Gastroenterol. 93, 1131–1135.

Pollock, I., Young, E., Stoneham, M., Slater, N., Wilkinson, J., Warner, J., 1989. Surveys of colourings and preservatives in drugs. Br. Med. J. 299, 649–651.

Poynton, L., Dowell, A., Dew, K., Egan, T., 2006. General practitioners' attitudes toward (and use of) complementary and alternative medicine: a New Zealand nationwide survey. Journal of the New Zealand Medical Association 119 (1247).

Price, S., 2000. The aromatherapy workbook. Thorsons, London.

Quevauviller, A., Panousse-Perrin, J., 1952a. Exaltation du pouvoir anesthétique local de la cocaïne par l'essence de Niaouli purifiée. Anesthésie 9, 421.

Quevauviller, A., Panousse-Perrin, J., 1952b. Influence du Gomenol sur l'activité in vitro de certains antibiotiques. Revue de Pathologie Comparée et Hygiene Générale 637, 296.

Ro, Y.-J., Ha, H.-C., Kim, C.-G., Yeom, H.-A., 2002. The effects of aromatherapy on pruritus in patients undergoing hemodialysis. Dermatol. Nurs. 14 (4), 231–238.

Rose, J., 1992. The aromatherapy book. North Atlantic Books, Berkeley.

Rossi, T., Melegari, M., Bianchi, A., Albasini, A., Vampa, G., 1988. Sedative, anti-inflammatory and antidiuretic effects induced in rats by essential oils of varieties of Anthemis nobilis: a comparative study. Pharmacol. Res. Commun. 5 (December 20), 71–74.

Roulier, G., 1990. Les huiles essentielles pour votre santé. St-Jean-de-Braye, Dangles.

Salji, J.P., et al., 1971. The antithyroid activity of Allium volatiles in the rat – in vitro studies. Eur. J. Pharmacol. 16, 251–253.

Schilcher, H., 1985. Effects and side effects of essential oils. In: Baerheim Svendsen, A., Scheffer, J.J.C. (Eds.), Essential oils and aromatic plants. Martinus Nijhof/Junk, Dordrecht.

Schmidt, P.W., 1936. Zentralblad für Bakteriologie. Parasitenkunde und Infektionskrankenheiten 138, 104.

Schmiedeberg, O., 1913. Grundriss der Pharmakologie, seventh ed Pharmakologie, Leipzig.

Schneider, G., 1975. Pharmazeutische Biologie. In: Wissenschaftsverlag, Mannheim, p. 128.

Schnitzler, P., Schumacher, A., Astani, A., Reichling, J., 2008. Melissa officinalis affects infectivity of enveloped herpes viruses. Phytomedicine 15, 734–740.

Seth, G., Kokate, C.K., Varma, K.C., 1976. Effect of essential oil of Cymbopogon citratus Stapf. On the central nervous system. Indian J. Exp. Biol. 14 (3), 370–371.

Shaikh, B.T., Hatcher, J., 2005. Complementary and alternative medicine in Pakistan: prospects and limitations. Evidence Based Complementary and Alternative Medicine 2 (2), 139–142.

Shemesh, A.U., Mayo, W.L., 1991. Tea tree oil – natural antiseptic and fungicide. J. Altern. Complement. Med. 9 (12 December), 11–12.

Sherry, E., Boeck, H., Warnke, P.H., 2001. Am. J. Infect. Control 29, 346.

Skoula, M., Harborne, J.B., 2002. The taxonomy and chemistry of Origanum. In: Kintzios, S.E. (Ed.), Oregano – the genera Origanum and Lippia. Taylor and Francis, London, pp. 67–108.

Stewart, D., 2005. The chemistry of essential oils made simple. Care Publications, Marble Hill, Missouri.

Szalontai, M., Verzar-Petri, G., Florian, E., 1976. Acta Pharm. Hung. 46, 232.

Szalontai, M., Verzar-Petri, G., Florian, E., 1977. Contribution to the study of antimycotic effect of biologically active components of Matricaria chamomilla L. Parfümerie und Kosmetik [Hungary] 58, 121.

Szalontai, M., Verzar-Petri, G., Florian, E., Gimpel, F., 1975a. Pharmazeutische Zeitung 120, 982.

Szalontai, M., Verzar-Petri, G., Florian, E., Gimpel, F., 1975b. Dtsch. Apoth. Ztg. 115, 912.

Taddei, I., Giachetti, D., Taddei, E., Mantovani, P., Bianchi, E., 1988. Spasmolytic activity of peppermint, sage and rosemary essences and their major constituents. Fitoterapia 59, 463–468.

Thiemer, K., Stadler, R., Isaac, O., 1973. Arzneimittelforschung 23, 756.

Thompson, D.P., Cannon, C., 1986. Toxicity of essential oils on toxigenic and nontoxigenic fungi. Bull. Environ. Contam. Toxicol. 36 (4), 527–532.

Tisserand, R., Balacs, T., 1995. Essential oil safety. Churchill Livingstone, New York.

Trease, G.E., Evans, W.C., 1983. Pharmacognosy, twelfth ed. Baillière Tindall, London.

Valnet, J., 1980. The practice of aromatherapy. Daniel, Saffron Walden.

Verdet, 1989. Why phytotherapy? Aromatherapy Study Trip Lecture notes. In: Price Publishing, Hinckley, p. 10.

Verhoef, M.J., Sutherland, L.R., 1995a. Alternative medicine and general practitioners. Opinions and behaviour. Canadian Family Physician 41, 1005–1011.

Verhoef, M.J., Sutherland, L.R., 1995b. General practitioners' assessment of and interest in alternative medicine in Canada. Soc. Sci. Med. 41 (4), 511–515.

Viaud, H., 1983. Huiles essentielles. Présence, Sisteron.

Vichkanova, S.A., Dzhanashiya, N.M., Goryunova, L.V., 1973. Antiviral activity displayed by the essential oil of Eucalyptus viminalis and of some frost-hardy eucalypti. Farmakol. Toksikol. 36 (3), 339–341.

von Braunschweig, R., 1999. Powerful contents of the angelica root: the monoterpenes. Forum E1.

Wagner, H., Wierer, M., et al., 1986. In vitro Hemmung der Prostaglandin Biosynthese durch étherische Öle und phenolische Verbindungen. Planta Med. 184–187.

Warnke, P.H., Becker, S.T., Podschun, R., Sivananthan, S., Springer, I.N., Russo, P.A., et al., 2009. The battle against multi-resistant strains: Renaissance of antimicrobial essential oils as a promising force to fight hospital-acquired infections. Journal of Craniomaxillofacial Surgery 37 (7), 392–397. Epub 2009 May 26.

Warnke, P., terheyden, H., Açil, Y., Springer, I.N., 2004. Tumour smell reduction with antibacterial essential oils [letter]. Cancer 100, 879–880.

Weiss, R.F., 1988. Herbal medicine. In: Arcanum, Göteborg, p. 296.

Wharton, R., Lewith, G., 1986. Complementary medicine and the general practitioner. Br. Med. J. (Clin. Res.) 292 (6533), 1498–1500.

Zara, M., 1966. Association atoxique de dérivées terpéniques d'huiles essentielles possédant une triple action en hépatologie (cholérétique, antispasmodique, lipotrope). Vie Médicinale 47 (10), 1549–1553.

Zondec, B., et al., 1938. Phenol methyl ethers as oestrogenic agents. Biochem. J. 32, 641–645.

Section 2

The foundations of practice

Section contents

Hydrolats – the essential waters

5

Len Price

CHAPTER CONTENTS

Introduction

The subject of aromatic waters is intriguing, yet not one on which very much has been written. It has been necessary to search many books on herbalism and aromatherapy to glean snippets of information. Even then the quality of information is not always very good, and very little would stand up to rigorous examination (save for the information on kekik water (Aydin, Baser & Öztürk 1996)). Most has been found in the French literature, as France is the country that most uses hydrolats, although even there not to a great extent today.

Water has the remarkable capability of picking up information relating to the vibrational energy found in a living plant, of storing this information and, under certain circumstances, of transferring it to the human body. This means that distilled hydrolats pick up and store not only physical plant particles (Roulier 1990) but possibly also subtle energetic information; consequently, such products have an almost homoeopathic aspect.

There are several kinds of water-based aromatic product used in therapies, including infusions, teas (it has been estimated that over 1 000 000 cups of chamomile tea are taken every day worldwide (Foster 1996)), tisanes, wines, vinegars and aromatic waters, which may be distilled or prepared. Distilled aromatic waters – hydrolats – contain the water-soluble compounds of the plant, but not the tannic acid and bitter substances, and make an excellent complement to that other product of distillation, the powerful essential oils. They are, however, very different in nature from the volatile essential oils, albeit obtained from the same plant, in as much as they are without aggression and are active on a different level; these 'gentle giants' are subtle, safe and effective, although any treatment must be carried out over a longer period of time than when using essential oils.

Some plants, whether containing essential oils or not, are distilled specifically for the hydrolat and not for the essential oil; when plants are distilled specifically for the hydrolat the quality of the water used is of great importance. Although there may be no volatile or aromatic molecules in these plants, and hence no aromatic oil, all water-soluble molecules within the plant are taken up by the steam; thus the hydrolats stand intermediate between, and to some extent represent a fusion of, aromatherapy and herbalism, containing as they do some of the useful plant molecules from both worlds. Hydrolats are used in conjunction with both essential oil treatments and herbalism, as well as on their own.

As these valuable products of the distillation process are so safe in use, they deserve to be much better known and far more widely used, especially by aromatherapists already familiar with the essential oils. Hydrolats last featured in the French *Codex* in 1965.

Terminology

In France the term hydrolat is used to describe the condensed steam which has passed through the plant material; the translation of hydrolat is given as 'aromatic, medicated water' (Mansion 1971) and this is the nomenclature adopted by Price and Price (2004 p. 31–34) to describe distilled plant waters, but many names are in use, some more accurate than others.

Terms used for these products are:

- Aromatic water – this term does not imply distillation and so is inaccurate.
- Floral waters – this is inaccurate and incomplete, as by no means all distilled waters are from flowers.
- Hydrosol – this is inappropriate, as it is a generic term applied to a wide range of products (including hydrolats) and is not specific: a hydrosol may be defined as a colloidal solution (i.e. a dispersion of material in a liquid, characterized by particles of very small size, of between 0.2 and 0.002 μm) where water is the dispersant medium.
- Essential water – this is an ancient name and aptly describes the aromatic distilled water from the still.
- Prepared water – this is an assembly of products to simulate a natural product.

Prepared aromatic waters

These are not produced by the distillation process but are put together in a laboratory. They consist of distilled water with the addition of one or more essential oils; these oils may be genuine plant extracts (volatile oil, absolute or concrete) or they may be partly or wholly artificial or synthetic. Essential oils are not generally soluble in water – probably on average only about 20% of any given oil is water soluble – but many can be 'knocked' into solution by shaking to produce a saturated solution. For each litre of distilled water 2–3 g (40–60 drops) of essential oil can be added; this must be shaken frequently and vigorously for 2 or 3 days and then stored in a cool place; it can be stored successfully at 10–15°C for several months. Essential oils suitable for use by this method are anise, basil, Borneo camphor, caraway, chamomile, cinnamon, citron, coriander, cypress, eucalyptus, fennel, garlic, geranium, hyssop, juniper, lavender, lemon, marjoram, melissa, niaouli, nutmeg, orange, origanum, peppermint, rosemary, sage, savory, tangerine, tarragon, verbena and ylang ylang (Lautié & Passebecq 1979 p. 91).

Prepared waters may be used for gargles, mouthwashes, bathing wounds and for ingestion, where 20 mL of the made water contains one drop of essential oil and therefore one teaspoonful contains about a quarter of a drop (about 0.25% concentration). Many essential oils exhibit significant bactericidal power at a concentration of 0.25%, as found in prepared waters, e.g. in a concentration of 0.18% clove essential oil kills the tubercle bacillus in a few minutes without causing any tissue damage or risk of toxicity, in contrast to some other preparations and antibiotics (Lautié & Passebecq 1979 p. 92).

Prepared waters do not have the same make-up as essential (distilled) waters, and therefore cannot have the same therapeutic properties. Some prepared waters are made with alcohol, and these are not recommended for use alongside aromatherapy. The main volume of sales of prepared waters is to skincare manufacturers for use in 'natural' skin toners, refreshers and washes. Water which has had essential oil(s), synthetics or alcohol added to it is not a hydrolat, and the two should not be confused. To achieve a genuine plant water, distillation alone is the true method.

What are hydrolats?

Hydrolats are a product of distillation and can be considered as true partial extracts of the plant material from which they are derived. They may be byproducts of the distillation of volatile oils, e.g. chamomile water and lavender water, or of the distillation of plant material which has no volatile oil, e.g. elderflower, cornflower, plantain. Their method of preparation, by definition, necessitates that they be totally natural products with no added synthetic fragrance components. Hydrolats are obtained from aromatic and other plants by steam distillation, and during this process a proportion of the water-soluble compounds of the essential oil contained in the plant matter is absorbed by and retained in the water. As some essential oils have a relatively high proportion of water-soluble compounds, much of the essential oil can be lost to the water during the distillation process, e.g. *Melissa officinalis* [lemon balm]; in such cases it is imperative to use cohobation. This is a system whereby the water/steam in contact with the biomass during distillation is continuously recirculated, giving maximal opportunity for the water-soluble elements of the essential oil and the plant to pass into the water. Eventually this water reaches saturation point, when no more of the essential oil components can pass into solution (it is at this stage that the complete essential oil is gained); thus a water is produced that is rich not only in some essential oil molecules but also in other hydrophilic molecules found in the plant which are not usually part of the essential oil. When distilling for hydrolats, it is important that the water used in the distillation process should be of good quality, preferably from a non-polluted spring, and free of any chemical cleansers that may have been used to clean the still.

Aromatic waters contain about 0.02–0.05% (or perhaps more, depending on the plant) of the water-soluble parts of the essential oil freely dispersed in an ionized form; this is equivalent to up to approximately 10 drops per litre of hydrolat (Price & Price 2004 p. 47). They may have similar properties to the parent oils but not to the same degree, and often their properties are different.

Which plants yield a hydrolat?

Many aromatherapists think that only plants containing an essential oil are distilled, but this is not so. Many plants containing very little or no essential oil at all are processed, primarily to gain the hydrolat. The hydrolat from each plant, like the essential oil, is unique and reacts according to its constituents. *Hypericum perforatum*, often macerated in olive oil to obtain its therapeutic properties (see Carrier oils in Ch. 8), is an example of a plant that contains an essential oil but which is rarely distilled for this on account of the minute yield, which would cause the price to be prohibitive; it is therefore distilled for its hydrolat. *Plantago*

lanceolata [plantain] is an example of a non-aromatic plant which is distilled only for its hydrolat. This illustrates that water-soluble molecules other than volatile essential oil molecules can be taken into the steam, yielding a therapeutic water at the end of the process.

Yield

It is not possible to obtain an almost unlimited or even a large quantity of water from a small amount of plant material. The quantity of hydrolat is proportionately limited to the plant weight, and therefore hydrolats of excellent quality are obtained when cohobation is an integral part of the distilling process. This method is used to produce a number of hydrolats, e.g. rose, and yields a saturated hydrolat; *Melissa* is another case where a whole essential oil cannot be achieved until the steam water is saturated with the water-soluble molecules of the essential oil, thereby preventing the loss of these from the essential oil.

Yields of distilled waters usually lie between the limits of 1–1.5 and 2–5 L/kg of plant matter, and vary according to the particular plant. The waters of thyme, savory and rosemary require a smaller quantity of plant than do waters of lettuce, hawthorn, yarrow or hemp agrimony. Some waters are known as 'weight for weight' products, as the quantities of plant matter and water product are equal, e.g. 100 lb of roses are distilled with sufficient water to yield 100 lb of fragrant rose water (Poucher 1936).

Appearance and aroma

Distilled waters are not strongly coloured and are clear, with the exception of cinnamon water, which is always opalescent; for the most part they have only slight, delicate coloration (Viaud 1983 p. 23). Their smell may be generally reminiscent of the original plant material, but this is not always the case; an example is distilled lavender water, which often disappoints (Price & Price 2004 p. 58–59)

Keeping qualities and storage

Waters need to be stored at a temperature of less than 14°C, and in the shade. At higher temperatures certain waters tend to show flocculation. The maximum storage period under the conditions given must not, in general, exceed 1 year, as some hydrolats are fragile and break down after a relatively short time. They are best purchased in small quantities, although Rouvière and Meyer (1989) say that the plant waters resulting from the distillation process of essential oils have a life of 2–3 years, owing to the presence of soluble compounds from the essential oils, which inhibit bacterial growth: this has been confirmed by the authors (Price & Price 2004 p. 56–57). Those hydrolats that have a good content of antiseptic phenols keep well; the distilled waters of *Satureia hortensis* and *Origanum vulgare* can be kept for more than 2 years with no discernible change.

Composition

It is known that, besides certain volatile compounds (isovalerianic, cyanhydric, benzoic and cinnamic acids), distilled plant waters can contain many other volatile principles, although these are rarely properly identified. Analysis of three hydrolats (*Lavandula angustifolia*, *Salvia officinalis*, *Matricaria recutita*) showed that they contain substances present in the plant (Montesinos 1991 p. 24, Price & Price 2004). The pH of a hydrolat is closely linked to the concentration of alcohols and phenols present and to the degree of dissociation; they are sometimes neutral, but usually have a weak acid reaction (Price & Price 2004 p. 58).

Quality

The basic criteria for obtaining a good-quality hydrolat are the same as those for the procurement of a genuine essential oil, i.e. using a known botanical species, grown organically or wild, with a known chemical make-up; a distillation of sufficient duration and at low pressure; and a hydrolat that itself has had nothing added and nothing extracted. It is imperative that only products obtained during steam distillation and without colouring matter, stabilizers and preservatives be used. Products procured from a high-street chemist's shop do not usually conform to this high standard, often containing synthetic materials; alternatively, they may be entirely artificial.

As with an essential oil, it is difficult to judge the quality of a distilled water from the smell: a true distilled water does not necessarily smell the same as the oil from the same plant because it has a different chemical make-up; when freshly distilled it may have an odour and taste of the still, although this is not long lasting.

Unfortunately, most hydrolats from plants distilled for their essential oils are discarded, and are saved only if ordered beforehand. It is generally thought that because hydrolats are often thrown away, they should be inexpensive; unhappily this is not the case, as the cost of transporting the bulk (volume and weight) of the product is reflected in the final cost.

Uses of hydrolats

> A nice attention, however, is certainly necessary in the use of them.
>
> John Farley (1783), principal cook at the London Tavern, Dublin, referring to the water and infusions of bay.

Waters are ultramild in action compared to essential oils and are useful for the treatment of the young, the elderly, and those in a state of delicate health. The less volatile odorous molecules are integrally dispersed in the water in ionized form, therefore irritation of the skin and mucous surfaces is avoided. Hydrolats have a higher concentration of volatile elements than do teas and so are more efficacious and quicker acting, with a very easy method of use, i.e. drinking small quantities.

Hydrolats work synergistically with essential oils and so they can be prescribed as a complement to either phytotherapy (Streicher 1996) or aromatherapy. Herbalists in France do not use these waters on their own to any great extent, but they are used as a complement to other phytotherapeutic treatments, both internally and externally; they are used both singly and as ready-prepared mixes.

General

Being non-aggressive, waters can be used safely for disinfection of open wounds and on mucous surfaces; they have been mentioned for use in cases of eczema, ulcers, bronchitis, tracheitis, colitis, burns and pain, whether local or generalized (e.g. *Chamaemelum nobile* [Roman chamomile] is said to ease post-zoster pain). They are used in gargles, nasal sprays, skin sprays, compresses and vaginal douches.

Skin care

Hydrolats are nearly free of irritating components, and their mild action and lack of toxicity make them ideal for use as skincare products; they have long

Case study 5.1

Severe burns

A. Hanson – Aromatherapist

Client assessment

One day, when Harry, 36, lit a ring on his gas stove, the whole space exploded into flames, burning his face and neck. Although he managed to put some cold water on his face, he had to extinguish the fire and comfort his four children. The aromatherapist arrived half an hour after the burning occurred and Harry was in great pain. The hospital was over 25 km away, the burn needed immediate treatment, and Harry was reluctant to go to the hospital anyway.

Intervention

Day 1 – afternoon: Burnt hair was sticking to Harry's face and neck and he was in shock. First, he was asked to stand in the shower for 10 minutes with cold water pouring over his face and neck. Meanwhile, three basins were prepared as follows:

1. Ice cubes, 200 mL of lavender hydrolat (*Lavendula officinalis* – all the therapist had with her) and 50 mL of peppermint hydrolat (*Mentha* x *piperita*) to help cool the skin.
2. 0.5 L of cold water, 5 mL lavender essential oil and 50 mL of peppermint hydrolat.
3. Ice cubes and cold water.
- A clean teatowel was torn in half, wrung into basin 1 (keeping it fairly wet) and applied to Harry's face and neck.
- The second piece was dipped into basin 2 and applied; these two applications were repeated many times, as the towel immediately turned warm on his burn. Ice cubes were continually added to the first and second basins – plus another 50 mL peppermint hydrolat to basin 1 and another 5 mL lavender essential oil to basin 2.

This went on for 2 hours, during which time Harry was given a strong painkiller.

As the skin had cooled down somewhat, the following gel was prepared and thickly but very gently applied to the whole area:
- 25 mL fresh aloe vera (direct from the plant)
- 10 drops *Lavandula officinalis* – analgesic, anti-inflammatory, antiseptic, cicatrizant
- 20 drops *Melaleuca alternifolia* [tea tree] – analgesic, anti-infectious, anti-inflammatory

Harry felt immediate relief and after 5–10 minutes the pain lessened. After 1 hour the gel had formed a strong film (stronger than that on healthy skin) and the pain was gone.

His eyes and lips were very swollen, his face red, and on his upper lip blisters were forming where he had licked off the gel. More was applied there, after which Harry went to bed and slept soundly.

Day 2 – morning: The whole face was sore, the nose having an open wound where the skin was burned off. It was not bleeding, although it was weeping and swollen. There were brown dry patches under his eyes, his eyelids were swollen and red, his lips swollen and cracked, and his cheeks streaked in red and white.

The whole area was sprayed with rose hydrolat (*Rosa damascena*), a very wet compress was made with the hydrolat to try and help remove the burnt hair still stuck on his skin. When it was removed and the skin was dry the gel blend was applied again to the whole face, upper lip and neck. Photographs were taken.

Day 2 – evening: During the day the brown patches had paled somewhat. His chin and neck were still painful. The nose had dried up and a scab was forming around the edges of the wound. Harry had slept during the day.

The spraying and compress treatments were repeated with the rose hydrolat, and more burnt hair came away. As the emergency was over, a weaker gel blend was then made, using 25 mL aloe vera gel with only 5 drops each of *Lavandula officinalis* and *Melaleuca alternifolia*.

Day 3 – morning: The skin was cleansed again with rose hydrolat to remove the last of the burnt hair; the nose and lip had started to dry up, the area was less swollen and the patches under the eyes were almost gone. The whole area was still sensitive.

Day 3 – evening: The nose and lip had started bleeding slightly, but as the face and neck showed only a faint redness by then, the gel blend was applied only to the nose and lip, and carrot oil, which is anti-inflammatory and helpful to burns, to the rest of the area.

Day 4 – morning: This was the turning point! No pain, only itching. Harry's nose and lip had small scabs and looked clean, with no suggestion of impending infection. A doctor representing the insurance company arrived and said that the nose and lip had second-degree burns, the face and neck first-degree. He did not believe the burn had been as bad as reported, until he was shown the photographs.

Harry took a lukewarm shower, the gel dissolving in the water. Carrot oil was then applied to the whole area except the nose and lip, which was given the gel blend again. The procedure was repeated in the evening.

---

been used in this way in the form of cleansers, toners (all skin types, especially sensitive skin), conditioning creams and lotions. They are also used in baby care, bath preparations, hair rinses, aftershave preparations and facial sprays.

Children

Hydrolats produced for therapeutic use should not contain added alcohol as a preservative and so are suitable for children, especially as they may be sweetened with honey or sugar. They are recommended for young children for both external and internal use because they do not irritate the skin or mucous surfaces (note: care must be taken when procuring the hydrolat: concentrated waters do contain alcohol (Price & Price 2004 p. 38)).

Eye care

Some hydrolats are used in preparations for eye-washes, e.g. *Myrtus communis* [myrtle], *Centaurea cyanus* [cornflower] and *Chamaemelum nobile* [Roman chamomile] soothe pains resulting from inflammatory states in the eyes.

Traditional medicine

Hydrolats are often prescribed by some complementary practitioners to adjust the 'energy balance' and the 'environment' (both internal and external) of the person, for instance according to Chinese medicine. The conditions treated include disorders of the digestive system such as constipation; rheumatism, migraine (from liver irritation), parasites, and ear, nose and throat problems.

Routes of absorption

First there is the oral route through the walls of the digestive tract. The culinary aspect is attractive here, as hydrolats are easily added to foods and are palatable (Price & Price 2004 pp. 173–177).

The rectal route using an enema is also used, and the active substance is here absorbed across the mucous surfaces of the large intestine.

Finally there is the skin; here the substance is absorbed from the whole surface of the body.

Methods of use and dosages

- Put 50 mL of hydrolat into a bath to aid relaxation and promote a soothing effect.
- Use it on a cottonwool pad as a skin tonic after cleansing.
- Use it as a mouthwash or gargle.
- Put a teaspoonful (5 mL) into tea (without milk), fruit juice or fruit salads, coffee (petitgrain or orange flower water is delicious

in coffee and fruit salads) or in a morning glass of water.
- Oral (internal) use may safely be recommended where appropriate; up to three teaspoonfuls (15 mL) per day may be ingested.

The duration of treatment is dependent on the particular organ and person being treated:

- For treatment of the liver, two teaspoonfuls should be taken before supper or before going to bed.
- For treatment of the kidneys and bladder, three teaspoonfuls should be taken between 3 pm and 7 pm.
- For treatment of the lungs, six teaspoonfuls should be spread throughout the day in acute cases, or three teaspoonfuls for chronic cases.
- For gargles hydrolats may be used neat, but in general use they should be diluted, up to 1 in 10 depending on the water.

Table 5.1 lists the properties and indications for the use of hydrolats for general conditions, skin conditions and emotional states: in the absence of any other kind of proof these are based almost wholly on anecdotal evidence. There is a general table giving the properties of these waters in Price and Price (2004). Waters have certainly been in continual use for three and a half centuries, and perhaps longer, in cooking, for medicine and for personal cleanliness (Genders 1977).

Cautions

It should be noted that preservative is often added to shop-bought natural hydrolats to improve their shelf-life, and these should be avoided for culinary or therapeutic purposes. When purchasing waters it may also be necessary to obtain a certificate from the supplier to ensure that the proper conditions of harvesting, processing and stocking have been observed.

Like other partial plant extracts, hydrolats will possess the claimed activity of the plant only if its constituents giving this activity are contained within that fraction of the plant forming the partial extract. Many partial plant extracts, particularly distillates, have the advantage of being virtually colourless, making them easy to incorporate into a range of products. Unfortunately, over the years this has led to the production of distillates from a wide range of plant materials which are not suitable for this form of processing, and

Table 5.1 Properties and indications: essential waters

Essential water	General	Skin	Emotion
Achillea millefolium [yarrow]	Circulatory problems (women)		
Calendula officinalis [marigold]	Emmenagogue, hypertension, staphylococcus	Eczema, skin drainer, pyodermatitis	
Centaurea cyanus [cornflower]	Skin problems of intestinal origin		
Chamaemelum nobile [Roman chamomile]	Cardiac calmative? Healing, ophthalmic	Antiiinflammatory, infections	Calming
Citrus sinensis [orange flower]	Cardiac calmative, anticollibacillus		Seasonal nervous depression, uplifting
Cupressus sempervirens [cypress]	Haemorrhoids, broken veins		
Eucalyptus globulus [Tasmanian blue gum]	Bronchi, kidneys, pancreas, antidiabetic	Acne	
Foeniculum vulgare [fennel]	Galactogen, antiseptic		
Helichrysum angustifolium [everlasting]	Diabetes, aerophagy, pulmonary depurative	Bruises, abscesses, couperose skin, cicatrizant	Nervous depression, sedative
Hypericum perforatum [St John's wort]		Soothing	
Hyssopus officinalis [hyssop]	Low dose – clears the lungs; high dose – antiepileptic		
Juniperus communis [juniper]	Diuretic, kidney deflocculant, rheumatoid arthritis	Skin astringent, oily skin, refreshing	
Lavandula angustifolia [lavender]	Intestinal antibiotic, rheumatism	Soothing, pimples, burns, insect bites	
Lavandula x *intermedia* [lavandin]		Acneic skin, herpes	
Melissa officinalis [lemon balm]	Blepharitis, conjunctivitis, digestive, headaches	Irritated skin, insect bites, herpes	Sedative, relaxing, uplifting, depression
Mentha x *piperita* [peppermint]	Eupeptic, antiseptic	Itching, inflammation, cooling	Refreshing
Myrtus communis [myrtle]	Soothing antiseptic		
Ocimum basilicum [basil]	Carminative, digestive		
Origanum majorana [marjoram]	Clears the liver, gallbladder		
Origanum onites [kekik]	Cardiovascular stimulant		

Continued

Table 5.1 Properties and indications: essential waters—cont'd

Essential water	General	Skin	Emotion
Pinus sylvestris [Scots pine]	Balsamic, diuretic		
Rosa damascena [rose]	Mouth ulcers	Toning all skin types, dermatitis, wrinkles, couperose	Mental strain, calming, sedative
Rosmarinus officinalis [rosemary]	Emmenagogue, rheumatism, circulation stimulant	Toning oily and mixed skins	Stimulating, alertness
Salvia officinalis [sage]	Emmenagogue, pelvic congestion, diuretic, rheumatism, ulcers	Astringent, oily skin, acne, eczema	
Salvia sclarea [clary]	Sore throat, period pain	Astringent, oily skin, acne, inflamed, mature skin	Depression, anxiety
Satureia montana [savory]	Revitalizing		
Thymus serpyllum [wild thyme]	Intestinal antiseptic, Gram −ve		
Thymus vulgaris (population) [thyme]	Intestinal antiseptic, Gram +ve	Acne, dermatitis, insect bites, eczema	Stimulating, revitalizing
Thymus vulgaris ct. *alcohol* [sweet thyme]	Eye problems		

Case study 5.2

Menopausal problems

P. Price – Aromatologist

Client assessment

Norma, aged 52, suffered from menopausal symptoms, such as sleepless nights, hot flushes and restless legs. Occasionally she had migraines or severe headaches. She felt tired all the time and was forgetful. The worst symptom was the flushing, which Norma had been suffering from for over 4 years, the problem being so severe that during that time she had not been able to have a cover on her, otherwise she woke up drenched with sweat, needing to change the bed.

Intervention

After a thorough consultation, the following was advised:
* Cut down on processed foods and alcohol.
* Walk rather than drive whenever possible.
* Go to her GP for a thyroxin level check – this can fall during menopause, thereby being a contributory factor to tiredness, memory loss and headaches.

The following hydrolats were blended together 50/50:
* *Rosa damascena* [rose]
* *Ribes nigrum* [blackcurrant]

Both are beneficial for menopausal symptoms, in particular hot flushes, and help to balance the natural hormone levels in the body. Norma was asked to drink 25 mL of this three times a day, in 25 mL warm water, and to contact the therapist in 7 days to let her know how she was coping. She was also reminded about starting her lifestyle changes.

Outcome

After 5 days an excited Norma phoned to say that she had just had her first good night's sleep for years, and that she had slept with a sheet over her. She was delighted and amazed that the hydrolats had worked so quickly – as was the therapist! She had not had time to make any serious lifestyle changes – just increase her walking time and practise deep breathing.

Within the month, her intake of hydrolats was reduced to twice a day and the next month to once a day, by which time Norma was sleeping with a duvet and the headaches had notably improved.

Norma enjoyed the taste and was happy to continue the treatment, which she is still on at the time of writing.

Her thyroid test showed that she needed slight supplementation, and within 3 months her tiredness had improved.

therefore little credence can be given to any claimed activity of the plant material or to its extract (Helliwell 1989).

Summary

Continued use of hydrolats over centuries indicates that these substances have a potential for therapeutic use and are worthy of investigation. Physically they contain some water-soluble molecules known to be therapeutic, in common with essential oils and some compounds found in other types of herbal preparation, and it may be that they also carry information and energy in a manner somewhat analogous to homoeopathic remedies. They are gentle in use and may safely be used in some cases where the use of the more powerful essential oils would be inadvisable, and may also be used to complement other forms of treatment; they have the advantage of being relatively inexpensive.

References

Aydin, B., Öztürk, 1996. The chemistry and pharmacology of origanum (kekik) water. In: 27th International Symposium on Essential Oils, September, Vienna.

Farley, J., 1783. Handbook on the art of cookery and housekeepers complete assistant, p. 307.

Foster, S., 1996. Chamomile: *Matricaria recutita* & *Chamaemelum nobile*. In: Botanical series 307. American Botanical Council, Austin, p. 6.

Genders, R., 1977. A book of aromatics. Darton, Longman and Todd, London, p. 13.

Helliwell, K., 1989. Manufacture and use of plant extracts. In: Grievson, M., Barber, J.,

Hunting, A.L.L. (Eds.), Natural ingredients in cosmetics. Weymouth, Micelle, pp. 26–27.

Lautié, R., Passebecq, A., 1979. Aromatherapy; the use of plant essences in healing. Thorsons, Wellingborough.

Mansion, J.E., 1971. Harrap's new standard French and English dictionary.

Montesinos, 1991. Eléments de reflexion sur quelques hydrolats. Study written for Ecole Lyonnaise de Plantes Médicinales, Lyons.

Poucher, W.A., 1936. Perfumes, cosmetics and soaps vol. II, Chapman & Hall, London, pp. 34–35.

Price, L., Price, S., 2004. Understanding hydrolats: the specific hydrosols for aromatherapy. Churchill Livingstone, Edinburgh.

Roulier, G., 1990. Les huiles essentielles pour votre santé. Dangles, St-Jean-de-Braye, p. 115.

Rouvière, A., Meyer, M.-C., 1989. La santé par les huiles essentielles. M A Editions, Paris, pp. 82–83.

Streicher, C., 1996. Hydrosols – the subtle complement to essential oils. Plexus 1, 22.

Viaud, H., 1983. Huiles essentielles – hydrolats. Présence, Sisteron.

Sources

Claeys, G., 1992. Précis d'aromathérapie familiale. Equilibres, Flers, p. 74.

de Bonneval, P., 1992. Votre santé par les plantes. Equilibres, Flers.

Grace, U.-M., 1996. Aromatherapy for practitioners. Daniel, Saffron Walden, pp. 84–85.

Price, S., 1997. Aromatic water. The Aromatherapist 3 (2), 44–47.

Price, L., Price, S., 1999. Essential waters. Riverhead, Stratford upon Avon.

Rose, J., 1994. Hydrosols: the other product of distillation. Aromatherapy correspondence course notes, California.

How essential oils enter the body

6

Len Price

CHAPTER CONTENTS

Introduction

Essential oils follow three main pathways to gain entry to the body: ingestion, inhalation and absorption through the skin (Fig. 6.1). Ingestion is little used in the UK. Of the two remaining pathways, inhalation is a very effective method and indeed is regarded by some (e.g. Buchbauer 1988) as the only method truly deserving the name aromatherapy. However, topical application via the skin has also been found to be effective – the route selected depends on the problem being helped.

Inhalation

Access via the nasal passages is a speedy and effective route in the treatment of emotional problems such as stress and depression (and also some types of headache). This is because the nose has direct contact with the brain, which is responsible for triggering the effects of essential oils regardless of the route they use to gain access to it. The nose itself is not the organ of smell, but simply modifies the temperature and humidity of the inhaled air and collects any foreign matter that might be breathed in. The first cranial (olfactory) nerve is responsible for the sense of smell and serves the receptor cells, of which there are two groups of about 25 million, each occupying a small area (about 4 cm^2) at the top of the nostrils (Van Toller 1993).

Inhalation and the mucous membranes

When any vapour is inhaled, some molecules from it inevitably travel down the pathway to the lungs where, if they are appropriate essential oils, they can have an immediate and beneficial impact on many breathing difficulties. In the nose the endothelium is thin and the site is close to the brain, therefore it must be assumed that essential oil molecules reach the local circulation and the brain fairly easily and quickly. On their journey to the lungs some molecules are undoubtedly

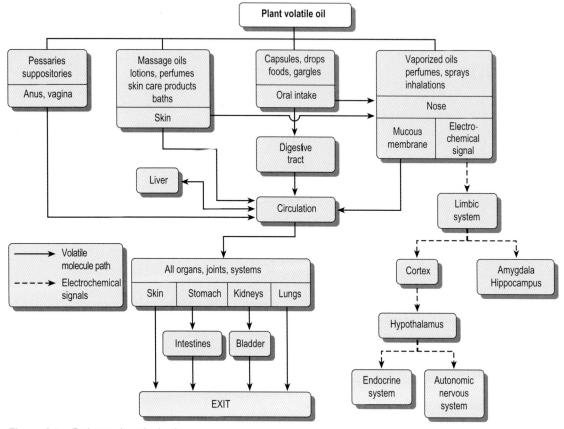

Figure 6.1 • Pathways into the body

absorbed by the mucous linings of the respiratory pathways, the bronchi and multitudinous bronchioles, where access is very easy. Arriving at the point of gaseous exchange in the alveoli, the molecules are transferred to the blood circulating in the lungs. It can be seen that deep breathing will increase the quantity of any essence or essential oil taken into the body by this route. Ill effects due to inhalation of essential oils normally used in aromatherapy are rare.

Methods of inhalation

Inhalation is an unobtrusive way of using essential oils in a healthcare setting. They may be given via a tissue, drops on the hands (in an emergency) a vaporizer etc., and all are effective in the appropriate situation. To select oils for particular conditions, see the tables in Ch. 4 and Appendix B.9 on the CD-ROM.

Tissues

Inhalation from a tissue with five to six drops of essential oil (three drops for children, the elderly and pregnant women) is most effective for immediate results, requiring two or three deep breaths to ensure good contact with the cilia. To give further benefit, and easier with children and the elderly, the tissue can be placed inside the shirt, blouse or nightwear so that the effects may continue as the heat of the body causes the oil molecules to evaporate and float upwards to the nose. Firm tissues such as kitchen towels hold the aroma longer than do paper handkerchiefs.

Q-tips

This method uses less essential oil than does a tissue. The Q-tip is held against the dropper and one drop allowed to wet it. Unlike a crumpled tissue it cannot be placed next to the skin, but has the advantage of slower evaporation, so it can be used for longer.

Hands

This is an excellent method but should be confined to emergencies only, and is not suitable for children. A solitary drop of essential oil (single, or from a mix) can be put into one of the patient's palms, which is then rubbed briefly against the other palm to disperse and warm the oil. With eyes closed, the patient places the cupped hands over the nose, avoiding the eye area, and takes a deep nasal breath. It is usually respiratory or stress conditions that require this sort of help.

Steamers

Allowing a patient to hold a basin of hot water is not acceptable in many hospital situations because of health and safety regulations. Even if the nurse holds it there is always the possibility that some people, especially those with learning difficulties, may strike out (involuntarily or otherwise) and knock the hot water over themselves or the nurse. Home-visiting health professionals may find that this method can be used safely with people whose movements are stable. Dry inhalation is safer for those not enjoying full health and living alone. A proprietary brand electric diffuser can be used.

Nebulizers are safer, but essential oils, especially if undiluted, can attack some kinds of plastic, so care must be taken not to damage the equipment. A precautionary test is advisable for any plastic that might come into contact with essential oils. This applies also to facial steamers. These methods are normally used for respiratory problems and the common cold, though any problem that can benefit from inhalation will obtain speedier relief when steam is used. The heat of the water evaporates the oil molecules more quickly, increasing the strength of the vapour, and for this reason only half the number of drops are needed than for inhalation from a tissue (three drops for an adult and one to two drops for a child, elderly person or pregnant woman). The following cautions may be helpful:

- Ensure the patient's eyes are kept closed and watch carefully for any adverse reaction, such as choking or coughing, which can happen if too many drops have been used or too deep a breath is taken.
- One drop only – with water of not too high a temperature – is adequate for asthmatics because the overpowering effect of the vapour (stronger because of the speedy evaporation referred to above) may have an adverse effect.

Baths

Treatment by putting oils into the bath is effective because not only do they come into gentle contact with the skin, they are also inhaled at the same time; thus a double benefit is derived. Note that undiluted essential oils can attack a plastic bath. For details, see Methods of percutaneous absorption, below.

Spray bottle

A quick way of freshening the air when dressings are being changed for patients with bed sores, gangrene etc. is to use 10–12 drops of essential oil in 250 mL of water, shaking the bottle well before spraying the room. The essential oils to use in this case are *Pinus sylvestris* [Scots pine], *Thymus vulgaris* [thyme] (all chemotypes, though phenolic thymes are the most powerful antiseptics), *Syzygium aromaticum* [clove], *Eucalyptus smithii* [gully ash], *Mentha* × *piperita* [peppermint].

Vaporizers and diffusers

Possibly the most favoured way of using inhalation in a healthcare setting at present is from a vaporizer. A slight drawback is that the lightest molecules are liberated first from the oil, the heavier ones being released progressively. Although there are many different types of vaporizer available, only electric ones are considered safe where patients are concerned (the British Safety Standard mark should be looked for on the model to be used). Electric vaporizers should be thermostatically controlled at a low temperature, preventing the essential oils from becoming too hot. If this occurs, not only are they used up too quickly to be economical, but the heaviest molecules burning off last may produce an unpleasant acrid smell.

Box 6.1

Use of fragranced cleaning materials

When lecturing abroad, the authors' room in the hotel was on the 24th floor.

They stepped into the lift and began to ascend. After one or two breaths, Len's breathing began to be laboured. I could smell immediately that the lift had just been cleaned with a synthetic lavender product and it was this that was affecting Len's lungs.

At the 10th floor his breathing was noticeably worse, so I placed his handkerchief over his mouth and nose, telling him to hold his breath as long as he could. I also pressed the 12th floor button, but the lift was already programmed for its first stop at the 24th.

When we reached the 24th floor, Len stumbled out of the lift and tried to take a breath. However, he was now in the throes of an asthma attack and breathing was very difficult.

Fortunately, our room was near the lift, and as soon as we entered I took out the bottle of Len's 'Rescue' blend of undiluted essential oils, which I carry everywhere with me.

Putting a few drops on his handkerchief for his nose and mouth, I quickly removed his shirt and applied about 20 drops down his spine, rubbing them well into his spinal column and across each side of his back in the area of his lungs, adding more drops to ensure full coverage.

With my first and second fingers, I then 'drew' firm lines several times in the spinal channel, repeating these together with the rubbing of the lung area for several minutes.

Almost immediately Len's breathing began to improve, his shoulders more relaxed – and without heaving.

The essential oils in this blend are equal quantities of:

- *Abies balsamica* [Canadian balsam]
- *Aloysia triphylla* [verbena]
- *Boswellia carteri* [frankincense]
- *Eucalyptus smithii* [gully gum]
- *Hyssopus officinalis* [hyssop]
- *Pinus mugo* var. *pumilio* [dwarf pine]

Diffusers (units with a small blown-glass container for the essential oils) are more efficient in that they push out all the differently sized molecules at the same time. Unlike vaporizers, which use heat, there is no burning of residue when the essential oil is used up. Their only disadvantage is cost: the oils are used up fairly rapidly and the equipment cost can be up to three times greater than an electric vaporizer. A recent development on the market uses a new technique to deliver evenly and economically all sizes of molecule contained in the essential oils into the atmosphere. The essential oils are released in a regulated manner so that the air does not become overloaded; there are time switches for selecting both operating and rest times, making this method suitable for clinical use.

Ethical considerations

When the effects required for a whole ward are the same for each occupant, e.g. keeping a ward free from infection or perhaps conducting a trial, the method is viable and effective; it can also be useful in the reduction of stress and insomnia, as well as in the destruction of germs. A few hospitals use vaporizers and diffusers in single-occupancy rooms only and not in general ward areas, as it is felt by some to be unethical to impose aromas (which may be disliked or unwanted by some) on other occupants. The same consideration should be given to the wearing of perfume and the use of scented cleaning materials, both of which can adversely affect the health of some people. Large vaporizer units used in hotels and offices are often run on commercial-grade essential oils and aromas to keep costs down, without taking into account the effect long-term exposure may have on people. It is already known that artificial perfumes and adulterated essential oils cause sensitivities in asthmatics and skin reactions in those susceptible to such effects (Box 6.1). 'Environmental fragrancing', as this practice is termed, is most advanced in the USA, where there is growing concern at the use of synthetic aromas. The liberty of the individual is an important consideration and, unlike shoppers irritated by 'muzak' or 'fragrancing' designed to alter their mood, hospital patients are not free to walk away from an unwanted environmental influence.

Absorption via the skin

Until the second half of the 20th century the skin was thought to be almost impermeable (Maibach & Marzulli 1977, Stoughton 1959). This idea still persists, even though the skin has been known for more than half a century to be a poor barrier to lipophilic substances (Brun 1952) and it has been shown that essential oils in a base oil applied to the skin are absorbed into the bloodstream (Jäger et al. 1992). Most chemicals are absorbed to some degree, and this is made use of in patch therapy, e.g. glyceryl trinitrate must penetrate the skin to reach the blood vessels and heart to treat angina, and many other substances – including oestradiol, scopolamine and nicotine – are administered in this way (Cleary 1993).

Transdermal delivery

Many drugs are unsuitable for use in therapeutic transdermal delivery systems owing to their low ability to permeate the skin, so the use of penetration-enhancing agents is advantageous; various studies suggest that essential oils offer a useful selection of safe penetration enhancers to aid topical drug delivery. Eucalyptus and chenopodium essential oils caused a 30-fold increase in the drug 5-fluorouracil (5-FU) permeability coefficient using excised human skin; animal studies showed enhanced skin penetration for some drugs with eucalyptus oil, camphor and limonene; and in laboratory tests on excised human skin the penetration of 5-FU was increased with aniseed oil (2.8 times), ylang oil (7.8 times) and eucalyptus oil (34 times) (Williams & Barry 1989).The skin permeation of the neuroleptic drug haloperidol was increased in the presence of cineole and (+)-limonene, but that of chlorpromazine was not; in fact (+)-limonene reduced it (Almiral et al. 1996); terpenes have been shown to have an enhancing effect on the transdermal permeation of hydrophilic drugs, and chlorpromazine is more lipophilic than haloperidol. The principal component of eucalyptus oil was investigated to determine whether 1,8-cineole could be detected in effective amounts in skeletal muscles after dermal application; the bioavailability of 1,8-cineole was 320% greater when using an applicator than with an occlusive dressing (Weyers & Brodbeck 1989).

Takayama and Nagai (1994) studied the promoting effects of terpenes present in essential oils on the percutaneous absorption of indomethacin from hydrogels in rats in vivo and found that absorption was remarkably enhanced by cyclic monoterpenes such as limonene, terpinene and terpinolene. It was noted that the terpenes had a strong fluidizing effect on the lipid bilayer structure,

and (+)-limonene in the presence of ethanol changed the barrier structure of the skin, accelerating the transfer of ethanol, and thus the permeation of indomethacin was promoted because of its affinity with alcohol.

Sesquiterpenes also have been shown to increase 5-FU absorption across human (cadaver) skin; the increase was thought to be brought about by disrupting intercellular lipid bilayers and by forming complexes with 5-FU: sesquiterpenes with polar functional groups produced the greatest improvements in absorption (Cornwall & Barry 1994). The mechanisms by which penetration enhancers increase the permeability of the stratum corneum are discussed by Cornwall et al. (1996).

Cinnamon oil, clove oil and galangal were studied as percutaneous enhancers for benzoic acid and it was found that skin penetration was significantly enhanced by all three volatile oils (Shen et al. 2001). in vitro tests with cajuput, cardamom, melissa, myrtle, niaouli and orange oils on the permeation of estradiol through hairless mouse skin showed that niaouli was the best permeation enhancer. The whole oil of niaouli was a better activity promoter than its single isolated compounds, and the data demonstrated complex terpene mixtures to be potent enhancers of transdermal penetration for moderately lipophilic drugs such as estradiol (Monti et al. 2002). Clove oil tested on the transdermal delivery of ibuprofen in rabbits showed significant enhancement in vitro and a lesser effect in vivo; the enhanced delivery was attributed to the principal components eugenol and acetyl eugenol (Shen et al. 2007). Basil oil was found to be a promising penetration enhancer for the drug labetolol (Jain et al. 2008).

The skin as a water barrier

Water comprises 90% of any cell, and therefore the skin has developed as a barrier specifically to resist water; nevertheless, it is slightly permeable to water-soluble substances, to water itself and to lipids (Riviere 1993). The absorption of drugs and poisons through the skin was studied by Macht (1938) and there has been a considerable amount of research on pesticides and the skin. Pesticides, which dissolve in essential oils, are lipid-like and can therefore penetrate the skin – every farmer is aware of this health hazard and many people are killed each year by pesticides, mostly in developing countries. The amount absorbed through human skin varies enormously: for example, less than 1% of cypermethrin pesticide is absorbed, whereas up to 65% of the antifungal agent benzoic acid may penetrate the skin (Hotchkiss 1994).

The skin's success as a barrier is due in the main to the stratum corneum, the tough and durable, self-repairing keratinized layer, which is 20 layers of dead cells thick. Once a chemical gets past the epidermis – the only great obstacle – the rest of the journey into the body is easy, because of the presence of lipids in all cell membranes. For example, the antibacterial substance hexachlorophene is absorbed through the skin and was shown in 1969 to cause microscopically visible brain damage in rats (Winter 1984 p. 138) and chloasma in humans; in the 1970s hexachlorophene was used as an antiseptic in baby soaps and talcum powders, causing brain damage and even death in some babies after it had penetrated the skin (Jackson 1993). The lipid solubility of essential oil components allows these compounds to cross the blood–brain barrier (where certain substances are held back by the endothelium of cerebral capillaries) and make contact with the fluids around the brain (Anthony & Thibodeau 1983).

Many factors dictate the rate and quantity at which any given substance penetrates the skin, but it is now generally recognized that the skin is a semi-permeable membrane susceptible of penetration by substances to a greater or lesser degree (Lexicon Vevy 1993a). The physicochemical properties of the molecules, such as the molecular weight, spatial arrangement, polarity, optical activity, liposolubility, coefficients of diffusion and dissociation, are fundamental to skin penetration. Mills (1993) states that an advantage of the percutaneous route for remedies is the avoidance of the 'first-pass liver' effect, i.e. they are not subject to immediate metabolization by the liver as they are with oral administration.

The skin as a gateway

Because of their solubility in the lipids found in the stratum corneum, lipophilic substances (such as essential oils) are considered to be easily absorbed. The absorption of organic compounds with anionic or cationic groups (weak acids and alkalis) takes place when they are found in undissociated form – then they are more lipophilic than when dissociated; it

also depends on their dissociation constant and on the pH of the substance and of the skin. The majority of essential oils and their components pass through the skin and the organism (Valette 1945) and can be detected in exhaled air within 20–60 minutes (Katz 1947). Some examples of the times recorded are: 1,8-cineole and α-pinene take 20 minutes; eucalyptus, eugenol, linalyl acetate, geranyl acetate, anethole and thyme oil take between 20 and 40 minutes; bergamot, aniseed and lemon oils take between 40 and 60 minutes; true lavender, pine, geranium and citronella oils and cinnamaldehyde take between 60 and 80 minutes; coriander, rue and peppermint oils, geraniol and citrals take up to 2 hours.

Once the essential oil constituents have passed the epidermis and entered the complex of lymph and blood vessels, nerves, sweat and oil glands, follicles, collagen, fibroblasts, mast cells, elastin and so on (known as the dermis), they are then carried away in the circulation to pervade every cell in the body.

The main factors affecting the penetration of the skin by essential oils are detailed below.

Intrinsic factors

- **Area of skin.** The very large area of the skin – in the region of 2 m^2 – makes it possible for a significant quantity of essential oils to be applied and so taken into the body. If a set quantity of essential oil in a carrier is applied to a small area of skin, then less will enter than if the same quantity were to be applied to a greater area.
- **Thickness and permeability of the epidermis.** On palmar and plantar skin sites where the epidermis is quite thick and there are no oil glands, the time taken to cross the skin is longer, especially for any lipid-soluble components. There is less resistance to water-soluble components, however, e.g. garlic placed on the feet is soon detected on the exhaled breath. Easy penetration may occur on parts of the body where the skin is thinner, e.g. behind the ears, on the eyelids and inside the wrist. The skin regions of the legs, buttocks, trunk and abdomen are less permeable than are those of the soles, palms, forehead, scalp and armpits (Balacs 1993).
- **Gland openings and follicles.** Hydrophilic molecules can find a path through the skin using the sweat glands; lipophilic molecules may use the sebaceous glands as a pathway, also travelling between the cells through the fatty cement and through the cells themselves, all of which contain

lipids (Lexicon Vevy 1993b). The skin of the forehead and scalp contains numerous oil glands, and here the epidermis is thinner. This again makes for easy penetration of lipophilic substances, although the water layer on the skin must present a partial barrier for the lipophilic molecules. The number of follicles and sweat glands is another factor: generally speaking, the more openings the speedier the access. When sweating, because of a fever or after a sauna, for example, the body is exuding and ingress of essential oils is hindered.

- **Reservoirs.** Essential oils, being lipid soluble, gain access to lipid-rich areas of the body (Buchbauer 1993), therefore it is possible that they may be sequestered (stored apart) in the body, as happens in the plants that produce them. If so, there may be reservoirs of essential oils (or at least of some of their constituent molecules) in the outer layers of the epidermis and subcutaneous fat, and these may persist for some time. It is considered that lipophilic components can, at least temporarily, be retained in this layer and consequently will not be available for rapid diffusion to other adjacent levels (Lexicon Vevy 1993b). Subcutaneous fat has a poor blood supply, and although essential oils are slow to enter they probably tend to stay there for a long time. A Dutch Government Commission report in 1983 showed that many MAC (maximum acceptable concentrations) for toxic chemicals failed to take into account the significant physiological differences between the sexes. Women's skin is more permeable to toxic chemicals than that of men, and because they carry more fat, their body levels of fat-soluble chemicals are generally higher and take longer to disperse (Eisberg 1983).

- **Enzymes.** Enzymes in the skin can activate and inactivate many drugs and foreign compounds. They can also activate and inactivate the body's own natural chemicals, such as hormones, steroids and inflammatory mediators. The activities of these skin enzymes may vary greatly between individuals and with age (Hotchkiss 1994). The skin contains many enzymes and therefore provides a 'laboratory' where metabolism can take place. Certainly some enzymes will effect a change in some essential oil molecules, and even a slight change in molecular shape will mean a change in the effect on the body. In the case of some phthalic esters, enzymatic action effects complete metabolization during skin absorption; enzymes in the skin can either activate or inactivate drugs and other alien compounds, and there is great variation between individuals and with age. Bacterial action breaks down the triacylglycerides in sebum to organic free fatty acids and incompletely esterified glycerol derivatives, and it is reasonable to suppose that similar sorts of processes may happen with the essential oils.

- **Damaged skin.** Broken, inflamed and diseased skin is a poor barrier and ingress is rapid through cuts, abrasions, ulcers, psoriasis, burns etc. Aged skin and skin dehydrated through exposure to sunlight does not accept substances easily: some dermatological problems (e.g. ichthyosis) may also have this same effect.

Other physiological factors

- **Rate of circulation.** Where there is an increase in the rate of blood flow, perhaps due to rubbing (massage) or inflammation, there is an increased rate of absorption. Massage not only increases the speed of blood flow (causing hyperaemia) but also raises the local skin temperature slightly, hence we can expect an increased rate and degree of absorption of essential oils owing to the lowering of the viscosity and dilation of the blood vessels (Pratt & Mason 1981). Proof that essential oils in a base oil applied to the skin are absorbed into the bloodstream has been provided by Jäger et al. (1992) by the detection of linalyl acetate and linalool in a blood sample taken 5 minutes after the oil was applied.

- **Rate of distribution.** Concerning distribution, the speed of the lymph and blood circulation is a limiting factor because the circulation is slower in the capillary loops than in the veins. The speed may be increased, for example, by massage or by warmth (e.g. infrared). Both these methods may be used to increase the rate of distribution of essential oils. It has been proved that the blood vessels constantly resorb and expel terpenes so that a balance of flow results (Römmelt et al. 1974, Schilcher 1985).

External factors

- **Hydration.** Hydrated skin is very permeable, hence the effectiveness of what the editors term aromabalneotherapy (the use of essential oils in a bath). It has been shown that in a bath the essential oils penetrate the skin 100 times faster than does water and 10 000 times more quickly than do the ions of sodium and chloride (Römmelt et al. 1974). Conversely, if the stratum corneum is dehydrated its permeability is decreased.

- **Degreased skin.** Although detergents, degreasants, soaps etc. increase the permeability of the skin to essential oils, they are not necessarily recommended.
- **Warmth.** A warm room, warm oils, warm hands and warm body all help to speed up absorption. If the body is too warm (e.g. after exercise) it is exuding and eliminating, making ingress of oils difficult.
- **Occlusion.** Occlusion due to a covering, e.g. a compress, has a sealing-in effect and reduces the ability of the essential oils to volatilize, and aids warming. Oils applied under occlusion, as with all other substances, have an enhanced effect because of the increase in the quantity absorbed, due to local warming and reduced loss of molecules from the site of application due to evaporation: as evaporation is reduced, absorption may be increased (Bronaugh et al. 1990). Clothing may be regarded as being partially occlusive.

Oil-related factors

- **Viscosity.** All essential oils have a low viscosity, but some oils with a relatively high viscosity, e.g. sandalwood, which comprises 90% sesquiterpenols, will still cross the skin at a rate similar to other oils. Viscosity plays a more important part with regard to the carrier oils because some, such as hazelnut, are quite viscous and others, such as grapeseed and sunflower, are less so.
- **Molecular size.** If a substance's molecular weight exceeds 500 it is unlikely to pass the skin. Essential oils, being products of distillation, are limited to a maximum molecular weight of 225 (rarely reaching 250). In some cases it may be worth considering the use of a carrier that is partially hydrophilic (e.g. wheatgerm oil, walnut oil), even if to a small extent. The size and shape of the individual essential oil molecules also have a bearing on the speed at which they penetrate the skin. Small molecules pass easily down the follicular and sebaceous ducts, and the smaller the molecule the faster it penetrates. Dissociation may also be relevant. When dissolved in a carrier the essential oil molecules may split into ions, thereby becoming even tinier. The larger

molecules, being less volatile, are less likely to be lost to the atmosphere; they stay on the skin longer and therefore have a greater opportunity for penetration. Even though essential oils are quite volatile and evaporate from the warm surface of the skin, absorption may be 20–40% of the oil applied and up to double that, depending on the extent of occlusion.

- **Frequency of use.** There is some evidence that repeated use of the same oil makes the skin more permeable.
- **Carriers.** The carrier medium can have a significant effect on the absorption of essential oils (see Phototoxicity, Ch. 3 Part II). In a laboratory test using rat skin, the absorption of phenol was enhanced when a barrier cream was used; in humans, penetration of fragrance chemicals was increased when mixed with ethanol (Hotchkiss 1994). Saturated oil carriers such as lard, wool-fat and mineral oil (including some baby oils) all prevent or seriously delay absorption; the higher the degree of unsaturation of a fat the easier the absorption process becomes. Zatz (1993) found that when phenol was applied to the skin in a saturated fat the antiseptic effect was inhibited.

Methods of percutaneous absorption

Many of the techniques used on the skin entail the use of water, vegetable oil or a bland lotion to dilute and spread the essential oils.

Compresses

Compresses are sometimes required on open wounds such as leg ulcers, bedsores, boils etc., and on bruising or areas of severe localized pain such as arthritis, stomach pain, fractures etc. A non-adherent silicon dressing should be used on ulcers, and a low-adherent absorbent dressing on open wounds. The size of compress, number of drops of essential oils and amount of water used are dependent upon the size of the area to be treated. A septic finger requires only a minuscule square of the dressing material chosen, and an eggcupful of water to which two drops of essential oil have been added, whereas a swollen rheumatic knee would require a piece of cloth large enough to cover the swelling, and a small basinful of water (about 200 ml) containing five to six drops of essential oils. As always, the quantities of essential oil should be halved for children and the elderly.

Case study 6.1

Back and menstrual pain

A. Windsor – Aromatherapist

Client assessment

Edna had suffered lower back pain during the last 3 months of her first pregnancy, and this had recurred since the birth, albeit less intense and not so frequent. When her periods recommenced, they were usually preceded by a headache and accompanied by menstrual pain for the first 2 days. She did not want medication, but approached her GP, whom she knew accepted aromatherapy for certain disorders; after showing her the proposed treatment plan, the GP was happy for Edna to go ahead, so long as she reported back after a month, whether or not the results were beneficial.

Intervention

Back massage, abdominal massage and compress were the treatments decided upon, the abdomen being massaged first, after which a compress was placed under Edna's abdomen, on a warm towel, while her back was massaged – her weight keeping the compress in place.

Equal quantities of the following oils were chosen for both massage and compress treatments:

- *Angelica archangelica* rad. [angelica] – antispasmodic, sedative
- *Chamaemelum nobile* [Roman chamomile] – anti-inflammatory, antispasmodic, calming, menstrual (dysmenorrhoea), sedative

- *Pelargonium graveolens* [geranium] – analgesic, anti-inflammatory, antispasmodic, decongestant
- *Salvia sclarea* [clary] – decongestant, hormone regulator

For the massage, 2 drops of each were used in 10 ml sweet almond oil and 3 drops of each in 200 ml warm water for the compress.

Edna was given 4 drops of each of the above oils in 50 ml carrier oil for her husband to apply to her back, and herself to her abdomen each night. Edna herself was shown how to prepare a compress to use the 3–4 nights before her period was expected, being given a 10 ml bottle of the blended essential oils she needed for this.

- Treatment 2: 1 month later, Edna said she had felt more relaxed and the headache she had had at the start of her period had been less intense, as had her period pain.
- Treatment 3: 1 month later, there had been no headaches or back pain, so the compress was omitted from the treatment and the next appointment was made for 2 months' time.

Outcome

After 4 months there was still no pain during menstruation and the backache had not recurred.

The chosen material should be immersed in the mixture (well stirred) of water and essential oil, squeezed gently and placed over the required area. It should be covered in the normal manner, and a piece of Clingfilm can be ideal as a first layer to prevent evaporation of the essential oils. The compress should be left on for about 2 hours, or overnight if practicable. Some therapists apply essential oils diluted in a vegetable oil, if the skin is unbroken, and then cover it. During the 1914–1918 war other media used for wet dressings on large wounds with considerable tissue loss were ether and ointment bases, into which the essential oils were mixed (Valnet 1980 p. 67). For open wounds a cream or lotion base can be applied directly to the dressing.

Sprays

The spray method mentioned above can also be used as a method of application when the client cannot be touched, e.g. severe burns, zoster or wounds. A higher

concentration is needed when treating burns this way, e.g. 15–20 drops in 50 ml of distilled or sterilized water. Appropriate essential oils in this case are *Citrus limon* [lemon], *Lavandula angustifolia* [lavender], *L. x intermedia* 'Super' [lavandin], *Matricaria recutita* [German chamomile], *Melaleuca viridiflora* [niaouli] and *Pelargonium graveolens* [geranium].

Baths

A valuable method of use involving water and inhalation is the addition of six to eight drops of essential oils to the bath water after running it to the correct temperature. This amount in a bathful of water can appear to be too little, but it must be borne in mind that skin penetration is increased 100 times in this method and that inhalation also plays a significant part. Some advise adding the essential oils to another medium first, such as vegetable oil, dried milk, high-proof vodka, bubble bath mix etc. Albeit useful for certain skin conditions, vegetable oil is not necessary in most circumstances (and it can leave an oily ring on the bath which is difficult to remove).

Case study 6.2

Leg ulcers

P Price – Aromatologist

Client assessment

Joe, a widower aged 91, was retired and lived alone. He had few hobbies except cleaning his house and working in his garden, taking little exercise apart from these activities. His diet was simple yet sufficient.

Joe had a leg ulcer which was being treated with compression bandages by a community nurse once a week. She was reluctant to give information on the dressing used.

Presenting symptoms

The ulcer was 3 inches in diameter, situated on the outside calf of the left leg. Joe had been told that he could not expect any improvement because everything possible was being done for him, and the condition had remained static for some considerable time.

Intervention

For the first week of treatment essential oils were to be used in distilled water in a spray. The four oils selected were:
- 15 drops *Citrus bergamia* [bergamot] – anti-infectious, cicatrizant
- 20 drops *Commiphora myrrha* [myrrh] – anti-inflammatory, antiseptic, cictrizant
- 25 drops *Lavandula angustifolia* [lavender] – analgesic, anti-inflammatory, antiseptic, cicatrizant
- 10 drops *Melaleuca alternifolia* [tea tree] – analgesic, anti-inflammatory
- 100 ml warm water

The oils were selected very carefully for their constituent properties, which collectively addressed the pain, the infection and the healing.

After consultation with the doctor it was agreed that for the aromatherapy intervention the bandage could remain off for 3 days during the daytime, being replaced at night.

First visit (morning): Joe's wound was sprayed when the nurse removed his bandage (shaking the bottle well before use), Joe himself spraying the leg himself at intervals six times during the day (thereby becoming involved in his own care) until the nurse replaced the bandage at night. This was repeated each day.

Second visit (evening 3 days later): after these 3 days the commencement of healing was evident. Wearing protective gloves, the same synergy of essential oils was applied directly to the wound (in a 3% dilution using Calendula as a carrier) before the nurse applied the compression bandage. This was to be left for a week until the next bandage. During this week Joe's feet were massaged every day with the same blend, resulting in a noticed improvement in the circulation.

Third evening visit: The above procedure was repeated.

Outcome

After 3 months the ulcer was closed, the only evidence of it having been there being a small area of discoloured skin, which later improved.

Joe was consistent in the use of his oil blend once a day for the rest of his life and the ulcer did not recur. The quality of Joe's life was greatly improved as a result of the treatment – not least because his improved mobility meant he could work again in his beloved garden.

Although the essential oils are not completely soluble in water, it is a simple matter to disperse them by agitating the water vigorously (efficiently, so no globules can get into the eyes). For water births the essential oils are best dissolved first in a small amount of powdered milk (adding enough water to make a thin paste). Blend three to four drops in honey or dried milk for children and the elderly. For maximum benefit, the patient should remain in the bath for 10 minutes.

Foot, hand and sitz baths

It is sometimes easier to use a washing-up bowl for bathing individual areas – the sitz bath, for example, is ideal for haemorrhoids and stitches after childbirth. Three to four drops of essential oils are needed and hot water should be available to keep the bath warm during the 10 minutes. Arthritic hands and ankles can be treated in this way.

Topical application

Application means the 'putting on' of oils, either for self-use or via a third party. Treatment by massage employs an organized routine using specific movements to achieve specific aims, e.g. lymph drainage, relaxation etc. Aromatherapists mostly employ essential oils with massage, covered in Ch. 7 together with massage techniques suitable for nurses to administer without having qualified in whole-body massage.

There is not usually time for a nurse to spend an hour or more giving a patient an aromatherapy treatment but they do have time to apply a prepared oil or lotion on the relevant area daily. It takes no longer than giving other forms of medication and adds the magic of touch and care to the prescription.

The normal dilution is 15–20 drops in 50 ml of suitable carrier oil or lotion, but for the very young, the elderly, heavily medicated or those with learning difficulties half this amount is advised. When essential oils are to be applied daily, it is less messy to dilute them in a non-greasy lotion base of emulsified oil and water (garments and bed linen can become permanently soiled by vegetable oil). A number of rheumatology wards apply an aromatherapy lotion as part of the daily treatment, resulting in a reduction in the use of painkillers. For effectiveness in certain conditions, e.g. lowered immune system activity or toxic build-up, an essential oil lotion should be applied liberally to the lymph node areas such as the armpits and groin.

The significance of macerated carrier oils

It is worth taking care to select a carrier oil which is of holistic and/or symptomatic use, e.g. one of the macerated oils. Lime blossom carrier oil can help to induce sleep or soothe rheumatic pain; carrot or hypericum oils will help to reduce skin inflammation or accelerate the healing of burns; calendula or hypericum oils will help to soothe and heal bruising; and calendula, hypericum or rosehip carrier oils will relieve skin rashes etc. (Price 2000, Price et al. 1999). The quantity of essential oil added should be the same as when using a basic carrier oil.

Fixed oils and skin penetration

It has generally been considered that triacylglycerol molecules are too large to penetrate the skin, but tests on rat skin suggested that oils of linseed, safflower and avocado were of interest in carrying active substances into the skin (Valette & Sobrin 1963).

Essential fatty acid deficiency is recognized as a complication of long-term fat-free parenteral nutrition, and consideration has been given to the use of cutaneously applied vegetable oils as a way of avoiding this problem. Sunflower seed oil was used on three patients who had developed essential fatty acid deficiency after major intestinal resections (Press,

Hartop & Prottey 1974, Prottey, Hartop & Press 1975). The deficiency was corrected by topical application of 2–3 mg of the oil per kg of body weight per day for 12 weeks. Friedman et al. (1976) reported the correction of essential fatty acid deficiency in two infants given 1400 mg/kg per day of topically applied sunflower oil. In order for the essential fatty acid to be made available the molecules of triacylglycerol have to undergo hydrolysis. This implies that the topically applied oil has been metabolized and so skin penetration has taken place. In a report assessing the safety of sweet almond oil it is stated that pharmacological studies reveal that sweet almond oil is slowly absorbed through intact skin (Expert Panel 1983). Sweet almond oil has been used as a solvent for parenterally administered drugs (Hizon & Huyck 1956).

Miller et al. (1987) examined the use of safflower oil on five patients and deduced that topical application may improve plasma fatty acid profiles, but the adequacy of tissue stores remained unanswered. However, other investigators have reported that essential fatty acid deficiency cannot be influenced by cutaneously applied vegetable oils (Hunt et al. 1978, McCarthy et al. 1983, O'Neill, Caldwell & Meng 1976).

Clearly, uncertainty remains. However, there is evidence that oils rich in bonded essential fatty acids do benefit the skin. A deficiency in essential fatty acids increases transepidermal water loss, resulting in dryness; this may be corrected by the topical application of borage and evening primrose oils for 14 days, with a resulting 2% increase in the level of γ-linolenic acid in the stratum corneum (Hoffmann-La Roche 1989) (see Fixed oils in Ch. 8).

Internal pathway

Ingestion

There is no research comparing percutaneous absorption with the gastrointestinal route (Torii et al. 1991); however, ingestion is the main route employed by aromatologists and doctors in France for essential oils to enter the body, but it is not widely used by aromatherapists in other countries. Most aromatherapists are cautious about using ingestion because of the increased danger of an excessive dose reaching the liver than by external application. Further, there is the possibility of the essential oil molecules being changed by digestive enzymes, strong acids and metabolization. Nevertheless, the editors have used essential oils in this way for three decades for sore throats, stomach upsets, cystitis and constipation, with no reported adverse effects. The potential effectiveness of essential oils can be increased because the digestive system extends from the mouth to the anus. The digestive system is the source of many skin, lung and ENT problems and aromatherapy can have useful effects when administered in this way, and an aromatherapy treatment should, on occasion, include a blend for the digestive route. Repetitive antibiotic treatments and some food diets cause an imbalance in the intestinal flora and essential oils serve to redress this.

In the UK and elsewhere there are wide variations in training standards, ranging from those designed for simple beauty therapy to that enabling a therapist to practise clinical aromatherapy/aromatology. Therapists who have successfully completed an advanced training in aromatic medicine (aromatology) are in a position to advise the use of essential oils by this method.

Using the internal pathway, every drop of oil used reaches the body systems, unlike inhalation, when only a tiny amount of essential oil vapour enters the body, and unlike external application, where a proportion of the essential oils is lost by evaporation.

Methods of ingestion

By mouth (see also Ch. 3 Part I)

When essential oils are taken by mouth, knowledge of the constituents of the oils used is of paramount importance. This is not to say that an oil containing a potentially hazardous component cannot be ingested – these components are sometimes effective for certain disorders. It means that it is essential to determine the strength of concentration, the nature of any diluent used and the length of time for which it is to be taken. Alcohol and honey water are the most usual diluents (Valnet 1980), though vegetable oils (such as hazelnut and olive oils) are excellent for this purpose and are preferred by many doctors and naturopaths practising in France who have studied phytotherapy and are experienced in prescribing essential oils for internal use. Special dispersants are available for use to ensure that essential oils dissolve thoroughly in an excipient, including water. A rough

guide to the maximum safe dose is three drops, three times a day, for 3 weeks (see Ch. 3 Part I), although the client and the particular oils used must be considered. As mentioned above, all the oil is taken into the body via ingestion, so **extra training is essential**. This method is not harmful, but ingestion continued for too long can eventually lead to toxic build-up in the liver: this is particularly true of the powerful oils. It is for this reason that after 3 weeks a rest from the oils is advised to allow the liver the opportunity to eliminate any accumulated toxic matter.

The digestive pathway is of major importance in the treatment of serious conditions and indications for use of this route given by Franchomme and Pénoël (2001 p 317) are:

- diseases and infections of the digestive organs and tissues
- liver diseases and urinary tract (enterohepatorenal)
- diseases and infections of the pelvis (rectal)
- cardiopulmonary (orally: lymphatic circulation, and rectal: enterohepatic cardiopulmonary)

Case study 6.3

Spondolytis

Sarah Gelzer – Aromatologist

Client assessment (self)

S was hospitalized with complete bed rest for 8 weeks with inflammation of the spinal vertebrae and discs caused by *Staphylococcus* infection, which literally ate away pieces of the lumbar vertebrae. She was given 6 g antibiotics intravenously every day.

Intervention

Being an aromatologist, S made an essential oil mix to compensate for – and support – the effects of the antibiotics. Equal quantities of the following essential oils were mixed and 3 drops blended with honey were taken in a cup of herbal tea three times a day for 8 weeks:

- *Melaleuca alternifolia* [tea tree] – analgesic, antibacterial, anti-infectious, anti-inflammatory, immunostimulant
- *Origanum vulgare* [origanum] – anti-infectious, immunostimulant
- *Satureia montana* [savory] – analgesic, antibacterial, anti-infectious, immunostimulant
- *Syzygium aromaticum* [clove bud] – analgesic, antibacterial, anti-infectious, anti-inflammatory, immunostimulant

Case study 6.3

Spondolytis—cont'd

- *Thymus vulgaris* ct. *phenol* [thyme] – antibacterial, anti-infectious

Two other forms of treatment were followed:

- Application of a lotion daily to the part of the back S could easily reach, containing:
- *Melaleuca alternifolia*, properties as above
- *Thymus vulgaris* ct. *geraniol* – anti-infectious, anti-inflammatory, neurotonic
- *Ravensara aromatica* [ravensara] – antibacterial, anti-infectious, anti-inflammatory, neurotonic
- *Eucalyptus smithii* [gully gum] – analgesic, anti-infectious, balancing
- Swiss Reflex Treatment – a Swiss Reflex cream using the same oils as for the lotion above was used daily to massage the spinal reflexes.

Outcome

S was taken off the oral antibiotics 2 months earlier than normal and the intravenous antibiotics were stopped 3 weeks earlier than in most spondylodiscitis cases.

The general vitality level was better throughout than previous cases treated by the hospital.

In addition there were no side effects and S was in very good spirits, which amazed the medical team. S was the first person who did not need valium, as she had virtually no pain.

- in long-term treatments, bearing in mind the above advice
- for rapid action (sublingual: honey, lozenges and alcoholic solutions)
- for people intolerant or allergic to essential oils on the skin and in aerosols.

Many conventional drugs are given by mouth because they are usually tasteless and do not cause irritation. The tongue enables access to the venous circulation on its lower surface, and here the essential oils must be used in trace amounts. The advantage of the sublingual route is that the aromatic molecules pass directly into the bloodstream, bypassing the liver filter. If the taste is tolerable and there is no risk of irritation, the aromatic preparation (honey, Disper solution, vegetable oil etc.) can profitably be kept under the tongue for a few minutes. Some essential oils have an unpleasant odour, some taste quite bitter, and some may irritate the mucous lining; for this reason essential oils to be taken by mouth are frequently put into capsules.

Aromatherapists often advocate tisanes (herbal teas), and although these can be helpful they are not the same as essential oils in composition and do not have the same action. Whatever the occasional drawbacks, oral intake remains a major route in serious aromatherapy treatments, in particular with regard to action on the intestinal bacterial flora (Franchomme & Pénoël 2001 p 321).

Gargles and mouthwashes

After the removal of tonsils or complicated dental surgery, gargling with essential oils helps to relieve any pain or inflammation, stem blood flow and aid healing; at the same time the oils are antiseptic to the mucous surfaces. Two to three drops in quarter of a tumbler of water is all that is needed, the most important rule to follow being that the water should be well stirred before each mouthful to disperse the essential oils each time. For children, blend one drop only of essential oil in a teaspoonful of honey before adding the water. *Syzygium aromaticum* (flos) [clove bud] is the essential oil most used for pain in this context (see also Appendices on the CD-ROM).

Per rectum or per vaginam

Another method of internal use is by means of suppositories, which can be useful in cases of irritable bowel syndrome, haemorrhoids, pulmonary catarrh etc., and the use of pessaries for vaginal infections, candida etc. Suppositories, albeit not much favoured in the UK, allow the essential oils direct access to the bloodstream with little chance of metabolization. The maximum dose for suppositories and pessaries is six drops. Neurotoxic or irritant essential oils should not be used, and undiluted essential oils must on no account be used in the rectum. After aromatology training therapists should be confident in using this method.

Summary

This chapter has identified the principal routes by which essential oils can enter the body – and the principal hindrances. Detailed information has been given so that the aromatherapist can select the optimum pathway to achieve the desired therapeutic effect.

References

Almiral, M., Montana, J., Escribano, E.,
Obach, R., Berrozpe, J.D., 1996.
Effect of *d*-limonene, α-pinene and
cineole on the *in vitro* transdermal
human skin penetration of
chlorpromazine and haloperidol.
Arzneimittelforschung 46 (7),
676–680.

Anthony, C.P., Thibodeau, G.A., 1983.
Nervous system cells in anatomy and
physiology. Mosby, St Louis.

Balacs, T., 1993. Essential oils in the
body. In: Aroma '93 Conference
Proceedings. Aromatherapy
Publications, Brighton, pp. 12–13.

Bronaugh, R.L., Webster, R.C.,
Bucks, D., Maibach, H.I., Sarason, R.,
1990. In vivo percutaneous absorption
of fragrance ingredients in rhesus
monkeys and humans. Food Chem.
Toxicol. 28 (5), 369–373.

Brun, K., 1952. Les essences végétales en
tant qu'agent de pénétration
tissulaire. Thèse Pharmacie,
Strasbourg.

Buchbauer, G., 1988. Aromatherapy: do
essential oils have therapeutic
properties? In: International
Conference on Essential Oils,
Flavours, Fragrances and Cosmetics,
Beijing. International Federation of
Essential Oils and Aroma Trades,
London, pp. 351–352.

Buchbauer, G., 1993. Molecular
interaction. Int. J. Aromather. 5 (1),
11–14.

Cleary, G., 1993. Transdermal drug
delivery. In: Zatz, J.L. (Ed.), Skin
permeation: fundamentals and
applications. Allured, Wheaton,
pp. 207–237.

Cornwall, P.A., Barry, B.W., 1994. 456
Sesquiterpene components of volatile
oils as skin penetration enhancers for
the hydrophilic permeant 5
fluorouracil. J. Pharm. Pharmacol.
46 (4), 261–269.

Cornwall, P.A., Barry, B.W., Bouwstra,
J.A., Gooris, G.S., 1996. Modes of
action of terpene penetration
enhancers in human skin:
differential scanning calorimetry,
small angle X-ray diffraction and
enhancer uptake studies. Int. J.
Pharm. 127, 9–26.

Eisberg, N., 1983. Male chauvinism in
toxicity testing? Manufacturing
Chemist 3 (July), 3.

Expert Panel 1983. Cosmetic ingredient
review: 4 : Final report on the safety of
sweet almond oil and almond meal.
Journal of the American College of
Toxicology 2 (5), 85–89.

Franchomme, P., Pénoël, D., 2001.
L'aromathérapie exactement. In:
Jollois, Limoges (Eds.),
l'aromathérapie exactement.

Friedman, Z., Shochat, S., Maisels, M.,
Marks, K., Lamberth, E., 1976.
Correction of essential fatty acid
deficiency in newborn infants
by cutaneous application of sunflower
seed oil. Pediatrics 58, 650–654.

Hizon, R.P., Huyck, C.L., 1956. The
stability of almond and corn oils for
use in parenteral solutions. J. Am.
Pharm. Assoc. 45, 145–150.

Hoffmann-La Roche, 1989. Information
leaflet HHN–5379A/589.

Hotchkiss, S., 1994. How thin is your
skin? New Sci. 141 (1910), 24–27.

Hunt, C.E., Engel, R.R., Modler, S.,
Hamilton, W., Bissen, S.,
Holman, R.T., 1978. Essential fatty
acid deficiency in neonates: inability
to reverse deficiency by topical
application of EFA-rich oil. J. Pediatr.
92 (4), 603–607.

Jackson, E., 1993. Toxicological aspects
of percutaneous absorption. In:
Zatz, J.L. (Ed.), Skin permeation:
fundamentals and applications.
Allured, Wheaton, pp. 177–193.

Jäger, W., Buchbauer, G., Jirovetz, L.,
Fritzer, M., 1992. Percutaneous
absorption of lavender oil from a
massage oil. J. Soc. Cosmet. Chem.
43 (1), 49–54.

Jain, R., Aqil, M., Ahad, A., Ali, A.,
Khar, K., 2008. Basil oil is a
promisinbg skin penetration enhancer
for transdermal delivery of labetolol
hydrochloride. Drug Dev. Ind.
Pharm. 34 (4), 384–389.

Katz, A.E., 1947. Parfümerie Modern
39, 64.

Lexicon Vevy, 1993a. La peau: siége
d'absorption et organ cible. Skin Care
Instant Reports (Vevy Europe,
Genova). 10 (4), 35–41.

Lexicon Vevy, 1993b. La peau: siége
d'absorption et organ cible. Skin Care
Instant Reports (Vevy Europe,
Genova). 10 (6), 68.

Macht, D., 1938. The absorption of drugs
and poisons through the skin and

mucous membranes. J. Am. Med.
Assoc. 110, 409–414.

Maibach, H.I., Marzulli, F.N., 1977.
Toxicologic perspectives of
chemicals commonly applied to
skin. In: Drill, V.A., Lazar, P. (Eds.),
Cutaneous toxicity. Academic Press,
New York.

McCarthy, M.C., Turner, W.,
Whatley, K., Cottam, G., 1983.
Topical corn oil in the management of
essential fatty acid deficiency. Crit.
Care Med. 5, 373–375.

Miller, D.G., Williams, S.K., Palombo, J.
D., Griffin, R.E., Bistrian, B.R.,
Blackburn, G.L., 1987. Cutaneous
application of safflower oil in
preventing essential fatty acid
deficiency in patients on home
parenteral nutrition. Am. J. Clin.
Nutr. 46, 419–423.

Mills, S., 1993. The essential book of
herbal medicine. In: Penguin, London,
p. 333, 334.

Monti, D.P., Chetoni, P., Burgalassi, S.,
Najarro, M., Saettone, M.F.,
Boldrini, E., 2002. Effect of different
terpene containing essential oils on
permeation of estradiol through
hairless mouse skin. International
Journal of Pharmacy 237 (1–2),
209–214.

O'Neill, J.A., Caldwell, M.D., Meng, H.
C., 1976. Essential fatty acid
deficiency in surgical patients. Ann.
Surg. 185 (5), 535–541.

Pratt, J., Mason, A., 1981. The caring
touch. Heyden, London.

Press, M., Hartop, P.J., Prottey, C.,
1974. Correction of essential
fatty acid deficiency in man by
the cutaneous application of
sunflower- seed oil. Lancet 6
(April), 597–599.

Price, L., Price, S., 2008. Carrier oils for
aromatherapy. Riverhead, Stratford
on Avon.

Price, S., 2000. The aromatherapy
workbook. In: Thorsons, London,
pp. 162–172.

Prottey, C., Hartop, P.J., Press, M.,
1975. Correction of the cutaneous
manifestations of fatty acid deficiency
in man by application of sunflower
seed oil to the skin. J. Invest.
Dermatol. 64 (4), 228–234.

Riviere, J.E., 1993. Biological factors
in absorption and permeation.

In: Zatz, J.L. (Ed.), Skin permeation: fundamentals and applications. Allured, Wheaton, pp. 113–125.

Römmelt, H., Zuber, A., Dirnagl, K., Drexel, H., 1974. Münchner Medezin Wochenschrift 116, 537.

Schilcher, H., 1985. Effects and side effects of essential oils. In: Baerheim Svendsen, A., Scheffer, J.J. C. (Eds.), Essential oils and aromatic plants. Kluwer Academic, Dordrecht, p. 218.

Shen, Q., Hu, J., Xu, L., 2001. Effect of cinnamon oil and other colatile oils on percutaneous absorption of benzoic acid. Zhongguo Yiyuan Yaoxue Zazhi 21 (4), 197–199.

Shen, Q., Li, W., Li, W., 2007. The effect of clove oil on the transdermal delivery of Ibuprufen in the rabbit by *in vitro* and *in vivo* methods. Drug Dev. Ind. Pharm. 33 (12), 1369–1374.

Stoughton, R.B., 1959. Relation of the anatomy of normal and abnormal skin to its protective function. In:

Rothman, S. (Ed.), The human integument, normal and abnormal. American Association for the Advancement of Science, 3–24.

Takayama, K., Nagai, T., 1994. Limonene and related compounds as potential skin penetration promoters. Drug Dev. Ind. Pharm. 20 (4), 677–684.

Torii, S., Fukada, H., Kanemoto, H., Miyanchi, R., Hamauzu, Y., Kawasaki, M., 1991. Contingent negative variation (CNV) and the psychological effects of odour. In: Van Toller, S., Dodd, G. (Eds.), Perfumery: the psychology and biology of fragrance. Chapman & Hall, London, pp. 107–118.

Valette, C., 1945. Pénétration transcutanée des essences. Comptes Rendues Société Biologique.

Valette, G., Sobrin, E., 1963. Percutaneous absorption of various animal and vegetable oils. Pharmica Acta Helvetica 38 (10), 710–716.

Valnet, J., 1980. The practice of aromatherapy. Daniel, Saffron Walden.

Van Toller, S., 1993. The sensory evaluation of odours. Paper on clinical practitioner's course. Shirley Price International College of Aromatherapy, Hinckley.

Weyers, W., Brodbeck, R., 1989. Skin absorption of volatile oils. Pharmacokinetics. Pharm. Unserer Zeit 18 (3), 82–86.

Williams, A.C., Barry, B.W., 1989. Essential oils as novel human skin penetration enhancers. Int. J. Pharm. 57, R7–R9.

Winter, R., 1984. A consumer's dictionary of cosmetic ingredients. Crown, New York.

Zatz, J.L., 1993. Modification of skin permeation by solvents. In: Zatz, J.L. (Ed.), Skin permeation: fundamentals and applications. Allured, Wheaton, pp. 127–148.

Aromas, mind and body

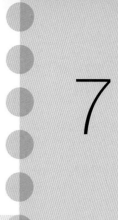

Len Price

Introduction

Smell is the most mysterious and evocative of our
senses: it is our chemical sense, informing us about
the surrounding environment and giving information
that is not tangible, visible or audible. This chapter
explores the connections between a person's thoughts,
feelings and immune status, and suggests that the ability
of essential oils to affect all these via the sense of smell
makes aromatherapy a truly holistic therapy.

The impact of the mind and emotions on the body

Throughout the ages people concerned with healing
have been aware that there is a connection between
thoughts, emotions and the state of health of the physical body. The *British Medical Journal* in 1884 observed
that 'the depression of the spirits at these melancholy
occasions (funerals) ... disposes them to some of the
worst effects of the chills' (Wood 1990a). These effects
can be real, and changes in blood chemistry have been
recorded even when the emotions are conjured up artificially, as in the case of superstition. Three thousand
years ago the impact and influence of the intangible human mind on the material body was recorded in the Old
Testament: 'A merry heart doeth good like a medicine;
but a broken spirit drieth the bones' (Proverbs 17: 22,
King James version).

In modern times this has been recognized not only
by psychotherapists and those in psychosomatic
medicine, but also in general medicine.

> The way we assess situations determines our emotional
> responses to them. Emotions release hormones and
> hormones can influence immunity. In the last analysis it
> is the way we think and feel that triggers the immune
> change.
>
> Wood (1990b)

Psychoneuroimmunology (PNI)

In the past the psyche, the nervous system and the immune system were studied more or less as independent systems functioning alongside each other, but without direct connections. The science of PNI attempts to understand how the brain and the immune system communicate with each other,

the intercommunicating system of chemical messengers,

the interconnections via nerve tissue and

the effects and interactions with one another.

PNI is also referred to as psychoendoneuroimmunology (PENI).

The immune system

Neuropeptide messengers produced by the immune system, brain and nerve cells provide two-way communication between the emotional brain and bodily systems via hormonal feedback loops. The limbic system (hypothalamus and pituitary), the spleen, the adrenal and thymus glands all have nerve interconnections. Thus emotions are capable not only of directing the body but also of receiving and being modified by information feedback from cells in the body.

Adrenalin and cortisol are two of the many chemical messengers whose release can be triggered by negative emotion in sudden or long-term stress: these two hormones influence the immune system directly to switch it off (Borysenko 1988 p. 14). Adrenocorticotrophic hormone (ACTH) suppresses pituitary action by stimulating the adrenal gland to produce adrenaline (epinephrine), which is a stimulator of the autonomic nervous system (ANS). The idea has gradually gained ground that emotional states can translate into altered responses in the immune system: negative thoughts and sad emotions can sometimes temporarily lessen the effectiveness of the immune system. Hence the body puts non-material thoughts and emotions into physical effect, either to produce a beneficial healing effect or to inflict self-damage. This idea is echoed by many writers.

The effect of the emotions on health

It has not yet been possible for anyone to show a link between a particular emotion and any specific physical disease – 'Pessimism is not linked to any particular disease' (Wood 1990b) – although pessimism or depression amplify symptoms of pain. It can probably be said that the course of nearly all disease is affected by thoughts, feelings, emotions and attitudes, which are in turn influenced by personality.

Fight-or-flight response

In the distant past people developed a response to dangerous situations designed to protect the body, known as the automatic primary stress response; the arousal system is located in the brain stem. When a person is presented with a threatening set of circumstances, the median hemisphere of the hypothalamus instantly puts chemical messengers (catecholamines) into the bloodstream. In conjunction with the sympathetic nervous system, these trigger an array of interconnected reactions – the release of steroids, glycogen and adrenaline, faster breathing, increased heart rate, raised blood pressure, dilated pupils and so on – all designed to prepare the body for instant action resulting from the awareness of danger. Today, this ancient inbuilt fight-or-flight response is evoked many times, not only in response to short-term acute physical risk (e.g. war, traffic, mugging etc.) but also to threats such as job security, divorce and money problems. Long-term stress conditions like these make the traditional response unsuitable: not only it is ineffective, but it can harm the body it is supposed to protect. The high-pressure lifestyle lived by so many people is responsible for many health-threatening situations, both chronic and acute, and it is now generally recognized that some physical problems in our society have a non-physical component in their aetiology. 'It is not a question of whether an illness is physical or emotional, but how much of each' (Dunbar 1954).

Anticipation stress

Why stress should have the effect of reducing the body's defences is not clear and is, as yet, unexplained, but it is known that students are prone to catch colds at examination times and that such times of stress reduce the efficiency of the immune system, as a result of lowered production of interferon leading to decreased function of natural killer cells. Some of the more ambitious students suffer a greater reduction in the immune system defences, perhaps because the examination represents a bigger threat to them (Borysenko 1988 pp. 12–16). The effects of stress of this kind are popularly recognized in the case of brides-to-be who may catch a 'bride's cold'.

Grief

Statistics exist for various stressful situations that make people more prone to accidents and poor health, e.g. divorce, marriage, holidays, death etc. Depression following the death of a spouse is likely to have an adverse effect on the protective immune system and the health of the survivor: there are 50% more deaths than would normally be expected in widowers during the first year after the loss.

Voluntary stress

Although repeated stressful situations may produce ill effects resulting in chronic illness, many people joyfully expose themselves to repeated stress with no apparent ill effect, e.g. mountaineering, car racing and skiing. It is when repeated stress is unwanted and creates unhappiness that it will have unwanted effects; on the other hand, if the repeated stressful situations are sought and enjoyed, they can bring beneficial effects. In sporting contexts the euphoria resulting from the release of endorphins is recognized, for instance 'runner's high'.

Thinking and healing

Using the mind to control pulse rate and breathing, and to bring about general relaxation of the body, has long been practised in different cultures. In the meditative state the brain waves drop from the β rhythm to the slower α rhythm; the blood circulation is diverted more to the brain and vital organs, with less going to the muscles, so that the heart rate is slower, blood pressure is lower and little oxygen is used.

Case study 7.1

Death and bereavement

M Cadwallader – Nurse aromatherapist

Client assessment

B, a 61–year–old man, was battling severe pain from cancer of the lung and he and his wife were but slowly coming to terms with the fact that his life would not be prolonged.

Intervention

The essential oils used to assist and comfort were put into a 10 mL dropper bottle:

- 2 mL (40 drops) *Boswellia carteri* [frankincense] – analgesic (to mental pain and fear also), antidepressive, energizing, immunostimulant
- 2 mL *Chamaemelum nobile* [Roman chamomile] – calming and sedative (easing anxiety, tension, anger and fear)
- 10 drops *Rosa damascena* [rose otto] – general tonic, neurotonic, balancing and calming to the mind

A few drops of this was applied to the soles of his feet and put on tissue to inhale. 15 drops were put into almond oil for hand, foot and back massages.

The therapist worked closely with him and his family in the hospital setting, his wife carrying a tissue with a drop of rose oil – she claimed it helped her accept the inevitable.

Outcome

His feeling of relaxation and peace was evident and he claimed he also slept well for a couple of nights after a treatment.

After he passed away – peacefully – the following blend was provided to help the family cope with the bereavement, oils to relieve grief being analgesic, calming, healing and stimulating to the heart and mind:

- 1 drop *Melissa officinalis* [melissa] – calming, sedative, uplifting to the emotions, a good pick-me-up after shock
- 3 drops *Origanum majorana* [marjoram] – analgesic, calming, neurotonic, strengthening to the mind
- 1 drop *Rosa damascena* [rose otto] – cicatrizant, as well as having the properties above
- 8 mL of lime blossom carrier oil – analgesic, relaxing

This blend was used by the family for self-massage around the neck and shoulders every night and morning. B's mother thanked the therapist, saying that she was sure it had helped her to accept and adjust.

All this is initiated by thought alone, effected via the hypothalamus. Hesse, experimenting on cats in the 1950s, found that when the hypothalamus was stimulated, increased activity or relaxation was produced (Hesse & Akerl 1955). Sometimes, in people suffering a terminal illness, this mind-to-body effect can make healing possible even though a cure is not.

It is now realized that for optimum healing the sufferer must be fully involved in all stages of the treatment, from diagnosis to final cure, and that all true healing comes from within. Healing is accomplished by mental and physical routes, with primary roles played by the patient, doctor and nurse, while family and friends take secondary supportive parts. As Plato wrote in the third century BC:

> The curing of the part should not be attempted without treatment of the whole. No attempt should be made to cure the body without the soul and if the head and the body are to be healthy, you must begin by curing the mind. . . . For this is the great error of our day in the treatment of the human body, that physicians first separate the soul from the body.

Trust and placebo

Another well-known example of the effect of thought on the physical body is the placebo effect. This happens when the cure or amelioration of an illness is due to the patient's trust and belief in a pre-scribed substance, to faith in the healer, or frequently a combination of both. Dummy painkillers are 56% as effective as morphine in the treatment of severe chronic pain (Chaitow 1991). This remarkable and much-used placebo effect is important in all healing: when people are made to feel better, positive healing thoughts, which encourage the healing process, are generated. If an aromatherapy treatment does no more than make people feel better in themselves, it puts the whole person into healing mode.

'Immunity is to some degree under mental con-trol' (Wood 1990a). Just as positive healing thoughts induce healing reactions in the body, the efficiency of the immune system is reduced by negative beliefs and thoughts. Immunity from disease appears to be enhanced or diminished by beliefs, and by the envi-ronment in so far as it affects our emotions. Fortu-nately, the human race is intrinsically optimistic, with a will to survive.

Where does aromatherapy fit in?

How can aromatherapy play an effective and worth-while part in the mental–physical sphere of healing? It is established beyond doubt that essential oils can have physical impact in that they are bactericidal, anti-inflammatory, antifungal, appetite stimulat-ing, hyperaemic, expectorant etc. (see Ch. 4 and Table 7.1). They possess properties which can affect the mind and emotions to sedate, calm and uplift; they also have effects on bodily systems, they evoke memories, change perception, calm agitation, relieve stress, activate cognitive responses and affect intercommunication (Cook 2008, Ouldred & Bryant 2008). They are therefore ideal tools for tackling not only physical problems but at the same time mental and emotional states, working via the sense of smell.

The placebo effect (expectations effect) is another factor that may influence the effect of an aroma on human behaviour, mood and health:

> People's beliefs that odours can influence their mood or health may lead them to perceive such consequences when they are exposed to an odorant and may even help trigger actual effects.
> The potential for placebo effects is high in an area such as aromatherapy where various essential oils are promoted as having specific beneficial mood and health effects and the individuals using the odorants desire such outcomes.
>
> Knasko (1997)

Table 7.1 Effects of essential oils used internally and externally (from Schilcher 1984)

External application	Internal application
Hyperaemic	Expectorant
Anti-inflammatory	Appetite stimulating
Antiseptic/disinfectant	Choleric, cholekinetic
Granulation stimulating	Carminative
Deodorizing	Antiseptic/disinfectant
Insecticide/insect repellent	Sedative
	Circulation stimulating

Relaxation response

When safe and calm, people experience the opposite of the stress response, in that tension, blood pressure, oxygen use and so on are reduced. This has been termed the 'relaxation response' (Benson 1975). It can be brought about by many means, including reading, listening to favourite music, contemplating nature – and aromatherapy.

When, during a massage, the touch of the therapist is combined with the mental and physical effects of the essential oils, the client is helped to achieve a temporary separation from worldly worries, somewhat akin to a meditative state. The massage itself induces the relaxation response, which activates the body's healing mode, and this, in conjunction with the essential oils, is outstanding for the relief of tension and anxiety, both physical and mental.

Whatever the method of application, the authors feel that in many cases most of the healing effect of essential oils is primarily through inhalation (see Ch. 6) via the mind and emotional pathways, and that a lesser part takes place via the physical body. There is no doubt that smelling plant volatile oils can affect the mood and general feeling of wellbeing in the individual. This is especially true when the essential oils are applied with whole-body massage: the physical and mental relaxation achieved during a massage session has to be experienced to be appreciated. To select essential oils to address the mental, emotional and physical needs of the client, the cause(s) of the health

Case study 7.2

Panic attacks and vertigo

Kate Stockbridge – Aromatherapist

Client assessment

A is in his mid-60s, referred for aromatherapy by a community psychiatric nurse as he had developed panic attacks and vertigo. She felt that aromatherapy would help in relieving his stress and therefore aid relaxation. His problems had arisen as a result of the long-term caring, full time, of a relative with Parkinson's disease.

A was physically and mentally tired and not sleeping well. He described himself as having a 'thickness of the head' and 'solid headaches'. Emotionally he was low – and tearful as he expressed his frustration at his condition. His arms and legs had large areas of 'shark's skin' – psoriasis and warts – and he complained of coldness and aching in his knees.

Intervention

This was aimed at easing anxiety and depression, promoting sleep, relieving headaches, and at the same time providing warmth and acceptable physical contact.

A was given six massage sessions, once a fortnight, remedial massage techniques being used around the patella where there were granular deposits, and around the scapula where there was much tension.

The oils chosen were one drop each of:

- *Citrus aurantium* var. *sinensis* [sweet orange] – antidepressant, calming, mildly sedative; also recommended for vertigo
- *Boswellia carteri* [frankincense] – analgesic, antidepressant, energizing, immunostimulant
- *Origanum majorana* (sweet marjoram) – analgesic, calming, nervous system regulator, neurotonic; also recommended for vertigo
- 10 mL sweet almond oil – emollient, helps relieve psoriasis
- 5 mL evening primrose oil – as above

For use in between treatments, A was given a 50 mL lotion containing:

- 10 drops *Citrus limon* [lemon] – anticoagulant, calming, immunostimulant
- 5 drops *Boswellia carteri* [frankincense] – analgesic, antidepressant, energizing, immunostimulant
- 5 drops *Chamaemelum nobile* [Roman chamomile] – anti-inflammatory, antispasmodic, calming and sedative, stimulant

This was to be applied twice daily to his shoulders, knees and psoriatic areas.

Outcome

After the first session A was more relaxed, although he still had some tension in the shoulder region. He appreciated the treatments, which relaxed and rejuvenated him.

By the third treatment the discomfort in his head had cleared and he began to feel brighter and more able to cope.

After his sixth and final session he no longer experienced vertigo, the headaches had gone, his skin was much improved and he felt less tense in his shoulders. Emotionally, he was better able to relax at home and felt more positive about the future.

Case study 7.3

Phobias

E Kell – Midwife/aromatherapist

Patient assessment

J attended the antenatal clinic at the Southern General Hospital in the early weeks of pregnancy and was extremely anxious and agitated. She was suffering from phobias, unable to enter a lift at any time and preferring very light rooms having windows with an open aspect. It became extremely difficult for J to attend the clinic because of her anxiety state, and her consultant suggested using aromatherapy.

Intervention

The first consultation took place in the antenatal clinic in a quiet bright room where, after an initial chat, J relaxed slightly and began to relate to – and trust – the aromatherapist.

She was offered a hand massage first, which was thought to be less threatening at the outset, allowing her to feel more confident with the therapist. She relaxed very well, so a shoulder and back massage was suggested, with J sitting astride a chair, her arms on a pillow placed on the chair back. The oils were chosen for their emotional effect, being confirmed in Price (2000) – *Aromatherapy and your Emotions*:

- 3 drops *Lavandula angustifolia* [lavender] – antispasmodic, cardiotonic, calming and sedative, tonic
- 2 drops *Chamaemelum nobile* [Roman chamomile] – antispasmodic, calming and sedative, stimulant
- 1 drop *Citrus aurantium* var. *amara* [neroli] – antidepressive, neurotonic
- 10 mL peach kernel carrier oil

After this first treatment she felt much more able to discuss her fears and worries and counselling was able to take place, after which ways were discussed as to how her partner could help her cope with her fears.

She was given a tape of simple relaxation techniques, such as breathing and visualization, to use daily, together with a blend of the oils above (9, 6, 3 drops in 50 mL peach oil), for her husband to massage into her shoulders every night.

It was decided that it would help allay J's fears to continue her aromatherapy treatments in a labour room, which enabled her to become familiar with both her surroundings and the midwives before she eventually arrived in labour.

In the early stages J was referred to a psychiatrist, but as she did not wish to take the medication prescribed at that point it was decided to continue with aromatherapy treatments, and her pregnancy progressed well.

When she was admitted to the labour suite, back and leg massages were given, using the blend above but with *Myristica fragrans* [nutmeg] instead of neroli. *Salvia sclarea* [clary] and lavender were given to her on a ball of cotton wool to inhale whenever necessary. She progressed well and surprised everyone – including herself – by remaining very calm throughout.

Outcome

Although she needed a forceps delivery, J coped extremely well with this, feeling that aromatherapy had had a great deal to offer her during both pregnancy and labour. She was delivered of a beautiful baby boy and both mother and baby did extremely well.

---

problem must be identified. All essential oils have an effect on both mind and body, although much research needs to be done in this respect.

Pregnancy and children

The influence of odours on humans begins even before birth; the odour of anise was presented to 24 neonates and it was shown that babies born to mothers who consumed anise during their pregnancy showed a stable preference for the smell, whereas babies born to non-anise consuming mothers showed aversive or neutral responses (Schaal et al. 2000).

A report by Nordin et al. (2004) showed that abnormal taste and smell was reported by 76% of 187 pregnant women tested, typically believed to be caused by their pregnancy. Increased smell sensitivity was common during the early stages of pregnancy (67%), occasionally accompanied by qualitative smell distortions (17%) and phantom smells (14%). Smell abnormalities occurred less in later periods of pregnancy and were virtually absent after delivery. Abnormal taste sensitivity was fairly commonly reported (26%), often described as an increase in bitter and a decrease in salt taste. Pregnancy smell and taste disorders relate to fetal protection mechanisms to avoid poisons and increase salt levels for the expanded fluid levels.

Anecdotal evidence indicates that during pregnancy olfactory sensitivity is increased, and the lack of scientific evidence to back this up was investigated (Cameron 2007). One hundred women who did not smoke were tested and the overall conclusion was that the effect of pregnancy was small and inconsistent, but interestingly the women felt that they had heightened awareness of smells during their pregnancy.

Adding the aroma of lemon to a classroom helps to involve all the senses in the learning experience, and Chu (2008) says that low-achieving school-children experienced success in a written task in the presence of an ambient odour (herbal tea), and when they experienced this same odour in a later task they were shown to be significantly better than a relevant control group. Chu claims that this is the first study to show a classic conditioning effect to influence human behaviour (but see Aromas, Memory and Mood, below).

The sense of smell is important in children with severe learning difficulties (see Ch. 13) who may have diminished hearing and sight, and essential oils can be used to make their life easier and more friendly. Fragrances have been used on wristbands to identify carers, each with their own aroma, to identify the child's possessions and to locate areas, rooms and facilities (Sanderson, Harrison & Price 1991). This technique can also be used to make a baby sitter acceptable to the child.

The elderly

Aromas are well accepted in homes for the elderly, where they can create a pleasant atmosphere, either stimulating or relaxing, and some aromas may create an ambience which will bring back memories, possibly sparking off nostalgic conversation between the residents, with obvious benefits (see Ch. 14).

Gender differences

There appears to be a gender difference in the impact on the mind of inhaled essential oils, as it seems that women are the more likely to derive beneficial results. One study indicating this was the use of *Citrus sinensis* [sweet orange] diffused into the waiting room of a dental practice, where the results of a questionnaire filled in by patients of both genders showed that sweet orange oil had a relaxant effect compared to non-odour controls. Compared to men, women had a lower anxiety state, a more positive mood and higher level of calmness. The typical smell of dental premises, eugenol, was associated with anxiety and fear, although this was masked for women by the orange aroma, lowering their

anxiety; for men this was only minor (Lehrner et al. 2000).

Another study set out to demonstrate the gender effect of odour on pain perception: 20 men and 20 women were exposed to pain by holding a hand in hot water while smelling previously selected odours. Separate analyses for men and women revealed a significant effect of odour on pain perception for women but not for men, and when the odour was found to be pleasant women demonstrated a significant reduction in pain perception (Marchand & Arsenault 2002). The gender difference was shown in a different light when subjects proofread pages of text containing misspelt words: all participants performed significantly better when aroma was present in the room; lavender produced the greatest effect on women, whereas peppermint had the greatest effect on men (Kliauga, Hubert & Cenci 1996).

Miyazaki, Motohashi & Kobashaya (1992a) investigated the effects on females of inhalation of orange oil (unspecified), *Chamaecyparis taiwanensis* lig. [hinoki] and menthol, and found an increase in speed performing a mental task and a decrease in the number of mistakes for all three aromas. Profiles of mood state (POMS) scores indicated that depression/dejection, anger/hostility and tension/anxiety decreased after inhalation of the oils, whereas fatigue scores tended to increase.

A similar study explored the effects of inhalation of orange oil (unspecified), *Chamaecyparis taiwanensis* lig. [hinoki] and eugenol on the mood of six male individuals, and POMS were monitored: blood pressure showed a decrease after inhalation of hinoki or orange oils, but an increased heart rate with eugenol. Eugenol was deemed to be unpleasant and scores indicated increases in fatigue, depression/dejection, confusion and anger/hostility and a decrease in vigour, whereas inhalation of hinoki oil had the opposite effect (Miyazaki, Motohashi & Kobashaya 1992b).

Pleasant smells give pleasure and feelings of self-esteem (Baron 1990, Nezlak & Shean 1990) and the effect on women may be greater because, according to Herz and Cupchik (1992), women have more intense odour memories than men.

Although it is understood that personality can bias sensory perception, Chen and Dalton (2005) say that the emotional state of a person has a similar effect. Subjects were exposed via video clips to prime happiness, sadness, negative/hostility and neutral feelings. The time taken to detect odours (suprathreshold odours of pleasant, unpleasant and neutral) and the intensity of the odours was recorded. It was found that females reacted faster to smells with emotional links than to neutral smells. Emotional states augmented the intensity of odours for males.

The skin of women is more permeable than that of men to toxic chemical molecules having a similar size to those of essential oil compounds, and they can retain more fat-soluble compounds in their body and so are affected more (Eisberg 1983).

It is interesting to note that almost all practising aromatherapists and users of aromatherapy products are women, only about 2% of men being involved: this is perhaps because the overall effects of essential oils on women are more significant than on men.

Anosmia – absence of the sense of smell

If a person has poor vision, it is obvious by the wearing of spectacles or using a white stick, but there is no easy means of recognizing a person's inability to smell. Aromas are made up of individual chemicals and each cilium is equipped with uniquely contoured depressions into which a single aroma molecule can fit, somewhat like a jigsaw puzzle. If the appropriate 'dock' for the molecule being inhaled is absent, that smell will not be registered.

Total, specific and temporary anosmia

Anosmia can be total (where nothing is smelt at all), specific (an inability to register certain smells) or temporary. Almost everyone suffers temporary anosmia at some time, and probably each person has about five specific anosmias. About 5% of people are insensitive to the sweaty smell notes, and whereas about 50% of people are anosmic to androsterone, musk is almost universally noticed. Some aromas have exceptionally low detection thresholds, for example grapefruit and green pepper. Individuals vary in their perception of aromas, even among young adults, who constitute the most consistent age group (Doty 1991), but these differences are due to more than genetic anosmias, as shown by experiments revealing that repeated exposures can alter detection thresholds (Wysocki, Dorries & Beauchamp 1989).

 Case study 7.4

Prolonged temporary anosmia

S Price – Aromatologist

Client assessment

Mr P had suffered from severe chronic sinusitis for several years, his sense of smell diminishing over the years. After an operation there was no improvement, and not being able to smell was upsetting him. His wife was an excellent cook and he was unable either to smell – or to taste – her cooking. His wife, having heard the therapist on the radio, persuaded him to travel the 60 miles to her clinic, to see if aromatherapy could help him.

Intervention

It was decided to carry out a treatment 'sandwich' once a week: massage of his face, including pressure points, a Swiss reflex treatment on the sinus reflexes of his feet (see Ch. 8), finishing with a repeat of the facial treatment.

Two of the essential oils in the selected blend have extremely strong aromas, yet Mr P was unable to smell them:

- 2 drops *Eucalyptus globulus* [blue gum] – anticatarrhal, anti-infectious, anti-inflammatory, expectorant
- 3 drops *Lavandula angustifolia* [lavender] – anti-inflammatory, antiseptic, calming

- 2 drops *Mentha x piperita* [peppermint] – anti-infectious, anti-inflammatory, soothing

After each treatment two spills, with eucalyptus and peppermint respectively, were held to his nose in the hope of a reaction.

He was also given 20 drops each of the same oils in 50 mL carrier lotion, to apply on his face every morning after shaving, instead of his usual astringent.

Outcome

At the third visit, when the peppermint spill was led to his nose, Mr P let out a delighted yell:'I can smell mint – it's faint, but it's definitely mint!'

After the next visit, Mr P showed enough improvement for him to visit the clinic only once a fortnight, still using his lotion at home very day.

After 3 months, the visits were altered to once a fortnight – and after 6 months from the commencement of treatment he had recovered his sense of smell sufficiently to appreciate some of the aromas from his wife's cooking – a happy result for her too!

Temporary anosmia may be caused by colds, rhinitis and sinusitis, and results in a loss of taste. There are four types of taste cells (salt, bitter, sour and sweet) although appreciation of food flavours does not depend solely on these but also on texture, acidity/alkalinity, hot/cold, the trigeminal nerve – and smell.

If a person is incapable of smelling an aroma, does this mean that aromatherapy will not be effective? Many aromatherapists believe that prolonged use of essential oils will restore the sense of smell in some cases.

The authors treated a case of chronic sinusitis (suffered for 17 years), when even after an operation the client was unable to smell his wife's cooking – his main cause for concern! After three treatments he was able to detect *Mentha* x *piperita* [peppermint], one of the essential oils in the mix used (which also included *Eucalyptus globulus* [Tasmanian blue gum] and *Ocimum basilicum* [European basil]). After 6 months of weekly treatments and daily self-care he had recovered his sense of smell sufficiently to recognize some of the gastronomic aromas greeting him on his return from work. This is in line with some surprising findings which indicate that in both humans and animals possessing specific anosmia, the sensitivity to some odours can be restored by repeated exposure to those odours (Holley 1993, Van Toller & Dodd 1992). There was an increase of cerebral blood flow in humans following inhalation of 1,8-cineole (found in eucalyptus and rosemary essential oils) and a similar result was obtained with an anosmic person (Nasel et al. 1994).

Fuji et al. (2002) claim that laryngectomy results in severe hyposmia (lowered smell ability) or anosmia. They tested olfactory acuity preoperatively and 3, 6, and 12 months postoperatively, and reported that olfactory acuity initially worsens but then improves to almost preoperative levels.

Polluted city air adversely affects the sense of smell: dwellers in Mexico City were found to have less olfactory ability than residents of Tlaxcala, where there is no pollution (Hudson et al. 2006). A later test showed that air pollution impairs olfactory and intranasal trigeminal sensitivity even in otherwise healthy young adults (Guarneros et al. 2009).

Does anosmia, sleep or unawareness negate aromatherapy?

- **Effect of aroma during sleep:** Aromas of essential oils have measurable physiological effects on humans during sleep. Ten participants were monitored to see whether any physiological changes occurred when they were subjected to 3-minute periods either of air alone or of peppermint aroma during stage two sleep. The results revealed conclusively that humans do react behaviourally, autonomically and centrally to the aroma of essential oil of peppermint administered while sleeping. Significant differences were found in responsiveness to periods with and without aroma for EEG, EMG and heart rate as well as behavioural changes (Badia et al. 1990).

- **Awareness:** Odour conditioning and physiological responses can occur even when people are not consciously aware of the odour (Lorig 1989, Lorig et al. 1988). Kirk-Smith and Booth (1990) used a fragrance at such a low level as to be imperceptible to the subjects, and found specific mood changes in both men and women compared to a non-odorous situation. In another study, half the subjects were exposed to a fragrance and the other half to no fragrance while working on stressful tasks. Days later all were exposed to the fragrance previously used, and those women previously exposed to the fragrance reported more anxiety, even though they were not consciously aware of an aroma on either day (Kirk-Smith et al. 1983). Degel and Köster (1999) revealed that unnoticed aromas can have an effect, showing that in certain circumstances odorants may influence attention performance in people who are not aware of their presence. A later investigation found that the unnoticed presence of odorants may affect everyday behaviour and cognitive functions (Holland et al. 2005).

From the results obtained in the above-mentioned tests, everything points to the fact that inhaled fragrances do have effects on humans even if:

- the aroma is at an imperceptible level and not noticeable
- the subject is anosmic or not
- the aroma is not being consciously registered
- the subject is asleep or awake.

Thus everyone, anosmic or not, conscious of the aroma or not, awake or not, is likely to benefit from aromatherapeutic treatment. See also Box 7.1 Smell adaptation.

Trials

When aromas are used therapeutically in clinical contexts they may be working in different ways at the same time. For example, lavender oil may:

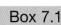
Box 7.1

Smell adaptation

It is a common assumption that the sense of smell is affected by adaptation as a result of continued exposure to a stimulus. An example of smell adaptation is that on entering a room there may be a noticeable aroma, but which is no longer apparent shortly afterwards. Presumably the aroma quickly disappears because receptors fatigue in the continuing presence of odorous molecules in the mucus (Engen 1982). The question arises whether, in these circumstances, aromas can bring about changes in the client. Engen goes on to say that, although olfactory adaptation is apparently commonly experienced, its effect has been exaggerated. He points out that animals using olfactory cues to find a mate would be frustrated if the cue should disappear halfway there.

A study investigating whether or not people with a professional interest in smell exhibited higher olfactory sensitivity showed that people working in an odorous environment showed no inferiority in terms of smelling ability. Working in an odorous environment for a full day had no major effect on general olfactory abilities, as indicated by measures performed at the beginning and end of a working day. Results do not support the idea that odorous environments are deleterious to general olfactory function (Hummel, Guel & Delank 2004).

Broad experience in the field of aromatherapy massage says that the aromas are indeed effective throughout the treatment, even though the quality of perception at the end of the treatment may well be different from that at the beginning.

- act pharmacologically as a light sedative
- be alerting, simply by being there as a stimulus
- create positive feelings because it is pleasant
- aid recall of past personal situations, positive or negative
- have social connotations of health or cleanliness (Kirk-Smith 1995).

The placebo effect must be taken into account when conducting trials using aromas, because the memory, attitude and expectations of the subject may modify the outcome, in addition to any effects of the aroma employed.

The use of olfaction in aromatherapy will increase and it is imperative that aromatherapy is put on a surer footing than at present; this can be achieved by the thousands of therapists currently in practice, who should not be deterred from embarking on clinical trials. With a little expert help in setting up a simple trial, much useful information could be gained in a relatively short time. Kirk-Smith (1995), in his review of therapeutic processes involving olfaction, agrees that further clinical evaluation of olfaction in therapy is needed, but trials involve many skills (therapeutic and scientific) and expectations or perceptions about the odour, as well as pleasantness, must be taken into account when predicting effects. It is not a simple matter to ascribe any reported benefits from the use of an aroma directly to that aroma. As mentioned above, it is imperative that the aromatic materials used in any future trials be precisely identified, otherwise the value of the tests will be diminished or negated.

Olfaction

Changes in thinking about odour reception have occurred following the identification of a very large family of genes responsible for coding olfactory receptors (Buck & Axel 1991).

People may have a sensitive sense of smell yet have poor perception and have difficulty in describing a smell; this is because olfactory input is widely distributed in the amygdala and the phylogenetically primitive cortex, without direct projections to the neocortex (Klemm et al. 1992).

The nose has two distinct functions:

- to condition the air inhaled for the lungs
- to act as the organ of the sense of smell.

An average human breathes in about 8 L of air each minute and more than a million molecules are taken in with each breath, yet even a remarkably small number of odorous molecules mixed in the air intake can be detected by humans (Engen 1987).

Inhalation

When essential oils are inhaled, the volatile molecules are carried by eddy currents to the roof of the nose, where delicate cilia protrude from the receptor cells into the nose itself. When the molecules lock on to these 'hairs' an electrochemical message is transmitted via the olfactory bulb and olfactory tract to the limbic system (amygdala and hippocampus). This may trigger memory and emotional responses,

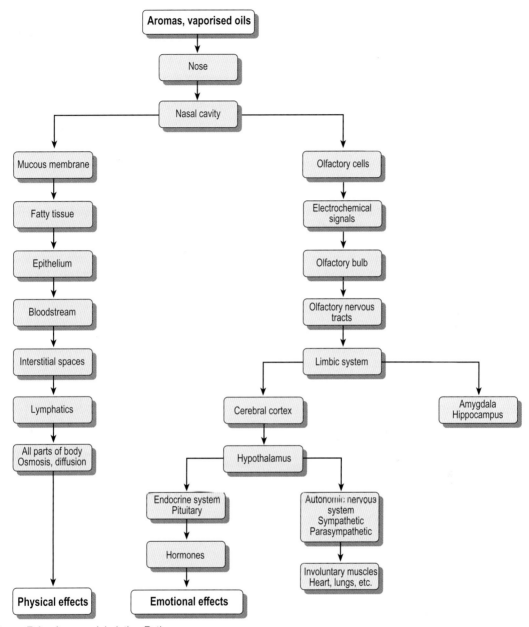

Figure 7.1 • Aroma – Inhalation Pathways

which can cause messages to be sent via the hypothalamus to other parts of the brain and the rest of the body (Fig. 7.1). Mainland and Sobel (2006) say that sniffing is necessary for olfactory perception and that a typical human sniff has a duration of 1.6 seconds, an average inhalation velocity of 27 L/min and a volume of 500 cm³. Sniffs are not merely a stimulus but are rather a central component of the olfactory perception, they also

- affect odour intensity perception and identity perception
- drive activity in the olfactory cortex
- are rapidly modulated by an olfactomotor system
- are sufficient to generate an olfactory perception even in the absence of an odour.

Humans recognize fewer molecules than other mammals, but can discriminate among 10,000 different odours (Menini et al 2004). The received messages are converted into action, resulting in the release of euphoric, relaxing, sedative or stimulating neurochemicals.

The limbic system, which developed 70 million years ago and used to be called the rhinencephalon (from the Greek *rhis* = nose, *enkephalon* = brain), is heavily implicated in the expression of emotion, although whether it generates emotions or merely integrates them is not clear (Stoddart 1990). The body can replace olfactory nerve cells, an unusual feature of human nerve tissue, which serves to emphasize their importance.

Fibres from the olfactory nerve carry impulses to two small but significant parts of the brain, the locus ceruleus (where noradrenaline (norepinephrine) is concentrated) and the raphe nucleus (serotonin) (Godfrey-Hardinge 1993 personal communication). It is suggested that sedative aromas such as *Origanum majorana* [sweet marjoram], *Lavandula angustifolia* [lavender], *Chamaemelum nobile* [Roman chamomile], *Matricaria recutita* [German chamomile] and *Citrus aurantium* (flos) [neroli] cause stimulation of the raphe nucleus, which then releases the neurochemical serotonin, whereas stimulating aromas such as *Rosmarinus officinalis* [rosemary], *Citrus limon* (per.) [lemon], *Ocimum basilicum* [basil] and *Mentha* x *piperita* [peppermint] will affect the locus ceruleus, which then releases noradrenaline.

The use of essential oil aromas in aromatherapy treatments is not too far removed from intranasal drug delivery in common use today, e.g. steroid inhalers for allergies, peptides and anaesthetics (Chen, Su & Chang 1989). Lavender, which has been used in the treatment of insomnia (Hardy, Kirk-Smith & Stretch 1995), consists largely of oxygenated terpenes, which interact with cell membranes to suppress cell action potentials (Teuscher et al. 1990) and might account for a sedative effect. Animal tests using 42 essential oils and their components showed linalyl acetate and linalool from lavender oil to have the most sedative consequences (Buchbauer et al. 1993): a serum level in line with intravenous injection was produced, possibly owing to ready absorption by nasal and lung mucosa (Buchbauer et al. 1991). The use of an essential oil for such a purpose has advantages, as lavender oil

- does not have unwanted side effects
- can be used to vary long-term treatment, giving relief from powerful drugs and their side effects
- masks malodours usually present in psychogeriatric wards.

Warren et al. (1987) patented the use of a stress-reducing fragrance which included nutmeg oil. Subjects were stressed, and with nutmeg oil present systolic blood pressure was reduced and subjects rated themselves as being calmer and less anxious. Nutmeg oil contains the phenolic ethers myristicin and elemicin, which convert to the hallucinogens TMA (trimethoxyamphetamine) and MMDA (methoxymethylene-dioxyamphetamine).

In their paper on the use of fragrances and essential oils as medicaments, Buchbauer and Jirovetz (1994) drew the conclusion that interaction between fragrance molecules and receptors in the central nervous system (in combination with reflectoric effects) is responsible for the sedation caused by the inhalation of fragrances or essential oils.

Many odorants stimulate not only the olfactory system via the first cranial nerve but also the trigeminal system via the fifth cranial nerve, which enervates the nasal mucosa. The trigeminal system is part of the body's somatosensory system and mediates sensations such as itching, burning or warmth and cooling: potent trigeminal stimulants such as ammonia and menthol have been used as smelling salts to arouse those who have fainted (Heuberger 2010).

Aromas affect emotions

Aromas are important in everyday life, though notoriously difficult to describe. We are surrounded by aromas, some natural but many synthetic. There are many natural aromatic messages, e.g. babies are able to recognize their own mother by her individual odour; also, synchronous menstruation occurs in groups of women living in close proximity, e.g. nuns.

Fragrances are added to almost everything from floor polishes to foods in order to

- improve sales
- manipulate the working environment, or in shops and hotels
- invoke a 'feel-good' factor in customers in shops or hotels
- reduce apprehension in airports and dentists' waiting rooms
- reduce traffic stress when used in cars.

These aromas are inflicted on us regardless of our wishes and feelings – like background music – and the short- and long-term effects on people are not always known, since the emotions produced can be strong and unforgettable. The psychosomatic effect of smell is experienced by most people: for example the unfamiliar mixture of odours encountered in hospitals can produce a feeling of dread, accompanied by physical manifestations such as sweating, nausea and fainting (in visitors as well as patients), and the memory of the smell of some school meals can affect the appetite throughout life.

Essential oils consist of natural molecules and at the very least are to be welcomed as a means of introducing a natural product into the synthetic hospital environment. The use of carefully selected essential oils makes good sense both therapeutically and financially, for they are simple and inexpensive to use and no costly equipment is required. (see Table 7.2)

The emotional and content qualities of autobiographical memories evoked by three memory-cue items (campfire, fresh-cut grass and popcorn) were presented in an olfactory, visual and auditory form by Herz (2004). The results showed that memories recalled by odours showed significantly more emotional and evocative content than those recalled by the visual or auditory forms. Herz argued that the data presented in his paper contributed to the growing body of evidence indicating a privileged relationship between olfaction and emotion during recollection.

Conditioning, pairing

Classic conditioning using a visual or an auditory stimulus requires many pairings, but in the case of olfaction sometimes only one pairing is needed, e.g. conditioning the body's production of natural killer (NK) cells, fever and cytotoxic T-lymphocytes (CTL) to camphor (see below). The connection between the olfactory and immune systems is important for species survival (Hiramoto et al. 1993). Taste and odour pair easily with illness, which is useful in some cases, but an odour may become associated with an unwanted state or an illness. Aversive conditioning using an odour has been used to control overeating and resulted in a significant loss of weight compared with a control group (Foreyt & Kennedy 1971).

Examples of pairing are:

- Schiffman and Siebert (1991) found that an apricot fragrance paired with a relaxed state later triggered the relaxed state; this conditioning was particularly useful in the treatment of lower back pain.

- Betts (1994) used olfaction to control arousal symptoms in epileptic seizures, not only in those who experience olfactory auras but in any patient having an aura long enough to give time to apply a countermeasure before the major seizure starts. Essential oils employed included lavender, chamomile, ylang ylang and lemongrass; rosemary oil was avoided **(see observations under Rosemary in** Appendix A on **the CD-ROM)**. Betts says that using the autohypnotic technique it is possible to train the patient to associate intense relaxation with the smell of the oil, so that the remembered aroma alone is sufficient to act as a countermeasure.

- Olness and Ader (1992) paired taste and aroma with an anticancer drug in the treatment of an 11-year-old girl who had a severe autoimmune disease. As a result of this pairing, the anticancer drug was needed in only six out of 12 treatments.

A neutral odour can be paired with an emotional state in a single session, so that it will evoke the same emotional state in different circumstances later. This effect is quite strong and it is not even necessary for the aroma to be perceived either during the pairing or when evoking the state; this is likely to be due to olfaction's relative lack of representation in the neocortex (Kirk-Smith, Van Toller & Dodd 1983). King (1988) has similarly paired a 'sea fragrance' with relaxation training, measuring the effects of fragrance alone with forehead EMG (electromyography). Rose and Behm (1994) found that inhalation of the vapour from an extract of black pepper served to reduce the withdrawal symptoms experienced on cessation of tobacco smoking; essential oils containing citral are also said to have this effect.

Sedative/stimulant influence of odours

It has long been known that aromas have an effect on the psyche; incense was used first as a calming agent to induce a state of contentment (Lee & Lee 1992) and there are many examples: in ancient Greece, the physician Galen recommended the use of aromatic herbs against hysterical convulsions; burning bay leaves were inhaled by the Oracle at Delphi to induce a trance-like state to enable communication with the gods. Later, aromatic woods were burned to drive out 'evil spirits'.

Table 7.2 Effects on the emotions mentioned by various authors. The figures indicate the number of times each is mentioned

Latin name	Common name	Arousal, alertness	Grief	Memory recall	Pain relief	Anger	Fear	Apathy
Achillea millefolium	Yarrow							
Aniba rosaeodora (lig.)	Rosewood							
Boswellia carteri	Frankincense							
Cananga odorata (flos.)	Ylang ylang					1		
Carum carvi (fruct.)	Caraway							
Cedrus atlantica (lig.)	Atlas cedarwood							
Chamaemelum nobile (flos.)	Roman chamomile				1			
Chamomilla recutita (flos.)	German chamomile							
Cinnamomum verum (cort.)	Cinnamon bark	2		1				
Citrus aurantium var. *amara* (flos.)	Neroli		1					
Citrus aurantium var. *amara* (fol.)	Petitgrain							
Citrus aurantium var. *amara* (per.)	Orange bitter							
Citrus aurantium var. *sinensis* (per.)	Orange sweet							
Citrus bergamia (per.)	Bergamot					1	1	
Citrus limon (per.)	Lemon	1				1	1	
Citrus reticulata (per.)	Mandarin							
Commiphora myrrha	Myrrh							
Coriandrum sativum (fruct.)	Coriander							
Cupressus sempervirens	Cypress		1				1	
Eucalyptus globulus (fol)	Eucalyptus							
Foeniculum vulgare var. *dulce*	Fennel							
Hyssopus officinalis	Hyssop							
Jasminum officinale	Jasmin				1			
Juniperus communis (fruct.)	Juniper berry						1	
Lavandula angustifolia	Lavender	2	1			1	1	

Table 7.2 Effects on the emotions mentioned by various authors. The figures indicate the number of times each is mentioned—cont'd

Latin name	Common name	Arousal, alertness	Grief	Memory recall	Pain relief	Anger	Fear	Apathy
Lavandula x *intermedia Super*	Lavandin	1						
Lippia citriodora	Verbena							
Melaleuca alternifolia (fol.)	Tea tree							
Melaleuca leucadendron (fol.)	Cajuput							
Melaleuca viridiflora (fol.)	Naiouli							
Melissa officinalis	Melissa		1			1		
Mentha x *piperita*	Peppermint	4		1	1	1		1
Myristica fragrans (sem.)	Nutmeg							
Ocimum basilicum	Basil					1		
Origanum majorana	Marjoram		1			1	1	
Pelargonium graveolens	Geranium					1		
Pimpinella anisum (fruct.)	Aniseed							
Pinus sylvestris (fol.)	Pine							
Ravensara aromatica	Ravensara							
Rosa damascena, Rosa centifolia	Rose otto		1					
Rosmarinus officinalis	Rosemary				1	1	1	
Salvia officinalis	Sage		1					
Salvia sclarea	Clary						1	
Santalum album (lig.)	Sandalwood							
Satureia hortensis, S. montana	Savory							
Syzygium aromaticum (flos.)	Clove bud							
Thymus serpyllum	Wild thyme							
Thymus vulgaris ct. *alcohol*	Sweet thyme							
Thymus vulgaris ct. *phenol*	Red thyme							
Valeriana officinalis	Valerian							
Vetiveria zizanioides	Vetiver							
Zinziber officinale	Ginger						1	

Almost a century ago a series of experiments on rats provided confirmation of the anecdotal sedative effects of some oils: when relaxing oils were dispersed in the air the rats took longer to perform tasks (Macht & Ting 1921): oils used included lavender, rose and valerian (common names only given). This method is effective because of the large area in the lungs available for the absorption of airborne oils into the bloodstream (Jirovetz et al. 1992).

Gatti and Cayola looked at the action of essences on the nervous system (1923a), the therapeutic effects of essential oils (1923b) and the use of valerian oil as a cure for nervous complaints (1929). They noted that the physical effects of the sedative/stimulant action of the oils were achieved more quickly by inhalation than by ingestion, and that opposite reactions could be obtained depending on whether the dose was small or large.

Since these early days more experiments have been carried out and knowledge of the psychotherapeutic effects of essential oils has grown, but nevertheless more research is needed; aromatherapy works, but it is necessary to find out how. Some interesting studies illustrating calming, stimulating and other effects are given below.

Many patients undergoing magnetic resonance imaging (MRI) body scans find them distressing and claustrophobic; this expensive procedure can be aborted by a stressed patient pressing the panic button, wasting both time and money. At the Memorial Sloan-Kettering Hospital in New York, a fragrance (constituents unknown) is used to calm patients receiving whole-body scans. Redd et al. (1994) administered bursts of heliotropine (a vanilla-like scent) to patients undergoing this procedure which reduced recalled anxiety by 63% in those who liked the smell. The calming brought about was thought to be attributable to the pleasing effect of the aroma, as pleasant conditions make stress more bearable.

According to Dember and Warm (*New Scientist* 1991), people do much better in a task that requires sustained attention if they receive regular puffs of an aroma. The test of concentration involved staring for 40 minutes at a pattern on a computer screen and hitting a key whenever the pattern changed very slightly. People generally did well to begin with, but performance eventually fell off and the fragrance effect was likened to a mild dose of caffeine. Peppermint was found to be stimulating and lily of the valley relaxing.

A traditional use of peppermint oil in aromatherapy was confirmed by Parasuraman (1991) when it was shown that peppermint aroma enhanced the sensory pathway for visual detection, allowing more control over attention; also rosemary (39% 1,8-cineole) was shown to be refreshing and to improve locomotor activity in mice (Buchbauer 1988).

The aroma of jasmine has been shown to stimulate mental function (Sugano 1989) and to shorten pentobarbital-induced sleeping time in mice (Kikuchi et al. 1989); *cis*- and *trans*-phytol were considered the stimulant-like compounds in a solvent-extracted oil. The sedative influence of lavender and the excitatory effect of jasmine in humans were confirmed by (Karamat et al. 1992). Sugano (1989) also showed that inhalation of lavender and the compound α-pinene had a sedative effect.

Aromas, memory and mood

Aromas can be employed easily and safely by using diffusers in rooms and cars, placing on tissues etc., and used in these simple ways they can improve sleep quality, change mood positively, alleviate stress and improve alertness. Aromas are able to remind people of past experiences, even from childhood, and when experienced during a learning process can aid recall of the information – this is sometimes known as 'context-dependent learning'. Much of this has been known anecdotally for some time, but there are now numerous studies showing that aromas do affect human conditions. In 1989, Rottman found that the aroma of jasmine in a room improved performance in problem-solving tests, and Schab (1990) found that the presence of an ambient aroma during a learning process brought about 50% better recall than when no aroma was present; Smith, Standing and Deman (1992) had a similar result. The effects of *Rosmarinus officinalis* [rosemary] and *Lavandula angustifolia* [lavender] were tested on 140 subjects divided into three groups, one being a control group. Either the lavender or the rosemary was diffused into a test cubicle prior to the test:

- Lavender produced a significant decrease in working memory and impaired reaction times for both memory- and attention-based tasks
- Rosemary significantly enhanced the quality of memory and alertness compared to the lavender and control groups.

The effects of aromatherapy on relaxation, alertness, mood, anxiety and EEG (electroencephalogram) were investigated in 40 subjects using lavender (unspecified) or rosemary (unspecified) essential oil diluted 10% in grapeseed oil and inhaled from a cotton swab. The rosemary group had increased alertness (decreased frontal α and β power) and were faster but not more accurate in mathematical computations. The lavender group performed the mathematics more quickly and more accurately, and the EEG recordings showed a stronger β power, suggesting increased drowsiness; both groups felt more relaxed, and it was concluded that aromas do affect psychological and physiological states (Diego et al. 1998).

Skamoto et al. (2005) investigated the effect of exposure to lavender aroma during rest periods at work. The workers carrying out a computer task requiring concentration (60 minutes' work interspersed with 30 minutes' rest) were divided into three groups:

• Group 1 was not exposed to odours in the break
• Group 2 was exposed to the aroma of jasmine
• Group 3 was exposed to the aroma of lavender.

The afternoon sessions when concentration was lowest showed a positive effect for lavender over the control and jasmine groups. This finding is interesting because although lavender is usually thought of as having a sedative effect (perhaps the lavender allowed for a more efficient rest period), it is known that it is amphoteric and can also have an arousing effect.

Moss et al. (2003) concluded that the aroma of essential oils produced objective effects on cognitive performance and subjective effects on mood: Zoladz and Raudenbush (2005) showed that cinnamon and peppermint aromas improved subjects' ability to pay attention, their recognition and working memory, visuomotor response speed, mood and energy. In a study to assess whether peppermint could increase the alertness of clerical workers in an office environment, typing accuracy, speed, increased performance and ability to alphabetize improved significantly (Barker et al. 2003).

Another study showed that aromas can influence the way people think and behave (Baron 1990). Subjects were put in a room that was intermittently fragranced with air freshener; under these conditions they set themselves higher goals, were more inclined to negotiate in a friendly manner and were able to resolve conflicts more successfully.

A study was carried out by Raudenbush, Corley and Eppich (2001) to determine whether physical tasks would be enhanced by the inhalation of peppermint aroma; athletes performed four tasks:

1. dynamometer hand grip
2. a 400-m dash
3. push-ups to exhaustion and
4. 20 basketball free-throw shots.

Participants performed the protocol twice under different odour conditions, first with a peppermint-odorized adhesive strip under the nose, and second with an odourless adhesive strip. The peppermint aroma resulted in increases in running speed, hand grip strength and number of push-ups, but had no effect on the skill-related basketball free-throw shots.

In a different study athletes performed a 15-minute treadmill stress test and at 3-minute intervals 50 mL of beverage (water with peppermint aroma added, unadulterated water, or a commercial sports drink) were consumed: in the control condition no beverage was consumed. Both the peppermint drink and the sports drink led to greater ratings of personal performance and increased mood (Schuler, Rawson & Raudenbush 2004).

Matricaria recutita [German chamomile] oil has been used to study the effects of olfaction on mood and imaging. When subjects were asked to visualize positive or negative phrases following exposure to either chamomile oil vapour or placebo, the oil significantly increased the time it took for images to be produced, suggesting either that enhanced neural processing was taking place or that the oil was sedative; it also shifted mood rating in a positive direction (Roberts & Williams 1992).

Psychophysiological effect of aroma

There can be no doubt that changes in physiological and psychological parameters can be caused by essential oil inhalation, and Miyazaki et al. (1991) reported that changes in mood due to inhalation could be measured using the light reflex of the pupil; they also found that orange oil (unspecified) increased the activity of the parasympathetic nervous system. Using encephalography (EEG) and psychological scoring to examine the effects of inhalation of various oils, it was found that bitter orange oil increased sleeping time significantly under conditions of mental stress. In psychophysiological studies of fragrance by Sugano and Sato (1991) it was concluded that lavender, orange and rose would elevate work efficiency and counter the effects of a stressful life; chamomile, jasmine and musk increased β-band microvibrations, suggesting mental stimulation.

These studies demonstrated that psychological and physiological parameters can be changed by the inhalation of essential oils, but the oils used in most of the tests cited in this section were not properly identified. Lavender was found to be unpleasant in some tests (Klemm et al. 1992, Lorig & Roberts 1990) but pleasant in others (Torii et al. 1988); there are similar findings with jasmine. It is hard to imagine that *Lavandula angustifolia* could consistently be rated as unpleasant, whereas it is entirely possible that *L. latifolia* or *L. stoechas* (among others) could merit this description: the ester content of lavenders grown in different regions can vary from 8% to 50%, altering the aroma considerably; jasmine oil is not distilled and contains traces of chemical solvent. It is astonishing that time and money can be spent in research without ascertaining what materials are being tested and studied, but this has happened, which tends to detract from the value of the whole exercise.

Klemm et al. (1992) studied the physiological responses of 16 young women to aromas from seven essential oils (birch tar, galbanum, heliotropine, jasmine, lavender, lemon and peppermint) assessed by EEG recordings from 19 locations on their scalps. Subjective responses to the odours differed, but the most consistently arousing and strong odours included galbanum, lavender, lemon and peppermint. The most pleasant were lemon and peppermint, whereas birch tar, galbanum and lavender were consistently

unpleasant. All aromas affected the EEG in at least some subjects, and all subjects responded to some.

It is not clear from studies carried out whether or not personal like or dislike of the odour has a real bearing on the effects of essential oil inhalation. Bulgarian rose, lavender and geranium oils were tested on 48 medical students by spraying a 1% solution into the room; there was an increase in concentration, attention span, work rhythm and a shortening of reflex times; these effects were independent of personal like/dislike of the aroma (Tasev, Toleva & Balabanova 1969). On the other hand, the study by Marchand and Arsenault (2002) came to the conclusion that if the aroma was found to be pleasant then mood perception was significantly increased, whereas unpleasant aromas significantly reduced mood perception. Practical experience shows that essential oils work in an aromatherapy treatment even if the aroma is not liked, although the client tends to be more relaxed and more ready to accept treatment with a positive outlook if the aroma is perceived as pleasant.

Summary

Great advances have been made in our knowledge of the interactions of the mind, emotions and nervous and immune systems, and there is growing recognition of their combined impact on general health. Essential oils have an effect on everyone and have an important role to play in bringing about a state of relaxation, thereby favouring healing – aromas are effective even during sleep or unawareness of their presence. Everyone is capable of deriving benefit from aromatherapy.

References

Badia, P., Wesensten, N., Lammers, W., Culpepper, J., Harsh, J., 1990. Responsiveness to olfactory stimuli presented in sleep. Physiol. Behav. 48 (1), 87–90.

Barker, S., Grayhem, P., Koon, J., Perkins, J., Whalen, A., Raudenbush, B., 2003. Improved performance on clerical tasks associated with administration of peppermint odor. Percept. Mot. Skills 97, 1007–1010.

Baron, R.A., 1990. Environmentally induced positive affect: its impact on self efficacy, task

performance, negotiation and conflict. Journal of Applied Social Psychology 20, 368–384.

Benson, H., 1975. The relaxation response. Morrow, New York.

Betts, T., 1994. Sniffing the breeze. Aromatherapy Quarterly 40 (Spring), 19–22.

Borysenko, J., 1988. Mending the mind, mending the body. Bantam, Toronto.

Buchbauer, G., 1988. Aromatherapy: do essential oils have therapeutic properties? In: Proceedings of the Beijing International Conference on Essential Oils, Flavours, Fragrances

and Cosmetics. International Federation of Essential Oils and Aroma Trades, London.

Buchbauer, G., Jirovetz, L., 1994. Aromatherapy – use of fragrances and essential oils as medicaments. Flavour & Fragrance Journal 9, 217–222.

Buchbauer, G., Jirovetz, L., Jäger, W., Dietrich, H., Plank, C., Karamat, E., 1991. Aromatherapy: evidence for sedative effects of the essential oil of lavender after inhalation. Z. Naturforsch. 46c, 1067–1072.

Buchbauer, G., Jirovetz, L., Jäger, W., Plank, C., Dietrich, H., 1993. Fragrance compounds and essential oils with sedative effects upon inhalation. J. Pharm. Sci. 82 (6), 660–664.

Buck, L., Axel, R., 1991. A novel multigene family may encode odorant receptors: a molecular basis for odour recognition. Cell 65, 175–187.

Cameron, E.L., 2007. Measures of human olfactory perception during pregnancy. Chem. Senses 32, 775–782.

Chaitow, L., 1991. Mind your immunity. Here's Health (October), 19–20.

Chen, D., Dalton, P., 2005. The effect of emotion and personality on olfactory perception. Chem. Senses 30, 345–351.

Chen, Y.W., Su, K.S.E., Chang, S., 1989. Nasal systemic drug delivery. Dekker, New York.

Chu, S., 2008. Olfactory conditioning of positive performance in humans. Chem. Senses 33, 65–71.

Cook, N., 2008. Aromatherapy: reviewing evidence for its mechanisms of action and CNS effects. Br. J. Neurosci. Nurs. 4 (12), 595–601.

Degel, J., Köster, E.P., 1999. Odors: implicit memory and performance effects. Chem. Senses 24 (3), 317–325.

Diego, M.A., Jones, N.A., Field, T , et al., 1998. Aromatherapy positively affects mood, EEG patterns of alertness and math computations. Int. J. Neurosci. 96 (3–4), 217–224.

Doty, R.L., 1991. Olfactory system. In: Gerchell, T.V. et al., (Ed.), Smell and taste in health and disease. Raven Press, New York, pp. 175–203.

Dunbar, H.F., 1954. Emotions and bodily changes, fourth ed Columbia University Press, New York.

Eisberg, S., 1983. Male chauvinism in toxicity testing? Manufacturing Chemist 3 (July), 3.

Engen, T., 1982. The perception of odours. Academic Press, New York.

Engen, T., 1987. Remembering odours and their names. Am. Sci. 75, 497–502.

Foreyt, J.P., Kennedy, W.A., 1971. Treatment of overweight by aversion therapy. Behav. Res. Ther. 9, 29–34.

Fuji, M., et al., 2002. Olfactory acuity after total laryngectomy. Chem. Senses 27, 117–121.

Gatti, G., Cayola, R., 1923a. L'azione delle essenze sul sistema nervoso. Rivista Italiana delle Essenze e Profumi 5 (12), 133–135.

Gatti, G., Cayola, R., 1923b. Azione terapeutica degli olii essenziali. Rivista Italiana delle Essenze e Profumi 5, 30–33.

Gatti, G., Cayola, R., 1929. L'essenza di valeriana nella cura delle malattie nervose. Rivista Italiana delle Essenze e Profumi 2, 260–262.

Guarneros, M., et al., 2009. Mexico City air pollution adversely affects olfactory function and intranasal trigeminal sensitivity. Chem. Senses 34, 819–826.

Hardy, M., Kirk–Smith, M., Stretch, D., 1995. Replacement of chronic drug treatment of insomnia in psychogeriatric patients by ambient odour. Lancet 346, 701.

Herz, R.S., 2004. A naturalistic analysis of autobiographical memories triggered by olfactory visual and auditory stimuli. Chem. Senses 29, 217–224.

Herz, R.S., Cupchik, G.C., 1992. An experimental characterisation of odour evoked memories in humans. Chem. Senses 17 (5), 519–528.

Hesse, W.R., Akerl, K., 1955. Experimental data on the role of the hypothalamus in mechanisms of emotional behaviour. AMA Arch. Neurol. Psychiatry 73, 127–129.

Heuberger, E., 2010. Effects of essential oils on the central nervous system. In: Başer, K.H.C., Buchbauer, G. (Eds.), Handbook of essential oils: science, technology and applications. CRC Press, Boca Raton, p. 283.

Hiramoto, R.N., Hsueh, C.M., Rogers, C.F., Demissie, S., Hiramoto, N.S., Soong, S.J., et al., 1993. Conditioning of the allogenic cytotoxic lymphocyteresponse. Pharmacol. Biochem. Behav. 44 (2), 275–280.

Holland, R.W., Hendriks, M., Aarts, H., 2005. Smells like clean spirit. Nonconscious effects of scent on cognition and behaviour. Psychol. Sci. 16 (9), 689–693.

Holley, A., 1993. Actualité du mécanisme de l'olfaction. In: 12èmes Journées Internationales Huiles Essentielles. Istituto Tetrahedron, Milano, pp. 21–27.

Hudson, R., et al., 2006. Effect of air pollution in residents of Mexico City. Chem. Senses 31, 79–85.

Hummel, T., Guel, H., Delank, W., 2004. Olfactory sensitivity of subjects working in odorous environments. Chem. Senses 29 (6), 533–536.

Jirovetz, L., Buchbauer, G., Jäger, W., Woidich, A., Nikiforov, A., 1992. Analysis of fragrance compounds in blood samples of mice by gas chromatography, mass spectrometry, GC/FTIR and GC/AES after inhalation of sandalwood oil. Biomed. Chromatogr. 6 (3), 133–134.

Karamat, E., Ilmberger, J., Buchbauer, G., Roblhuber, K., Rupp, C., 1992. Excitatory and sedative effects of essential oils on human reaction time performance. Chem. Senses 17, 847.

Kikuchi, A., Tsuchiya, T., Tanida, M., Uenoyama, S., Nakayama, Y., 1989. Stimulant like ingredients in absolute jasmine. Chem. Senses 14 (2), 304.

King, J.R., 1988. Anxiety reduction using fragrances. In: Van Toller, S., Dodd, G. H. (Eds.), Perfumery: the psychology and biology of fragrance. Chapman & Hall, London, pp. 147–165.

Kirk-Smith, M.D., 1995. Possible psychological and physiological processes in aromatherapy. In: Aroma 95 One body-one mind conference proceedings, .

Kirk-Smith, M.D., Booth, D.A., 1990. The effect of five odorants on mood and the judgement of others. In: MacDonald, D.W., Muller-Schwarze, D., Natynezuk, S.E. (Eds.), Chemical signals in vertebrates. Oxford University Press, Oxford, pp. 48–54.

Kirk-Smith, M.D., Van Toller, C., Dodd, G.H., 1983. Unconscious odour conditioning in human subjects. Biol. Psychol. 17, 221–231.

Klemm, W.R., Lutes, S.D., Hendrix, D. V., Warrenburg, S., 1992. Topographical EEG maps of human responses to odors. Chem. Senses 17 (3), 347–361.

Kliauga, M., Hubert, K., Cenci, T., 1996. Consumer panel study on the effect of peppermint and lavender fragrances on proof reading efficiency. In: Gilbert, A. (Ed.), Compendium of olfactory research. Kendall/Hunt, Dubuque IA, pp. 131–135.

Knasko, S.C., 1997. Ambient odour: effects on human behaviour. Int. J. Aromather. 8 (3), 32.

Lee, W.H., Lee, L., 1992. The book of practical aromatherapy. In: Keats, New Canaan CT, p. 125.

Lehrner, J., Eckersberger, C., Walla, P., Potsch, G., Deecke, L., 2000. Ambient odour of orange in a dental office reduces anxiety and improves mood in female patients. Physiol. Behav. 71, 83–86.

Lorig, T.S., 1989. Human EEG and odour response. Prog. Neurobiol. 33, 387–398.

Lorig, T.S., Roberts, M., 1990. Odour and cognitive alteration of the contingent negative variation. Chem. Senses 15, 537–545.

Macht, D.I., Ting, G.C., 1921. Experimental inquiry into the sedative properties of some aromatic drugs and fumes. J. Pharmacol. Exp. Ther. 18, 361–372.

Mainland, J., Sobel, N., 2006. The sniff is part of the olfactory perception. Chem. Senses 31, 181–196.

Marchand, S., Arsenault, P., 2002. Odours modulate pain perception: a gender specific effect. Physiol. Behav. 76, 251–256.

Menini, A., Lagostena, L., Boccaccio, A., 2004. Olfaction: from odorant molecules to the olfactory cortex. News Physiol. Sci. 19 (3), 101–104.

Miyazaki, Y., Motohashi, Y., Kobashaya, S., 1992a. Changes in mood by inhalation of essential oils in humans I. Mokuzai Gakkaishi 38 (10), 903–908.

Miyazaki, Y., Motohashi, Y., Kobashaya, S., 1992b. Changes in mood by inhalation of essential oils in humans II. Mokuzai Gakkaishi 38 (10), 909–913.

Moss, M., Cook, J., Wesnes, K., Duckett, P., 2003. Aromas of rosemary and lavender essential oils differentially affect cognition and mood in healthy adults. Int. J. Neurosci. 113 (1), 15–38.

Nasel, B., Nasel, C.h., Samec, P., Schindler, E., Buchbauer, G., 1994. Functional imaging of effects of fragrances on the human brain after prolonged inhalation. Chem. Senses 19 (4), 359–364.

Nezlak J B, Shean G D 1990 Social interaction and personal fragrance use. Perfumer & Flavorist 15, 43–45.

New Scientist, 1991. On the scent of a better day at work. 2 March, 18.

Nordin, S., et al., 2004. A longitudinal descriptive study of self-reported abnormal smell and taste perception in pregnant women. Chem. Senses 29, 391–402.

Olness, K., Ader, R., 1992. Conditioning as an adjunct in the pharmacotherapy of Lupus erythematosus: a case report. J. Dev. Behav. Pediatr. 13, 124–125.

Ouldred, E., Bryant, C., 2008. Dementia Care Pt 2: understanding and managing behavioural challenges. Br. J. Nurs. 17 (4), 242–247.

Parasuraman, R., 1991. Effects of fragrances on behaviour, mood and physiology. Paper presented at the annual meeting of the American Association for the Advancement of Science, Washington DC.

Plato, 3rd century BC. The Republic (D. Lee, Trans.). Penguin, Harmondsworth..

Price, S., 2000. Aromatherapy and your emotions. Thorsons, London.

Raudenbush, B., Corley, N., Eppich, W., 2001. Enhancing athletic performance through the administration of peppermint odour. Journal of Sport and Exercise Psychology 23, 156–160.

Redd, W.H., Manne, S.L., Peters, B., Jacobsen, P.B., Schmidt, H., 1994. Fragrance administration to reduce patient anxiety in MRI. J. Magn. Reson. Imaging 4 (4), 623–626.

Roberts, A., Williams, J.M.G., 1992. The effect of olfactory stimulation on fluency, vividness of imagery and associated mood: a preliminary study. Br. J. Med. Psychol. 65, 197–199.

Rose, J.E., Behm, F.M., 1994. Inhalation of vapour from black pepper reduces smoking withdrawal symptoms. Drug Alcohol Depend. 34, 225–229.

Rottman, T.R., 1989. The effects of ambient odour on the cognitive performance, mood and activation of low and high impulsive individuals in a naturally arousing situation. Doctoral Dissertation.

Sanderson, H., Harrison, J., Price, S., 1991. Massage and aromatherapy for people with learning difficulties.

Hands On Publications, Birmingham.

Schaal, B., et al., 2000. Human fetuses learn odours from their pregnant mother's diet. Chem. Senses 25, 729–737.

Schab, F.R., 1990. Odours and remembrance of things past. J. Exp. Psychol. Learn. Mem. Cogn. 16, 648–655.

Schiffman, S.S., Siebert, J.M., 1991. New frontiers in fragrance use. Cosmetics and Toiletries 106 (6), 39–45.

Schilcher, H., 1984. Ätherische Öle– Wirkungen und Nebenwirkungen. Dtsch. Apoth. Ztg. 124, 1433–1443.

Schuler, A., Rawson, A., Raudenbush, 2004. Effects of beverage flavour on athletic performance, mood, and workload. Journal of Sport and Exercise Psychology 26 (Suppl.).

Skamoto, R., Minoura, K., et al., 2005. Effectiveness of aroma on work efficiency: lavender aroma during recesses prevents deterioration of work performance. Chem. Senses 30, 683–691.

Smith, D.G., Standing, L., Deman, A., 1992. Verbal memory elicited by ambient odour. Percept. Mot. Skills 74 (2), 339–343.

Stoddart, D.M., 1990. The scented ape. In: Cambridge University Press, Cambridge, p. 132.

Sugano, H., 1989. Effects of odours on mental function. Chem. Senses 14 (2), 303.

Sugano, H., Sato, N., 1991. Psychophysiological studies of fragrance. Chem. Senses 16, 183–184.

Tasev, T., Toleva, P., Balabanova, V., 1969. The neuropsychic effect of Bulgarian rose, lavender and geranium. Folia. Med. 11 (5), 307–317.

Teuscher, E., Melzig, M., Villmann, E., Moritz, K.U., 1990. Untersuchungen zum Wirkungsmechanismus Ätherischer Öle. Zeitschrift für Phytotherapie 11, 87–92.

Torii, S., Fukuda, H., Kanemoto, H., Miyauchi, R., Hamauzu, Y., Kawasaki, M., 1988. Contingent negative variation and the psychological effects of odour. In: Van Toller, S., Dodd, G.H. (Eds.), 1988 Perfumery. The psychology and biology of fragrance.

Chapman & Hall, London, pp. 107–120.

Van Toller, S., Dodd, G. (Eds.), 1992. Fragrance: the psychology and biology of perfume. Elsevier, Barking, pp. 99–101.

Warren, C.B., Munteanu, M.A., Schwartz, G.E., et al., 1987. Method of causing the reduction of

physiological and/or subjective reactivity to stress in humans being subjected to stress conditions. .

Wood, C., 1990a. Sad cells. J. Altern. Complement. Med. (October), 15.

Wysocki, C.J., Dorries, K., Beauchamp, G.K., 1989. Ability to perceive androsterone can be acquired by ostensibly

anosmic people. Proc. Natl. Acad. Sci. USA 86, 7976–7978.

Zoladz, P.R., Raudenbush, B., 2005. Cognitive enhancement through stimulation of the chemical senses. North American Journal of Psychology March 01.

Sources

Kirk-Smith, M.D., 1995. Possible psychological and physiological processes in aromatherapy. In: Aroma 95 One body–one mind conference proceedings. Aromatherapy Publications, Brighton, pp. 92–103.

Schiffman, S.S., Siebert, J.M., 1991. New frontiers in fragrance use. Cosmetics and Toiletries 106 (6), 39–45.

Stevenson, C.J., 1994. The psychophysiological effects of

aromatherapy massage following cardiac surgery. Complement. Ther. Med. 2, 27–35.

Wood, C., 1990b. Say yes to life. In: Dent, London, p. 60.

Touch and massage

8

Shirley Price   Len Price

CHAPTER CONTENTS

Introduction

In certain countries the word 'massage' cannot be used by aromatherapists unless a massage certificate recognized by that country is held. In France and America a different name – 'therapeutic touch' – is often used which allows those not sanctioned by the government to carry out massage under a different name. The intention of the therapist is the same: to relieve tension and enable a beneficial result to take place.

Most aromatherapy schools teach their own specialized massage (or therapeutic touch); nevertheless, patients and clients can still benefit greatly from touch from an inexperienced or non-qualified person. Some massage movements are illustrated in this chapter for the benefit of those already qualified in aromatherapy and/or massage, and to encourage other nurses with a desire to use the simpler methods described. For the lay person or the busy nurse, knowledge of a few of the simpler techniques is an extremely valuable asset which can bring benefit to those needing care.

Touch and massage

Life takes it out of you, but massage puts it back.

Maxwell-Hudson (1999)

Massage begins with touch, which all of us need; it conveys a feeling of warmth, relaxation and security – all beneficial to good health. There are many empirical examples of massage therapy effects, including reduction of pain during childbirth and lower back pain (Field 2000 p. 45), even without essential oils. The addition of essential oils with analgesic properties enhances the relief obtained by massage alone.

Massaging babies and infants can reduce pain associated with teething, constipation and colic, as well as inducing sleep (Auckett 1981). Studies carried out on preterm infants showed without doubt that massage was beneficial to their growth and development (Field et al. 1987). The babies were massaged for 15 minutes three times a day for 10 days in an incubator. Compared with the control group, 47% of the treated infants gained more weight and were hospitalized for 6 days less.

Patient benefits

Whether the causes of ill-health are biomechanical, psychosocial, biochemical or a combination of these, massage seems to be able to exert a beneficial influence (Chaitow 2000). Touch itself is a basic human behavioural need (Sanderson, Harrison & Price 1991) and 'may be the only therapy which is instinctive; we hold and caress those we wish to comfort; when we hurt ourselves, our first reaction is to touch and rub the painful part' (Vickers 1996).

As research and scientific developments in the efficacy of drugs forged ahead, close patient contact diminished and by the 1960s massage had more or less lost its therapeutic status in medical care. However, in the late 1980s and 1990s there was renewed interest by nurses in the value of touch, and now many hospitals and hospices are using massage to benefit their patients; during this time massage has been enhanced by the addition of essential oils, transforming the treatment into aromatherapy (Buckle 1997) (see Box 8.1). The benefits are further enhanced by the choice of essential oils used (Wilkinson 1995) – increased energy levels, reduced side effects from drugs, symptoms not treated by the hospital relieved and emotional problems eased. The effects can last longer than those of massage alone, owing to the therapeutic action of the essential oil components (see Chs 10–15).

Patients can benefit from a massage (simple or involved) given by any of the following:

- a physical therapist – without essential oils
- a physical therapist using essential oils ready blended by an aromatherapist
- a nurse with no professional massage experience, but with a sound knowledge of essential oils
- a nurse using essential oils under the direction of an aromatherapist
- a nurse using touch and gentle non-manipulative massage movements, without essential oils (see Introducing massage, below).

The most important thing to remember is that nothing can replace hands-on, when the giver (whether or not a qualified masseur/se) is caring and works within his/her capabilities, combining gentle touch with a loving attitude. With the right approach, beginning with a small non-intrusive movement, both the giver and the receiver can come to enjoy the care they are sharing, making it easier for the receiver to open up and become more relaxed in body and happier in mind (Worrell 1997). Authors agree that it is not necessary to spend an hour on a massage for it to be effective – people also benefit from a short period of dedicated time.

Box 8.1

The Experiences and Meaning of Touch among Parents of Children with Autism attending a Touch Therapy Programme

Barlow and Cullen (2002) instigated a touch therapy programme aiming to enhance parents' perceptions of closeness with their children and provide them with an alternative to verbal communication to promote the latter. Parents of children with autism were taught simple massage techniques over 8 weeks. Having practised massage with their children, parents reported that the children tolerated the massage and not only were routine tasks such as dressing tolerated more easily, but the children appeared generally more relaxed. Parents reported feeling closer to their children and that touch therapy had opened a communication channel between them.

Physiological benefits

Massage increases the circulation of both blood and lymph, helping in the elimination of toxins from the body; it slows down the pulse rate, lowers blood pressure, releases muscle tension, tones underworked or weak muscles and relieves cramp.

Psychological benefits

Although these are perhaps not so easy to evaluate, they are significant and play their part in the holistic healing effect: relaxing an apprehensive mind, uplifting depression and despair, relieving panic or anger and, importantly, giving a person the feeling that

someone cares enough to spend time giving the specialized contact brought by touch and massage.

Massage and aromatherapy – therapies in their own right

Professional massage

Several colleges run short courses that are not sufficiently comprehensive to confer a recognized massage qualification. To meet professional standards and be competent to give a full, professional massage,

---

Case study 8.1

Anxiety

N Darrell – Aromatologist

Client assessment

Kay, a 42-year-old woman working in a family business, was referred for treatment by her GP, with severe anxiety and stress. Over the past 3 weeks, owing to business problems, she had become increasingly withdrawn and anxious. She was experiencing panic attacks (which left her clammy and freezing) in crowded places and also at night, which was disturbing her sleep pattern, thus she found it hard to wake up in the morning. She had extreme tension in her neck and shoulders, suffering headaches as a consequence. Her breathing tended to be shallow and rapid, and she had lost more than a stone in weight over the 3 weeks, partly due to lack of appetite.

Intervention

Because of the amount of anxiety she was experiencing she was taken through some breathing exercises before a full body massage, which was carried out using:

- 3 drops *Chamamaelum nobile* [Roman chamomile] – antispasmodic, calming, sedative
- 1 drop *Rosa damascena* [rose otto] – neurotonic
- 3 drops *Origanum majorana* [sweet marjoram] – analgesic, calming, neurotonic, respiratory tonic
- 10 mL grapeseed carrier oil

Kay opted for treatment twice a week and after the first treatment said she felt much calmer and more relaxed. She was standing upright rather than being bent over with the shoulder tension, and said that her head felt much clearer.

She was given a blend of the following neat essential oils to use at home in the bath, and as an inhalant if required:

1 mL *Valeriana officinalis* [valerian] – sedative, tranquillizing

1 mL *Chamaemelum nobile* – properties as above

2 mL *Lavandula angustifolia* [lavender] – analgesic, balancing, calming and sedative, tonic

2 mL *Origanum majorana* – properties as above

3 mL *Cananga odorata* [ylang ylang] – balancing, calming, sedative

On her next visit Kay reported that she found inhaling the oils when particularly anxious had relieved the hyperventilation and helped her to relax; she had also started to incorporate breathing exercises into her routine.

After six treatments over 3 weeks, Kay felt sufficiently confident to go shopping without anxiety. She had also been able to resolve some of the problems at work. She was beginning to put weight back on and her appetite had returned to normal.

She therefore decided to reduce her treatments to once a week, and after 3 more weeks she felt able to resume some of her work duties, when she reduced her treatments to once a month. She had not ceased taking her medication during her aromatherapy treatment time, but 6 months after first commencing aromatherapy, her doctor felt he could reduce her medication over the next 3 months.

At this time, she found she was able to carry out her normal work schedule and once again enjoy social activities. . . . She now goes for aromatherapy treatments when she feels the need.

the therapist must know anatomy and physiology, understand the relationship between the structure and function of the tissues being treated, and be knowledgeable in pathology, as well as being skilled in the proper manipulation of tissues (Beard & Wood 1964 p.1).

Massage and aromatherapy

It would prevent misunderstanding of the word aromatherapy if the qualification in massage were totally separate from that of essential oil knowledge. As Vickers (1996 p. 15) so rightly says, 'massage and aromatherapy should be judged on their own merits'. This 'combined' situation arose because aromatherapy was originally aimed at and studied by beauty therapists only, and massage is part of their training.

Aromatherapy schools in the 1970s taught their own specialized massage to beauty therapists; many placed too much emphasis on the massage and barely any on the essential oils. This situation has been regulated to a certain degree by the Aromatherapy Council (AC), which stipulates the number of hours to be spent on massage, anatomy and physiology and on essential oil knowledge in order for an aromatherapy course to be accredited by them (see Ch. 17).

Because the aromatherapy and massage are linked, neither is taken to its full potential: the massage training of aromatherapists is not as thorough as that of a physical therapist and the essential oil training is not as deep as that of an aromatologist (therapist qualified in aromatic medicine) and member of the Institute of Aromatic Medicine (see Ch. 9).

Beneficial effects of massage

Massage is widely recognized as providing the following benefits; it:

- induces deep relaxation, relieving both mental and physical fatigue
- releases chronic neck and shoulder tension and backache
- improves circulation to the muscles, reducing inflammation and pain
- relieves neuralgic, arthritic and rheumatic conditions
- helps sprains, fractures; breaks and dislocations heal more readily

- promotes correct posture and helps improve mobility
- improves, directly or indirectly, the function of every internal organ
- improves digestion, assimilation and elimination
- increases the ability of the kidneys to function efficiently
- flushes the lymphatic system by the mechanical elimination of harmful substances (especially toxins due to bacteria) and waste matter
- helps to disperse many types of headache (or migraine) originating from the gallbladder, liver, stomach and large intestine, and also those of emotional origin (including premenstrual syndrome or PMS)
- stimulates both body and mind without negative side effects
- helps to release suppressed feelings, which can be shared in a safe, confidential setting
- is a form of passive exercise, partially compensating for lack of active exercise.

These combined benefits not only result in increased body awareness, but also produce better overall health. Studies carried out in hospitals and private practice have shown that massage with essential oils greatly enhances and prolongs the health-giving effects.

Simple massage skills

The most easily acquired massage skills are:

- **Stroking**, which comes under the heading of *effleurage* movements (perhaps the most important for hospital use), for which the whole of both hands from fingertips to wrist should be used. Stroking is simply an extension of touch and, as well as being one of the simplest, is one of the most important movements in massage.
- **Frictions**, which come under the heading of petrissage (a deeper and more energetic series of movements than effleurage), and in which either the thumb or one or more fingers are employed. 'Rubbing it better' is a simple friction movement. The Hippocratic writings (from the Hippocratic collection 460–357 BC) remarks that 'the physician must be experienced in many things,

Case study 8.2

Depression

L Bischoff – Aromatherapist

Client assessment

After suffering a major depressive episode where she had brief reactive psychosis, Miss L was hospitalized for 1 week.

Shortly after her return from hospital she stopped taking her medication. She was advised against this, as it is possible for a relapse to occur, but she was adamant as she said it was making her feel worse. She also suffered from lower back pain through sitting for long periods at her knitting machine – an improved posture for knitting was suggested, although Miss L had not felt able to do any since leaving hospital. She used to do aerobics, but again, not since leaving hospital. She was not sleeping well and had PMS before her periods.

Intervention

It was felt important to tackle her emotional problems as well as the physical, and six weekly massage treatments were undertaken, using the following essential oils:

- *Boswellia carteri* [frankincense] – analgesic, antidepressive, anti-inflammatory, immunostimulant
- *Chamaemelum nobile* [Roman chamomile] – antispasmodic, calming, stimulant
- *Citrus aurantium* var. *amara* (flos.) [neroli] – antidepressive, neurotonic

- *Coriandrum sativum* [coriander] – analgesic, euphoric, neurotonic
- *Foeniculum vulgare* [fennel] – analgesic, anti-inflammatory, oestrogen-like

Miss L was given a full body massage at each treatment.

Outcome

She experienced great relief after the first massage and that night had a good night's sleep, feeling relaxed for several days afterwards.

After the second one her back felt much better – she was able to move more freely, although her sleeping pattern was not back to normal. It was therefore decided to give Miss L the same essential oils to use at home, in two blends:

1.5 mL of each oil in a 10 mL bottle, 6–8 drops of which was to be put into a bath at least 2–3 times a week

3 drops of each oil in 50 mL in oil of *Vitis vinifera* [grapeseed], to massage into her shoulders and neck every night before retiring

By the fourth treatment, Miss L had recommenced her aerobic classes, as her back felt so much better all the time. She was also sleeping as well as before her illness.

Because of this, a month was left before each of the remaining two treatments, the improvements remaining stable.

---

but assuredly also in rubbing, for rubbing can bind a joint that is too loose and loosen a joint that is too hard'.

Everyone has an innate ability to perform these two movements correctly and safely without the need for long training; both are taught thoroughly on aromatherapy courses.

Three further techniques, requiring greater skill and best learned on an accredited massage course, are:

- **Kneading** (a form of petrissage), involving use of the palm, the palmar surface of the fingers, the thumb, or thumb and fingers working together, is a squeezing and 'pulling' movement, often used on the shoulders and the thighs.
- **Percussion**, where the outside of the hands and fingers continually make and break contact with the body in a definite rhythm, is not normally used in aromatherapy.
- **Lymph drainage** is only briefly covered in an aromatherapy training programme. It is fully covered on a Vodder technique course.

Effleurage

Effleurage is the basis of all good massage. It can be used on its own, at the beginning and ending of a massage and also in between other types of movement. It consists of two types of stroking, using the whole hand or hands, which should mould themselves to the shape of the part of the body being massaged. The strokes are either deep (i.e. with pressure) or superficial (without pressure). Sometimes only part of the hand is used – perhaps only two fingers on a small area or on a baby.

Deep stroking with both hands is accomplished by moving up the part of the body being massaged with pressure towards the heart; its purpose is to assist the venous and lymphatic circulation by physical effect on the tissues.

Superficial stroking is effected without pressure and in any direction (the pressure is so light that the circulation is not directly affected). The perfection of this technique can require skill and long practice. In simple massage, superficial effleurage is mostly used as the return movement of deep effleurage, moving away from the heart back to the starting position.

Effleurage is used mainly to relax the recipient both mentally and physically and to improve the vascular and lymphatic circulation. Many different types of strokes come under this heading, but all should follow the basic principles above.

Frictions

Frictions are another form of compression massage, or kneading. They may be performed with the whole or the proximal part of the palm of the hand or with the thumb and fingers to carry out circular movements over a restricted area. There are two types of frictions:

1. **Fixed frictions** move the superficial tissues over the underlying structures, i.e. the part of the hand used is 'stuck' firmly to the client's skin, which is moved over the tissues beneath by making circles.
2. **Gliding frictions** move over a small area of the skin surface and may also progress along a specific path.

Frictions are primarily used to break down fibrous knots, loosen adherent skin, loosen scar tissue, relieve tension nodules in the muscles and increase the circulation in a specific area.

Other factors

Learning the different movements is only part of massage training. Equally important is the way in which these movements are performed. Essential factors to consider are contact, the direction of movement, the amount of pressure, the rate and rhythm of the movements, the medium used, the position of both patient and therapist, and the duration and frequency of the treatment (Beard & Wood 1964 pp. 37–40). Further factors include the need for full contact with the patient and complete relaxation of the masseur's own hands and arms because hard, tense hands transfer tension (and possibly pain) to the recipient. The mind should be cleared of any intruding, disruptive thoughts: the wellbeing of the client and how he/she can benefit must be uppermost.

The following principles need to be absorbed at the same time as the actual movements are learned.

Contact

No part of the human body is flat; nevertheless, when using effleurage (stroking movements) there should be full hand contact with every part of any large area to be massaged (Price 1999). Nothing breaks the relaxing effect of massage more than the repeated lifting off and replacing of hands. Fully relaxed hands and fingers maintain this contact by following the body's contours closely, draping themselves over the body like silk. The hands should remain in contact with the body for both outward and return journeys of all movements made in sequence: lifting off disrupts the flow of the massage as a whole (Price 2000 p. 203).

Pressure

In effleurage on a large area pressure should always be concentrated on the palm of the hand (Price 2000 p. 201). The fingers should be kept completely relaxed because pressure from fingers is not relaxing – finger pressure should be used in friction movements only. Normally, palm pressure should be applied only when moving towards the heart, with none on the return journey. One of the aims of massage is to stimulate the circulation (the return of venous blood is not easily accomplished by the heart – pressure towards the heart increases the rate of circulation. The lymphatic flow is also increased, ridding the body more quickly of any harmful substances.

Pressure in frictions using the thumb or finger pads needs to be firm, but care must be taken to use the whole finger pad and not to dig in with the tip.

Speed

This depends to a certain extent on the effects to be achieved. Generally speaking, massage is given to relax the recipient, and a rate of approximately 15 strokes a minute for a long stroke (e.g. hand to shoulder) is considered correct (Mennell 1945) or 18 cm (7 inches) per second (Beard & Wood 1964 p. 38). Anything faster than this is used only if the massage is intended to be stimulating.

Rhythm

Uneven or jerky movements are not conducive to relaxation and care should be taken to maintain a smooth, unbroken rhythm (Price 2000 p. 203). While massaging, relaxing music with a gentle rhythm can be of great help in sustaining continuous, fluent and flowing effleurage movements. Frictions also should be performed rhythmically (Beard & Wood 1964 pp. 10–11).

Continuity

Most massage is carried out to relax both mind and body, so the movements themselves (and the changeover from one movement to another) should be smooth and unnoticeable to the recipient. The whole area receiving massage should be covered without a break in continuity, contact or rhythm (except when carrying out percussion).

Duration

The duration of a massage session depends on how much of the body is to be massaged, the age of the individual, the size of the body and the enjoyment level of the recipient. Massage sequences suggested in this book last between 5 and 15 minutes depending on the area to be massaged. Ten minutes of massage normally provides sufficient relaxation to induce a good night's sleep.

Frequency

The frequency of massage treatment depends to a great extent on the pathological condition of the patient, as does the type of massage given. 'It is generally believed that massage is most effective daily, although some investigators have suggested that it is more beneficial when administered more frequently and for a shorter duration' (Beard & Wood 1964 p. 39).

Contraindications to massage

Contraindications to massage depend very much on the type of condition suffered. The lists below should be consulted to determine whether massage of any kind is appropriate or not.

Illness

Whole-body massage is not taught in this book and is contraindicated in the situations described below, but specific area massage (e.g. shoulders, hands and arms, feet and lower legs, face and scalp) is acceptable in most instances.

- **Infection.** The advice of the microbiologist or the infection control nurse should be sought.
- **Pyrexia.** If the client feels well enough an appropriate specific area could be massaged gently, using oils to give a cooling effect (e.g. include 0.5–1% peppermint in the blend).
- **Severe heart conditions.** Permission from the doctor or specialist must be obtained for whole-body massage.
- **Medication.** If the patients is on strong (and/or many types of) medication, specific-area massage only should be used.
- **Cancer.** There is some controversy regarding massage, and aromatherapists report that consultants can give conflicting advice. Some say that it is not advisable to encourage movement of the lymph as this may promote migration of the cancer to another area of the body; others say that moving the lymph and thereby encouraging the elimination of toxins (possibly some of the cancer cells also) could be beneficial (see Ch. 15). It is the opinion of Horrigan (1991) that, although surface massage will not cure cancer by natural means, it will not:
  - ○ make the cancer grow owing to an increased blood supply
  - ○ make the cancer spread
  - ○ interfere with chemotherapy and radiotherapy.

Localized damage

In the following situations the site of any trauma should be avoided, although other areas can be massaged:

- **Inoculations.** The site of an inoculation given within the previous 24 hours should not be massaged.
- **Recent fractures and recent scar tissue.** The healing of scar tissue can be hastened by the gentle application of essential oils in a carrier oil or lotion,

or spraying them in a water carrier on to the site if touch cannot be tolerated.

- **Bruises, broken skin, boils and cuts.** If small, these can be covered with thin transparent tape before proceeding with the massage.

Normal physiology

In the following situations whole-body massage is contraindicated, although specific-area massage is allowed:

- **Hunger.** If 6 hours or more have passed since any food intake, or if the patient feels hungry, fainting may occur with whole-body massage.
- **Digestion.** Immediately following a heavy meal, the digestive system is working full time and whole-body massage could cause either nausea or fainting.
- **Alcohol.** After recent alcohol intake, full body massage and certain essential oils can intensify the effects of alcohol, possibly causing dizziness, or a floating feeling. Specific-area massage does not have this effect and the amount of any essential oil used (in the recommended dilution) would be too small to contraindicate their use.
- **Perspiring.** Immediately after exertion, sport, a long hot bath or sauna, the body is excreting sweat and heat and absorbs essential oils with difficulty. It is advisable to wait 20–30 minutes before whole-body massage, although a 10–15-minute wait is adequate for specific-area massage.
- **Menstruation.** During the first 2 days of menstruation bleeding could be increased by whole-body massage. However, specific-area massage can help to relieve congestion and soothe any pain or discomfort.

Varicose veins and oedema

These two conditions are often believed to be unsuitable for massage. In fact, both can be alleviated by essential oils used in light effleurage. Special care is needed in the execution of the massage, and only gentle, almost superficial, *upward* effleurage strokes should be used.

- **Varices.** The area above the damaged valve should be cleared first with deep, firm, upward effleurage strokes, before commencing the light upward strokes on the affected area itself.
- **Oedema.** This condition must be treated by a precise technique. When present in an ankle the massage should begin with the upper leg, because it is important to clear this area first before attempting to relieve the oedema. Treatment of the lower leg should then be carried out, returning to the upper leg at intervals during the massage and to finish. The affected part must be elevated while giving the massage (Beard & Wood 1964 pp. 38, 60, 104).

Massage sequences

A technique for introducing massage and essential oils to a client or patient is given first, followed by some simple massage techniques, easily carried out after attending an introductory course on the subject.

Introducing massage

For some, close contact with patients can be 'a daunting commitment. Staff may need training to deal with the emotions massage may bring up' (quoted in Tattam 1992). In order not to take patients' anxieties on board, the therapist (or nurse) should endeavour to be empathetic, rather than sympathetic. Not everyone enjoys the thought of touching others (or being touched), but this can be overcome if a strong desire to help the patient and the pleasure of seeing a positive reaction makes it worth the effort.

The easiest part of the body to start with is the hand, as few people have a hang-up about shaking hands. The 'handshake technique' is also an excellent way of introducing the aroma of essential oils. Before going to see your patient, put a very small amount of carrier oil on your hand, add one or two drops of an essential oil – or one drop each of two (that you think the client may like) – and rub your hands gently together briefly, just to distribute the oils evenly.

1. Take your patient's right hand in yours as if to give a firm handshake (palm to palm – see Fig. 8.1A) and place your left hand over the top of the patient's hand, relaxing your fingers to 'cradle' his or her hand in a sandwich (Fig. 8.1B). While you are holding his or her hand, ask the usual

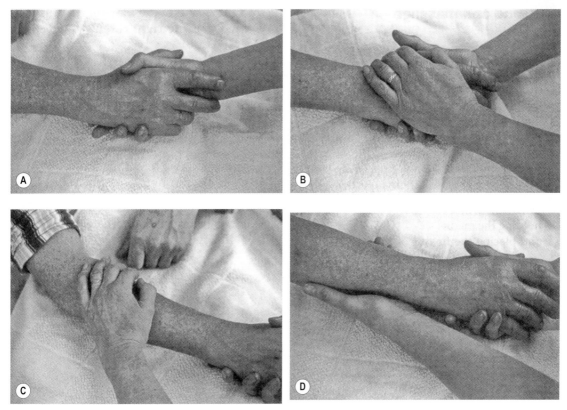

Figure 8.1 • (A–D) Handshake technique.

questions, such as 'Did you have a good night?' or 'How is your back this morning?' Your patient is bound to notice the aroma and comment on it. As you explain, you can say that essential oils are used for massage too; if the patient reacts well to the aroma – and shows interest – you can begin moving your left hand over the patient's hand in a stroking movement – even continuing over and around the wrist if the patient appears to like it. Ask if he/she would like the other hand to have a turn, and if so repeat the 'handshake', then follow steps 2 and 3 below.

2. Still holding the hand, gently raise the patient's forearm slightly, leaving the upper arm resting on the bed. Keeping your fingers in complete contact with the arm, begin to move your left hand firmly up the outer side of the lower arm (Fig. 8.1C); turn at the elbow, moving your palm underneath the arm and return gently to the wrist down the inner side of the arm (Fig. 8.1D). Turn your hand, bringing it back to the starting point.

3. Repeat the movement a few times, then suggest to your patient that you do the other hand to keep the body in balance.

Once you are confident and the patient is happy about being touched, the following sequences can then be carried out, allowing the essential oils to enter the bloodstream and give the desired benefits.

Hand and arm massage

1. Start with movements 1, 2 and 3 above, repeating three or four times. Where possible, take this stroke right up to and around the deltoid muscle and 'cradle' the whole shoulder, returning via the inner side of the arm, to finish at the wrist.

2. Still holding the patient's hand as in Fig. 8.1A, make large friction circles with the left thumb from wrist to elbow on the upper side of the arm, returning with a single

superficial stroke as in step 1. Repeat three or four times.

3.   Turn the arm over, now holding the patient's hand in your left hand: placing the fingers of the right hand on the lateral side of the forearm, make friction circles with the right thumb between the radius and ulna as far as the elbow, returning gently via the lateral side of the forearm to the wrist, with fingers underneath (Fig. 8.2A). Repeat three or four times.

4.   Leaving the fingers of both hands at the back of the wrist, push the thumbs firmly back and forth several times over the inside of the wrist in a zig-zag movement, (Fig. 8.2B).

5.   Slide the fingers down until they cover the back of the hand and stroke up the palmar muscles firmly, using the whole length of each thumb alternately, from finger level to wrist, several times (Fig. 8.2C).

6.   Turn the hand over and repeat wrist zig-zags as in step 4, on the dorsal side of the arm.

7.   Move your fingers down until they cover the patient's palm and stroke firmly between the metacarpals along their full length, right thumb between patient's thumb and first finger (returning via the radial side of the hand) and left thumb between third and fourth fingers (returning via the ulnar border of the hand). Repeat these strokes, this time with your right thumb between the patient's first and second fingers, and the left between the fourth and fifth fingers (Fig. 8.2D)

8.   With your right hand still supporting the patient's palm make friction circles with your left thumb up the little finger; at the base, turn your own palm uppermost and, using your first finger and thumb, slide down the sides of the finger to the tip (Fig. 8.2E,F). Move to the ring finger and repeat the frictions and return movement. Repeat on the other two fingers, using your right thumb to massage the patient's thumb.

9.   Push the fingers of your left hand through your patient's fingers (Fig. 8.2G) and, holding the patient's forearm with your right hand, rotate the wrist slowly and firmly anticlockwise, then clockwise.

10.   Smoothly change to the handshake hold and repeat step 1 several times.

To treat the patient's left hand, reverse the directions for 'right' and 'left' in the above text.

Foot and lower leg massage

When massaging the feet, it is very important to hold – and touch – the foot firmly. Many people have a dread of someone touching their feet, and in the majority of cases this can be attributed to having had their feet held so lightly that it felt ticklish or insecure – and thus unpleasant.

1.   Place your hands across the top of the right foot at toe level (Fig. 8.3A) and move them firmly up the lower leg to the knee. Separate them on each side of the leg, returning gently to the ankle (Fig. 8.3B); turn the hands as you reach the toes, ready to repeat the movement three or four times.

2.   When you have mastered this, incorporate the following 'sandwich' into the last part of the movement. As you approach the foot on the return journey, let the fingers of your right hand slide across the instep onto the sole of the foot, meanwhile turning the fingers of the left hand across the top of the foot towards the wrist of your right hand (Fig. 8.3C,D), squeezing both hands together as they move towards the toes. Lift off your right hand only, replacing it in front of (or behind) the left hand, ready to repeat the whole of movement 1 (with the sandwich) several times.

3.   On the last journey hold the foot firmly in the sandwich for a moment or two, before progressing to the next movement.

4.   Turn your hands so that your fingers are underneath the foot and with your thumbs carry out gentle frictions on the metatarsals – as in the hand massage (Fig. 8.3E). The frictions need to be gentle because this area of the foot is often tender, owing to poor lymphatic circulation or bronchial conditions (which the movement can help if done regularly).

5.   Bring your fingers back to the anterior surface of the foot and move them towards the ankle bone (Fig. 8.3F). Make firm circles round

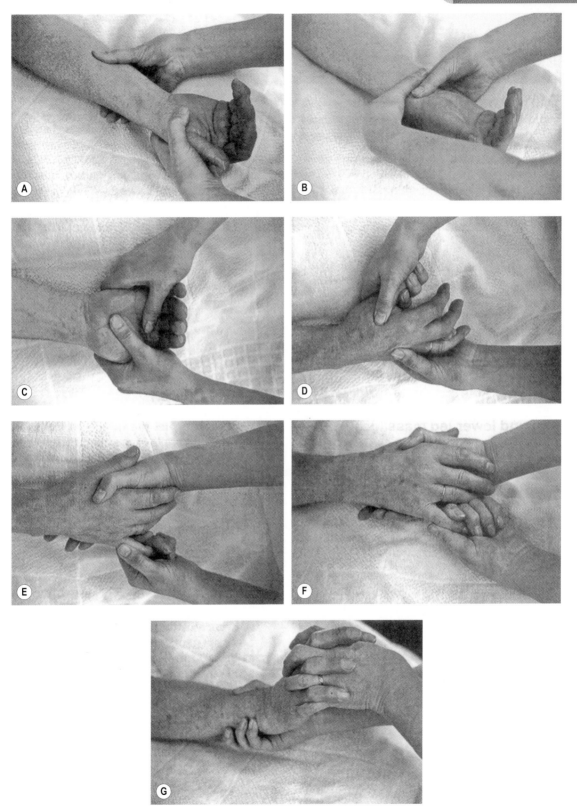

Figure 8.2 • (A–D) Hand and arm massage. (E–G) Hand and arm massage.

both sides of the ankle bone with the first and second fingers (Fig. 8.3G), relaxing the pressure as you come to the front of the foot. Repeat these circles several times. This movement covers the foot reflex point for the groin lymph and is ideal for relieving lymphatic congestion in the groin and increasing circulation in the legs generally.

6. Turn your hands into the position for movement 1 and repeat this movement (together with the sandwich, as in movement 2) several times, finishing by continuing the squeezing movement slowly until you are no longer in contact with the foot. For the left foot, reverse directions for 'right' and 'left' in the text. Should you wish to increase leg circulation further, ask the patient to bend her knee,

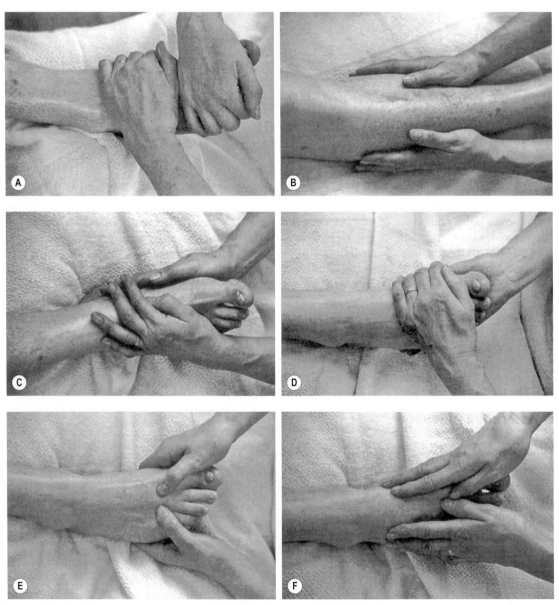

Figure 8.3 • (A–F) Foot and lower leg massage.

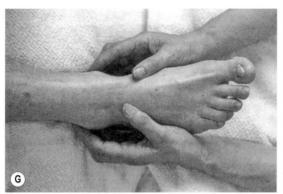

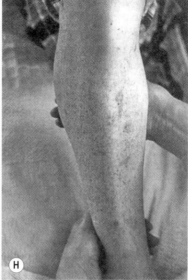

Figure 8.3, cont'd • (G–H) Foot and lower leg massage.

placing the foot flat on the bed. Sit on the toes (place a towel over them to protect your clothes from the oil if necessary) and continue as follows:

7. Carry out movement 1 several times, but only from ankle to knee.

8. Slide one hand to the back of the leg and move it with pressure up the gastrocnemius muscle, following with the other hand, then the first hand again, etc. – about 10 alternate strokes in all (Fig. 8.3H).

9. Repeat movement 5 around the ankle bones.

10. Finish with movement 1.

Shoulder massage

As a general rule, tensions and anxieties manifest themselves first of all as tension nodules in the trapezius muscle. This is not always apparent as continual pain, but can be felt immediately when someone presses firmly on the precise area of the taut muscular fibres (nodules).

The best time to give a shoulder massage (unless needed at any time to dissipate a headache) is just before retiring; this not only hastens sleep itself, but ensures a more relaxed body during slumber, which in turn puts the body into a healing mode.

If a special back and shoulder massage stool is not available, the best position for the patient is to sit straddled on a chair with a low back. There should be a pillow over the chair back, on which the arms and head can rest. This position is not always possible, and depends on the age and health of the patient. If it is impractical, the patient may sit normally on a stool or low-backed chair. Then proceed as follows:

1. Your feet should be about 45 cm apart, so that the knees can bend easily for carrying out movements effectively, without strain. Shake your hands to ensure that they are completely relaxed, before placing them gently, one over each shoulder (Fig. 8.4A).

2. Take your relaxed hands (you should be able to see a space between each finger) across the clavicles, cradling each deltoid muscle and across the latissimus dorsi to the base of each scapula – when your wrists will be pointing towards the spine; turn your hands until the fingers almost face one another (Fig. 8.4B). Move firmly with pressure up the back – one hand on either side of the spinal column – until you reach the clavicles again, with your fingers 'draping' over the shoulders as at the start. Repeat this three or four times.

3. Keeping your fingers on each clavicle, make friction movements with your thumbs across the upper trapezius from the neck to the point of the shoulder (Fig. 8.4C). Repeat this several times.

4. Keeping the fingers in the same position, stretch the thumbs down the spine as far as they will go without undue effort. Place them in the spinal channels and make friction circles up the channels as far as possible without exertion (Fig. 8.4D). Repeat this several times, circling several times on any one spot where you feel tension, before continuing.

5. Move round to the left side of the chair (keeping the left hand in contact with the patient), so that the patient's shoulder is directly facing the centre of your body. Feet should still be about 45 cm apart, as before. Open your hands as shown in Fig. 8.4E and, as you place the 'V' of the left hand on the point of the shoulder, bend your right knee (swinging the body to the right) and stroke up the deltoid to the hair line – your fingers will be in front

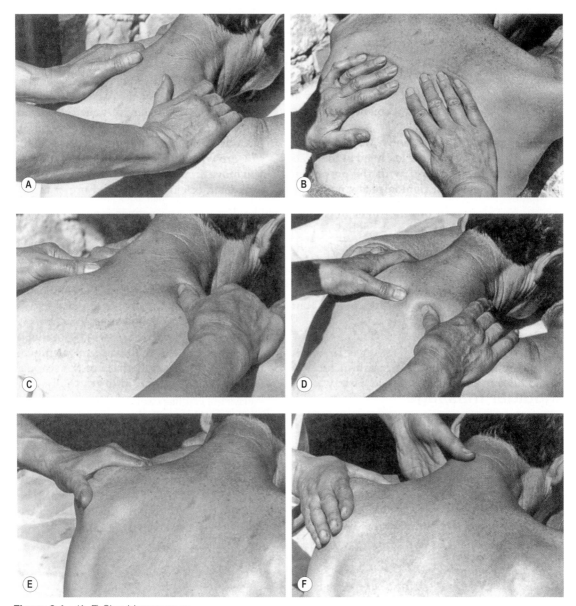

Figure 8.4 • (A–F) Shoulder massage.

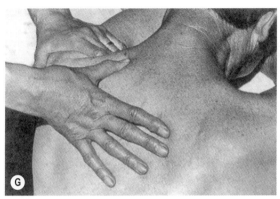

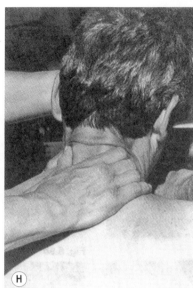

Figure 8.4, cont'd • (G–H) Shoulder massage.

of the shoulder and your thumb behind. As you reach the hair line, swing your body over to the left, bending your left knee, and stroke up the same area with your right hand as your left hand slides off the back of the neck (Fig. 8.4F). This time your thumb is in front of the shoulder and your fingers behind. Continue this alternate effleurage for a moment or two.

6. With your thumb, feel for painful tension nodules in the deltoid muscle. Firmly make friction circles over the knotty tissue with your thumb cushion (Fig. 8.4G). If the thumb tires too quickly, use the full length of both thumbs in single alternate strokes.

7. Repeat the shoulder effleurage described in movement 5.

8. Leaving your right hand on the shoulder, place your left hand on the patient's forehead and, keeping the fingers of your right hand separated from your thumb (as in movement 5), place the 'V' so formed at the base of the neck (Fig. 8.4H). Move firmly up the muscles of the neck, squeezing your thumb and fingers together as you move towards the hair line. Without lifting your hand from the patient, relax down to the base of the neck and repeat several times.

9. Keeping your hands on the patient, walk round to the back of the chair and repeat movement 2.

10. Keeping the left hand in contact, walk round to the right-hand side of the chair and repeat movements 4, 5, 6 and 7 on the other shoulder.

11. Without lifting your hands, walk round to the back of the chair and repeat movement 2, finishing at the base of the scapula with wrists together, and gradually and gently bring your fingertips to the centre and lift off.

Forehead massage

Standing behind the patient's head, lay your hand across the forehead with the fingertips of the left hand on the right temple and the length of the hand lying along the forehead (as in Fig. 8.5A). Move the hand slowly and gently across to the left temple (Fig. 8.5B), keeping contact as long as possible until the fingertips are almost on the hair. Before lifting off the hand, place fingertips of the right hand on the left temple, laying the length of the hand across the forehead and moving across to the right temple (Fig. 8.5C). Keeping the continuity and rhythm, repeat the two strokes with alternate hands for a few minutes. This stroke can also be done in an upward direction, but good contact must be maintained (Figs 8.5D–F).

Case study 8.3

Arthritic pain and mobility

A James – Aromatherapist

Client assessment

Mrs M, 75 years of age and in general good health, was positive and outgoing. She was very active and did not look or act her age. The pain from her neck and shoulder caused her some problems, as she found it difficult to get comfortable in bed and in the morning she was very stiff.

Intervention

A back massage was suggested, followed by a neck and shoulder massage. She attended the clinic on a weekly or fortnightly basis. The following oils were used for the massage:

- 2 drops *Eucalyptus citriodora* [lemon scented gum] – analgesic, anti-inflammatory, antirheumatic
- 2 drops *Piper nigrum* [black pepper] – warming, analgesic

- 2 drops *Zingiber cassumunar* rhiz. [plai] – anti-inflammatory
- 7 mL *Prunus amygdalis* var. *dulcis* [sweet almond]

Home treatment: 10 drops of each of the essential oils above were blended into 100 mL of white lotion, which she applied at bedtime and if the pain bothered her during the day.

Outcome

Over a period of 2 weeks there was a great improvement in the mobility of her neck; there was also much less pain. She noticed that if she did not have her massages regularly her neck and shoulders began to stiffen and her mobility reduced.

After six treatments she left a longer interval between treatments – a month to 6 weeks – but continued to use the home treatment prescribed.

Scalp massage

If you have been giving a forehead massage, scalp massage follows naturally. No further oil is needed because your hands will still be lubricated from stroking the forehead. When executed gently and firmly, massage of the scalp is exceedingly relaxing.

If the patient wishes to receive a scalp massage only, gently place under the nose a small amount of the diluted oil you would have selected had you been massaging part of the body. Then proceed as follows:

1. Place the hands on the scalp as shown in Figure 8.6A and, without moving the fingers through the hair, move the scalp firmly and slowly over the bone beneath.

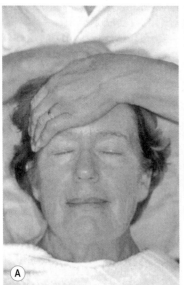
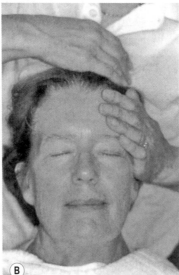
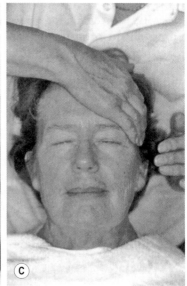

Figure 8.5 • (A–D) Forehead massage. (E–F) Forehead massage.

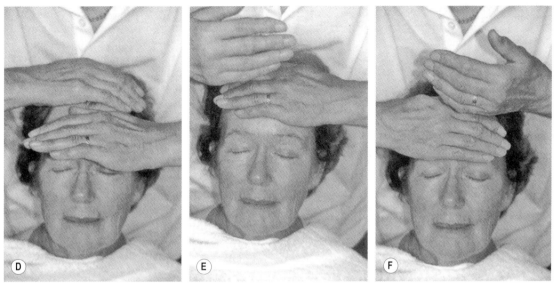

Figure 8.5, cont'd

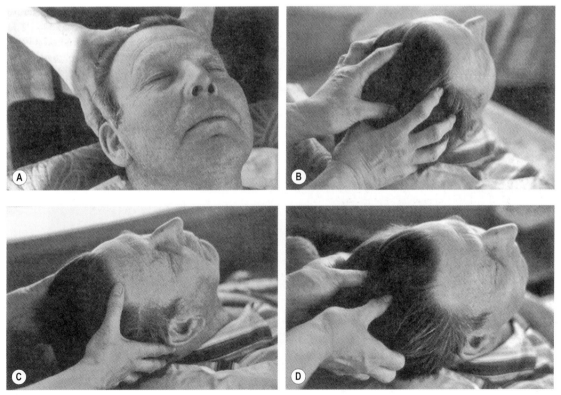

Figure 8.6 • (A–D) Scalp massage.

2. Place the hands as shown in Figure 8.6B and, once again, firmly and slowly move the scalp over the bone beneath.
3. Move the hands to another position and repeat.
4. Repeat movements 1, 2 and 3 several times.
5. Place the hands as shown in Figure 8.6C and bring the thumbs and fingers (stroking the scalp all the way) to meet each other at the centre of the scalp (Fig. 8.6D), then gently draw the fingers and thumbs through the hair to the ends.
6. Repeat this movement several times.

Simple back massage

In a hospital situation this should be kept reasonably brief unless it can be carried out on a massage bed of the right height, to ensure the correct posture of the therapist, thereby preventing backache. The feet should be approximately 45 cm apart, the rear foot facing in towards the bed, the front foot pointing - towards the patient's head. Stand level with the patient's hip, enabling you to reach the shoulders without strain. To follow the directions given here, it is necessary to stand on the patient's right-hand side.

1. Check that your hands are relaxed and use the whole hand, starting with hands on either side of the patient's spine at the level of the sacrum, fingers pointing towards the opposite shoulder (Fig. 8.7A). Effleurage up the back (covering as much as possible with relaxed hands), pushing upwards with both hands and then round the deltoid (Fig. 8.7B). Return with a superficial stroke right down the sides of the body before bringing the hands back to the starting point. Turn the hands and repeat the movement several times.
2. Repeat the same movement several times around the deltoid muscle only, finishing with the fingers over the shoulders.
3. Lift up your palms only, leaving your fingers lying over the top of the shoulder and, using the thumbs, make friction circles on the deltoid across the shoulders (Fig. 8.7C).
4. Place thumbs into the hollow channels on either side of the spine at the base of the neck, making small circles there with pressure on the upward half of each circle. The return journey of the circle should progress downwards so that the next circular movement will finish a little lower down the back. Extend the return of each circle until the thumbs are at waist line. Repeat movement 1 several times, then turn to face the patient, with your feet 45 cm apart and the

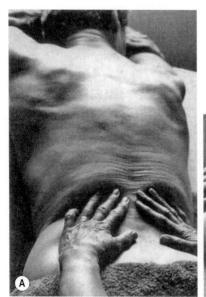
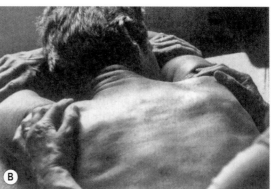

Figure 8.7 • (A–B) Back massage.

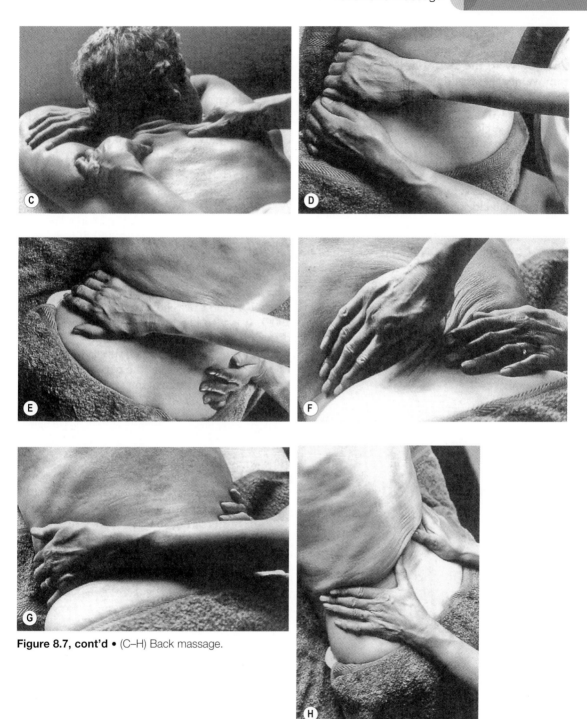

Figure 8.7, cont'd • (C–H) Back massage.

centre of your body opposite the patient's waistline.

5. Place both your hands on the gluteus maximus muscle farthest from you (Fig. 8.7D). Move your left hand straight across towards you with pressure on the initial lift (Fig. 8.7E). As your left hand returns to the left side of the body, move your right hand towards you to the right side of the body (Fig. 8.7F,G). As your right hand returns to the left side of the body, your left hand moves towards you again – to the right side. At every move, each hand is directed slightly higher up the body. Continue this two-way movement almost to the armpits, sliding both hands in a superficial movement down the lateral sides of the back, ready to repeat the whole movement several times.

6. Return to the position required for movement 1 and repeat that movement several times.

7. Using the whole of the length of the thumb and thenar muscle (Fig. 8.7H) push up firmly from the sacrum past the waist level, turning the thumb as the thenar muscle reaches the waist.

Take your thumb over to the fingers, then turn your hands towards the sides of the body until your fingertips touch the bed. Do not take your fingers around the body – when the fingertips make contact with the bed allow them to bend as the thenar muscle comes to meet them, making a fist on the bed.

8. Repeat movement 1 several times.

Abdominal massage

Abdominal massage has been well documented since the beginning of the 20th century as a natural method of relieving constipation (Hertz 1909). It is also used on people hospitalized for various reasons, such as the elderly, those with cerebral palsy, Parkinson's disease and those who are HIV positive etc. (Emly 1993). Movements that follow the peristaltic action of the colon are particularly important.

Stand at the side of the bed and place one hand on top of the other at the top of the patient's diaphragmatic arch (Fig. 8.8A). Check hands are relaxed and think 'palm' when directing the movement.

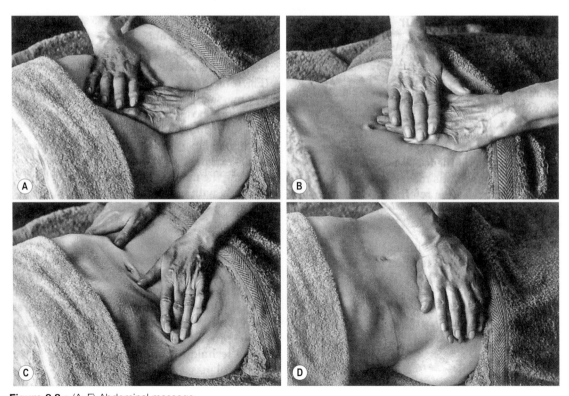

Figure 8.8 • (A–F) Abdominal massage.

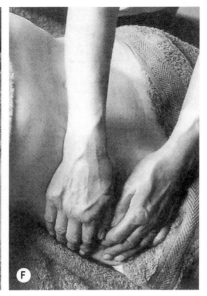

Figure 8.8, cont'd

1. Bring the hands gently down the centre of the body until you can see the patient's navel at the tips of your fingers (Fig. 8.8B). Turn your fingers outwards (Fig. 8.8C) and take them just under the waist. Lift both hands, keeping full contact and bringing them towards each other downwards (keeping palms down) to the pelvic bone. With your fingers in the original overlapped position, gently slide up the centre of the body to the sternum. Repeat the whole movement several times.

2. With overlapped hands at the right side of the body (Fig. 8.8D), move them slowly and gently in a clockwise circle up the ascending colon, across the transverse colon and down the descending colon several times, finishing where you began.

3. Keeping your hands reinforced and fingers relaxed, make small clockwise circles, in one big circle, with your palms, following the colon as in movement 2 (Fig. 8.8E).

4. Place both hands on the far side of the abdomen (Fig. 8.8F) and perform movement 5 from the back massage above, but gently, with less pressure.

5. Repeat movement 3. For severe constipation, the fingers of the underneath hand may be made into a fist in order to give a slower, more determined stimulus to the colon.

6. Repeat movement 2.

Pregnancy and labour massage

During pregnancy normal massage is encouraged up to the fifth month. As the pregnancy develops, the mother-to-be cannot lie comfortably on her tummy and the following special techniques show how the massage sequences above can be adapted at this stage.

Back massage is possible if the mother-to-be can adopt any of the following positions, whichever she finds most comfortable:

- Semi-prone, often referred to as Sims' position; on the left (or right) side and chest, the opposite knee and thigh drawn up so that it can rest on the bed, the trailing arm along the back (Fig. 8.9A).
- Sitting on the bed with legs in a squatting position, resting the top half of the body on the backrest plus pillows (Fig. 8.9B).
- Sitting straddled on a chair as suggested for shoulder massage, above.
- Sitting on a stool facing the side of the bed, resting arms and head on a pillow on the bed (Fig. 8.9C).

Leg massage can take place with the patient in a sitting position on the bed, supported by a backrest and pillows.

Abdominal massage should be very gentle and is excellent for calming the baby and relaxing the mother. Raise the upper half of the body with pillows. Movement 1 has been found to be very effective during a contraction (Fern 1992).

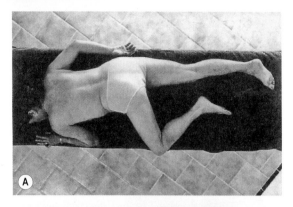

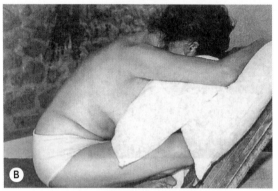

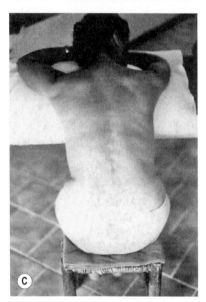

Figure 8.9 • (A–C) Massage during pregnancy.

Baby massage

For ease, the baby will be referred to as 'him' throughout the instructions.

New parents have no difficulty touching, stroking and cuddling their babies and it is a very small step from there to massage. However, as a baby's skin is delicate and rather 'loose', massage has to be gentle. Contact is particularly important for babies, so an excellent way to introduce massage is to sit on the sofa, supporting your back on cushions or pillows (Price & Price 2004). Place a warm soft towel over your abdomen and lay the baby there on his back – head away from you, drawing your knees up towards you to support him. The following movements can also be done on a baby mattress, covered with a warm towel and placed on a table (this is the best way for massaging the baby's back).

Put a little of the selected blend of oils onto warm hands, gently rubbing them together to distribute and warm the oil blend. Then carry out the following movements.

Tummy

Holding one of the baby's hands to make him feel secure and prevent him from 'thrashing' around (Price & Price 2004), place the fingers of the other hand gently on his tummy and, using as much of the finger lengths as possible, make gentle but firm clockwise circles around his navel (Fig. 8.10A). Repeat several times.

Scalp and forehead

1. Place the fingers of both hands firmly on the baby's scalp, so that it can be moved gently over the bone beneath (Fig. 8.10B). Move the fingers to a different position and repeat.
2. With fingertips on the baby's scalp, move the whole length of the thumbs alternately up his forehead several times. Repeat movement 1.

Feet and legs

1. Gently holding the baby's right thigh with your right hand, place the left hand fingers on top of his foot, and with as much of the length of the thumbs

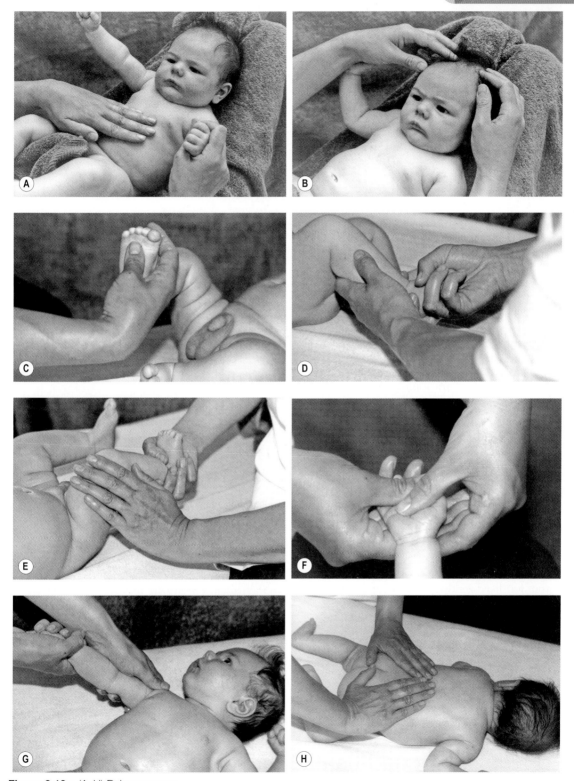

Figure 8.10 • (A–H) Baby massage.

Continued

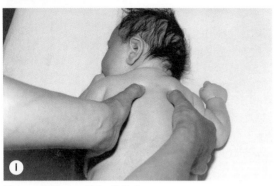

Figure 8.10, cont'd • (I) Baby massage.

as possible over the sole of his foot, move in slow circles over the middle area (Fig. 8.10C).

2. Hold the baby's foot with the right hand and move the left thumb in circles from ankle to knee, returning lightly (Fig. 8.10D). Repeat several times.

3. Gently but firmly take the curved lengths of the left fingers from the baby's ankle to his thigh, covering as much of the outside of his leg as possible in the one stroke, returning lightly underneath (Fig. 8.10E). Repeat several times.

4. Repeat movement 1.

5. Repeat movements 1–4 on the other foot and leg, reversing the handhold used.

Hands and arms

1. Placing the fingers of both hands on the back of the baby's hand, place your right thumb over his fingers and make circles on his palm with your left thumb (Fig. 8.10F).

2. Holding his hand with your right hand, take your left hand gently but firmly up his arm to the shoulder and around it, returning very lightly on the back of his arm (Fig. 8.10G). Repeat several times.

Repeat both movements on the other hand and arm, reversing the handhold used.

Back

The back is easier to do on a baby mattress (see above).

1. With fingers and thumbs making a triangle (Fig. 8.10H), move the whole finger length up baby's back, using as much of the hands as possible to

'cuddle' round his shoulders, before returning very gently down the sides of his body. Repeat 4–5 times.

2. Place your hands around the sides of the baby's body, with one thumb on each buttock. Making large circles with the flat of the thumbs and move slowly and progressively up his back, with slight pressure on the upward half of each circle. On reaching the shoulders (Fig. 8.10I), take the thumbs right round them, returning very gently down the sides of his body. Repeat 3–4 times.

3. Repeat movement 1.

Swiss reflex treatment

This technique was devised by Shirley Price in 1987 while in Switzerland (hence the name), and although it is based on reflex points it differs from reflexology, which is 'an ancient Eastern technique which makes use of somewhat mysterious connecting pathways or energy flow lines in the body' (Price 2000 p. 43). These culminate in various areas of the body, occurring in the feet, hands, ears and tongue, where reflexes representing every part of the body can be found. Foot reflex points can be used as a diagnostic aid; furthermore, massaging the relevant points with essential oils can treat the body via the energy flow lines. As with any therapy, an accredited training is necessary to understand the position, significance and connection between the bodily systems and reflex points.

Prior to treatment, the therapist must either be aware of the patient's problem areas or test each reflex for a reaction.

In a Swiss reflex treatment (SRT), reflexes specific to the patient's health are massaged, together with a precise dialogue between therapist and client. A bland cream base is used, to which are added essential oils selected by the same method as for an aromatherapy massage. The ratio of essential oil to cream is a minimum of 30 drops to 30 mL, as such a tiny amount is used. The treatment is much simpler to learn than the techniques involved in reflexology, although knowledge of the location of the representative reflexes is of primary importance before treatment can be carried out successfully. As with all practical subjects, attending a practical course is the best way to learn. However, the basic principles are described below.

SRT involves special client participation, including *daily* self-treatment (or treatment by partner or carer) at home. Without daily treatment, the results are approximately the same as in reflexology or normal massage; however, with daily SRT, positive results are gained much more quickly. Therapists trained in this method by the author before her business passed into other hands – and present students of the Penny Price Academy of Aromatherapy (see Useful addresses, p. 528) – have had some extraordinarily positive results (see Case Studies 8.4, 8.5).

Method of treatment

Having determined which reflexes are in need of treatment, always begin with the solar plexus reflex area (Fig. 8.11A) and finish on the kidney–bladder area (Fig. 8.11B).

1. Apply a very small amount of cream all over the dorsum and sole of the right foot.

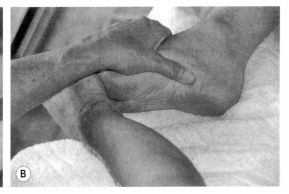

Figure 8.11 • (A–B) Swiss reflex massage.

Case study 8.4

Arthritic pain

S Price – Aromatologist

Client assessment

Mrs U, 58, had just recovered from a second attempt at a hip replacement, the healing of which was helped considerably by aromatherapy. Now, she was to undergo an operation to fuse her cervical vertebrae on account of the severe arthritic pain there. She was very anxious about this, as due to the death of her husband she needed to be able to continue driving. She wore a surgical collar, which she hated.

Intervention

Mrs U was given a Swiss reflex treatment using the following essential oils, added to a 30 mL jar of bland, non-greasy Swiss reflex cream base:

- 10 drops *Rosmarinus officinalis* [rosemary] – analgesic, anti-inflammatory
- 4 drops *Origanum majorana* [sweet marjoram] – properties as above
- 8 drops *Juniperus communis* [juniper berry] – properties as above

She was then shown how to massage the same areas herself at home every day, and given the jar of reflex cream.

At the second visit 2 weeks later no improvement had been made, and it was discovered that the client had been massaging the wrong reflex! This experience indicates the importance of giving the client a marked chart, illustrating exactly not only the sequence of the treatment but also the reflex points to be massaged (on this occasion it had been forgotten!).

Two weeks later, Mrs U was experiencing somewhat less pain and a slight improvement in neck mobility. The improvement continued over the next 2 weeks and at the fourth appointment she arrived smiling – wearing a collar homemade from firm foam sponge wrapped in a pretty scarf.

Outcome

Six weeks later, with only self-treatment and a visit every 2 weeks to confirm all was progressing well, she arrived without even the silk-wrapped foam collar. She had had her appointment with the consultant prior to the operation and he was so amazed at the change in her mobility and the lack of pain that he told her the operation would not now be necessary. He asked her what she had been doing, but unfortunately Mrs U was too embarrassed to say she had been rubbing her big toe!

Case study 8.5

Mining accident

D Moore – Aromatherapist

Client assessment

Frank had been in a mining accident 19 years previously. A roof beam had fallen on his shoulder, which was damaged, causing a rib to be broken which had pierced his lung. Apart from being unable to move his arm away from his side, he was having breathing difficulties and when walking could only move his feet 15–17 cm at a time.

He had been under a consultant for the whole 19 years and was becoming progressively worse, rather than better. His wife had heard Shirley Price speaking on the radio about aromatherapy and decided to try this treatment for Frank.

Intervention

When they arrived, it was obvious that an aromatherapy body massage would not be possible – the answer had to be Swiss reflex treatment.

This was given to him twice a week for the first week, once a week for 2 further weeks, once a fortnight for the next month, then once a month and eventually once every 2 or 3 months. The oils selected for Frank, in 30 mL of the bland reflex cream base, were:

- *Piper nigrum* [black pepper] – analgesic, antispasmodic, expectorant

- *Juniperus communis*. ram [juniper twig] – analgesic, anticatarrhal, neurotonic
- *Boswellia carteri* [frankincense] – analgesic, anticatarrhal, anti-inflammatory, expectorant, immunostimulant
- *Lavandula officinalis* [lavender] – analgesic, antispasmodic, calming, general tonic

Frank's wife was taught how to do the daily treatment and they returned in 4 days to check she was doing it correctly – which she was.

After 6 weeks it was obvious she had never missed a day, as Frank could raise his right arm about 10 cm; after another 2 months this had not only increased to 30 cm, but his shoulders and head were halfway to being erect and his feet were able to take steps of around 26–30 cm.

Outcome

After 6 months Frank was leaving the centre with his head erect and an almost normal, albeit slow, step. He had proudly shown the therapist how he could lift his arm almost up to his shoulder and was looking forward to the day he could comb his own hair with his right hand again.

---

2. Carry out foot movements 1 (but up to the ankle only) and 2 several times to warm the foot, then wrap in a towel.

3. Repeat these two movements on the left foot and wrap in a towel.

4. Place the palm of the left hand over the toes of the right foot and begin by massaging the solar plexus reflex area in a circular motion with the whole of the length of your right thumb (Fig. 8.11A) – as firmly as the individual patient will tolerante (if the patient is highly stressed, even gentle stroking will seem painful). The pressure should be just such that the patient feels slight discomfort ('pain'). Maintain this same pressure – and circling – until the client is able to tell you that the 'pain' is no longer evident. If the discomfort is still present after 1 minute, the original pressure was probably too strong and the movement should be repeated with just

enough pressure to take the patient to his/her lowest pain threshold.

5. Using the same method as in movement 4, massage any reflex area of which the representative organ is presenting a problem to the patient, e.g. lung area for bronchial problems, digestive system area for constipation (concentrating on the large intestine reflex areas, in a clockwise direction), spinal areas for rheumatism or arthritis (in three small sections if the whole spine is affected). Change your hand positions when necessary.

6. Placing your right hand across your body over the patient's toes, massage with the side length of the thumb in a firm circle, from kidney to ureter to bladder (Fig. 8.11B), relaxing the pressure on the return half of the circle.

7. Repeat movements 2 and 3 and rewrap in the towel.

8. Repeat movements 2–7 on the left foot, reversing 'right' and 'left' in the text.

Carrier oils

Vegetable carrier oils constitute the bulk of the material used in an aromatherapy massage. Their function is to 'carry' or act as a vehicle for administering the essential oils to the body, and also as lubricants, to make massage movements possible. This section briefly discusses the nature of carrier oils, and details the properties and applications of those more frequently used in aromatherapy.

Fixed oils

Carrier oils are also known as fixed oils, because they do not evaporate, in contrast to the volatile plant essential oils, which do. Fixed carrier oils constitute a different chemical family from essential oils, which is why their properties are so different. Because of their lubricating quality and non-volatile nature they leave a permanent oily mark on paper; essential oils do not leave an oily mark, although any colour present will leave a stain. All essential oils dissolve easily and completely in fixed oils in all proportions.

Chemically speaking, carrier oils are classed as lipids, which are a diverse family of compounds found naturally in plants and animals. Oils and fats have similar structures, but at room temperature (15°C) fats are solid and oils are liquid. For the detailed chemistry of carrier oils, see *Carrier Oils for Aromatherapy and Massage* (Price & Price 2008).

Vegetable oils contain a high level of unsaturated fatty acid units (>80%), which is why they are important for our health. The double bonds are less strong than single bonds and introduce an element of weakness into a compound. Once opened up they can absorb other molecules for transportation elsewhere in the body, and can also facilitate the natural digestive breakdown of the triacylglycerols. Oils with a high degree of unsaturation are less stable than those that are highly saturated, owing to the weakness of the double bonds; thus they are open to attack by oxygen and moisture, which can lead to breakdown and rancidity.

Cold-pressed oils

Carrier oils used in aromatherapy should, wherever possible, be cold pressed, although this term is a slight misnomer as the extraction process generates a certain amount of heat – and cooling is normally required. Temperatures are usually maintained below 60°C, and in this way changes to the natural characteristics of the oil are kept to a minimum.

Vegetable oils may be refined to meet the particular requirements of large-scale users such as the pharmaceutical industry, cooking oil manufacturers, food processors and cosmetics companies. Processing here frequently involves the use of high temperatures and chemicals, when many of the natural properties of the oil are lost, its character is altered and its use in aromatherapy is not desirable. This is the type of oil usually found on supermarket shelves.

Mineral oils are high molecular weight hydrocarbons, with very different properties from those of vegetable oils. They are oily and greasy, with a tendency to clog the pores, and are less able to be absorbed by the skin: because of this unsuitability they are not normally used in aromatherapy.

Types of carrier oil

There are three broad categories:

- **Basic oils.** These can be used with or without essential oils for body massage and are generally pale in colour, not too viscous, and have very little smell. They include sweet almond, apricot kernel, peach kernel (see page 193), grapeseed and sunflower.
- **Special oils.** These tend to be more viscous, heavier and more expensive. They include avocado, sesame, rose hip and wheatgerm. The extra-rich oils such as avocado and wheatgerm are seldom, if ever, used on their own: it is more normal to use them as 10–25% of a carrier oil blend.
- **Macerated oils.** As these have certain additional properties to the oils above, because of the way they are produced, they can be used on their own, although it is preferable to add one or two drops of appropriate essential oils to increase the effect on health conditions. Chopped plant material is added to a selected fixed oil (mostly sunflower or olive), agitated gently for some time, then left for some weeks before filtering. All the plant's oil-soluble compounds (including any essential oil compounds that may be present) are transferred to the carrier oil, giving them extra therapeutic effects.

There are more than 20 suitable carrier oils available (Price & Price 2008) – a small selection is detailed below. Table 8.1 gives a more complete list, including particular properties and indications for each.

Table 8.1   Properties and indications of carrier oils

Fixed oils (*indicates macerated)	Properties and indications – general										
COMMON NAME *Scientific name*	Analgesic (light)	Anti-inflammatory	Antipruritic	Arthritis	Astringent	Circulatory	Haemorrhoids	Laxative	Lowers blood cholesterol	PMT	Rheumatism
ALMOND SWEET *Prunus amygdalis* var. *dulcis*		X	X	X				X	X		
APRICOT KERNEL *Prunus armeniaca*			X					X	X		
AVOCADO *Persea gratissima*						X					
CALENDULA* *Calendula officinalis*		X			X						X
CARROT* *Daucus carota*	X	X									
EVENING PRIMROSE *Oenethera biennis*				X					X	X	
GRAPESEED *Vitis vinifera*											
HAZELNUT *Corylus avellana*			X		X	X					
JOJOBA *Simmondsia chinensis*			X		X	X					
LEMON BALM* *Melissa officinalis*										X	
LIME BLOSSOM, LINDEN* *Tilia europoea*										X	
MACADAMIA *Macadamia ternifolia*								X			
OLIVE *Olea europoea*				X			X				X
PASSIONFLOWER *Passiflora incarnata*			X								
PEACH KERNEL *Prunus persica*					X					X	X
ROSE HIP *Rosa canina, R. mosquetta*											
ST JOHN'S WORT* *Hypericum perforatum*	X	X				X				X	X
SUNFLOWER *Helianthus annuus*					X				X		
TAMANU *Calophyllum inophyllum*	X	X									
WALNUT *Juglans regia*					X		X				
WHEATGERM *Triticum vulgare*						X				X	

	Sprains/bruises	Varicose veins	Wounds	Acne	Broken veins	Burns	Eczema	Emollient, dry skin	Psoriasis	Scars	Shingles zoster	Sunburnt skin	Sun protection	Wrinkles, mature skin
Properties and indications – skin														
							X	X	X					
							X	X						X
	X			X	X					X				
	X	X		X	X	X								
		X	X			X	X							
			X				X	X	X					
							X							
			X										X	
	X				X				X	X	X			
									X					
												X	X	
		X					X					X		
							X						X	
	X				X	X				X				X
		X			X						X			
	X	X												
						X	X	X	X					
					X				?					
				X					X					

Basic oils

Almond sweet (*Prunus amygdalis* var. *dulcis*)

Sweet almond oil is one of the most-used carrier oils; pale yellow in colour, it is slightly viscous and very oily. Apricot kernel *(P. armeniaca)* and peach kernel *(P. persica)* oils are very similar – it can be very difficult to discriminate between them. Their advantage over some other base oils is that they have less tendency to become rancid. The unrefined oil has a delicate, sweet smell and a flavour with a hint of marzipan. Sweet almond oil is used in laxative preparations and is said to be effective in reducing blood cholesterol levels (Leung & Foster 1996). It is an excellent emollient and nourishes dry skin; it also helps to soothe inflammation (Stier 1990). Almond oil is beneficial in relieving the itching caused by eczema, psoriasis, dermatitis and all cases of dry scaly skin, and is absorbed slowly through the intact skin (Expert Panel 1983 p. 97). It is said to be non-irritant, non-sensitizing and safe for cosmetic use (Leung & Foster 1996), but a few people are allergic to cosmetics containing almond oil, suffering a stuffy nose and skin rash (Winter 1999 p. 88).

Grapeseed (*Vitis vinifera*)

Grape seeds cannot be cold pressed and the oil is produced commercially by hot extraction. If it can be 'rescued' before it is refined, it is suitable for aromatherapy as refining includes chemical processing. The oil is tasteless, almost odourless, and as it is very fine it is also used to lubricate watches. It is a gentle emollient and leaves the skin with a smooth satin finish without feeling greasy.

Sunflower (*Helianthus annuus*)

Much of the sunflower oil available commercially has been obtained by solvent extraction, so care must be taken to ensure that only cold-pressed oil, which is also available, is used in aromatherapy. Sunflower oil has slight diuretic properties; it is said to aid cholesterol metabolism and may be used to counteract arteriosclerosis (Stier 1990). It is expectorant and, as it contains inulin, it may be useful in the treatment of asthma. The oil is beneficial for skin complaints and bruises, and is effective on leg ulcers. It has been reported as being efficacious in the treatment of

multiple sclerosis (Anon 1990, Millar et al. 1973, Swank & Dugan 1990).

Special oils

Avocado oil (*Persea gratissima, Persea americana*) Lauraceae

True cold-pressed avocado oil (from the dried fruits) is a deep green colour and is comparatively rare. It keeps well but should not be chilled, as some useful parts of the oil would precipitate – it solidifies at 0°C. Occasionally it has a slightly cloudy appearance, occasionally with sediment, which can indicate that it has not been subjected to extensive refining. Refined avocado oil, used by the cosmetics industry, is bleached, leaving it pale yellow to colourless; it is widely available but should not be used therapeutically for obvious reasons.

Avocado oil is a good, penetrating emollient, useful for massage, where 10–25% is used in a base carrier oil. It is valuable in muscle preparations, has skin healing (Leung & Foster 1996 p. 54), moisturizing, and anti-wrinkle properties, and is recommended for dry skins. It has been used in Raynaud's disease (Stier 1990 p. 54). As far as is known, avocado oil is non-irritant and non-sensitizing (Winter 1999 p. 73). The ingested pressed oil is said to be helpful in constipation, liver and gallbladder problems and urinary infections (Price & Price 2008 p. 57 p. 40).

Evening primrose oil (*Oenothera biennis, O. glazioviana, O. nagraceae*)

Evening primrose oil, pressed from the seeds, includes 10% γ-linolenic acid (GLA), which is comparatively rare. This highly unsaturated oil is more reactive and less stable than most other oils. It oxidizes on exposure to air and light and is sensitive also to heat and humidity, therefore it should be stored in a cool, dark place. It is thought to be beneficial in the treatment of atopic eczema (Kerscher & Korting 1992, Lovell 1981), although this is contested by Berth-Jones and Graham-Brown (1993). It is known to be useful in the treatment of dry, scaly skin (Price & Price 2008 p. 100) and to benefit sufferers of psoriasis (Ferrando 1986). The oil improves dandruff conditions and accelerates wound healing

(Price & Price 2008 p. 100); for cosmetic use it is incorporated in anti-wrinkle preparations. Borage oil is sometimes added to increase the level of GLA. When ingested, evening primrose oil is said to control arthritis (Lovell 1981) and Horrobin (1983) claims it is helpful to PMS, though Collins et al. (1993) repudiate this claim.

Jojoba oil (*Simmondsia chinensis*, *Buxus chinensis*)

Jojoba oil is in fact a wax, not an oil; the seeds produce a liquid wax which does not become rancid, giving it a long shelf-life (it will solidify if stored in a refrigerator). It is very stable (indigestible to bacteria), so preservatives (often the cause of allergies or skin irritations) are not necessary. Jojoba contains the anti-inflammatory agent myristic acid, making it beneficial for arthritis and rheumatism. It is particularly useful in cases of acne, as its molecular structure is similar to that of sebum, and it is used to control the build-up of excessive sebum (Anon 1983). It is also used for nappy rash and chapped skin (Bartram 1996 p. 258), psoriasis, sunburn and eczema. Jojoba oil may cause an allergic reaction (Winter 1999 p. 265), and contact dermatitis has also been reported (Scott & Scott 1982).

Peach kernel oil (*Prunus persica*)

This oil, usually cold pressed, is chemically and physically similar to almond and apricot kernel oils, albeit more expensive, as it is not produced in large quantities. It is emollient and nourishing, so is beneficial for dry, sensitive and ageing skins. It is reputed to relieve itching and help eczema (Price & Price 2008 p. 151). The oil is often used in the cosmetic industry as a substitute for almond oil (Wren 1975) in facial massage oils and skin care creams. Culpeper (1616–1684) tells us that the oil brings rest and sleep when applied to the forehead, and when ingested it is said to relieve constipation and high blood cholesterol (Price & Price 2008 p. 151).

Rose hip (*Rosa mosquetta*, *R. rubiginosa*)

Rose hip oil, taken from the seeds within, is a golden-red colour and contains significant amounts of vitamin C. It also contains small quantities

of *trans*-retinoic acid, which contribute to its therapeutic properties. Studies in Chile have identified that the oil is a tissue regenerator and has an effect on the skin to minimize premature ageing and wrinkles, as well as reducing scar tissue. It is helpful on wounds, burns and eczema.

Wheatgerm (*Triticum vulgare*)

Wheatgerm is a rich orange-brown colour and very viscous. It is seldom used on its own, being commonly employed as 10–25% of the carrier oil mix. Because of its high content of vitamin E, a natural antioxidant, it is added to less stable oils to increase their useful life. The oil is rich in lipid-soluble vitamins and so is good for revitalizing dry skin. It is also said to be useful on ageing skin, where its natural antioxidants are an effective weapon against free radicals. The oil is beneficial for tired muscles and should be included in the mix for after-sports massage.

Macerated oils

Calendula (*Calendula officinalis*)

Calendula oil is obtained by macerating chopped plant material in sunflower oil, and the normal orange-yellow colour of the calendula flowers is reflected in the colour of the oil. Although calendula is sometimes referred to as 'marigold' it is a very different plant from *Tagetes patula* and *Tagetes minuta* [tagetes, French marigold], which are also known as marigold. Calendula extracts have been used to promote healing and reduce inflammation (Fleischner 1985), and it is most effective on broken veins, varicose veins, bruises etc. Calendula is specifically indicated for enlarged or inflamed lymph nodes, sebaceous cysts and acute or chronic skin lesions (Casley-Smith & Casley-Smith 1983).

St John's wort (*Hypericum perforatum*)

This plant is usually macerated in olive oil, the resulting oil being a deep red colour, owing to the presence of hypericin. An anti-inflammatory oil, hypericum is useful on wounds where there is nerve tissue damage and also for inflamed nerve conditions, hence it is used in cases of neuralgia, sciatica and fibrositis. A 20% hypericum tincture has been used in the treatment of suppurative otitis, and extracts are stated to have been used clinically in Russia to treat infection (Shaparenko et al. 1979). The use of hypericum in the treatment of vitiligo (Newall, Anderson & Phillipson 1996) has also been reported, as has its use as an astringent and diuretic (Martindale 1993). Hypericin, the red pigment, is being studied as a possible antiviral agent in the management of acquired immunodeficiency syndrome (AIDS) (Abrams 1990, Anon 1991).

Summary

Touch and massage have profound benefits, not only for the recipient but also for the therapist, and its recent neglect in official healthcare is slowly beginning to be remedied. This chapter has identified the main benefits, as well as the contraindications. It has also provided a basic grounding in simple massage techniques, and suggested some of the more useful massage sequences. Carrier oils comprise the major part of any blend used in an aromatherapy massage and should be selected with care, to augment the effects of essential oils on presenting symptoms.

References

Abrams, D.I., 1990. Alternative therapies in HIV infection. AIDS 4, 1179–1187.

Anon, 1983. Botanicals in cosmetics. Jojoba: a botanical with a proven functionality. Cosmetics and Toiletries 98, 81–82.

Anon, 1990. Lipids and multiple sclerosis. Lancet 336, 25–26.

Anon, 1991. Treating AIDS with worts. Science 254, 522.

Auckett, A.D., 1981. Baby massage. Newmarket press, New York.

Barlow, J., Cullen, L., 2002. Increasing touch between parents and children with disabilities: preliminary results from a new programme. J. Fam. Health Care 12 (1), 7–9.

Bartram, T., 1996. Encyclopedia of herbal medicine. In: Grace, Christchurch, p. 258.

Beard, G., Wood, E.C., 1964. Massage – principles and techniques. Saunders, London.

Berth-Jones, J., Graham-Brown, R.A.C., 1993. Placebo controlled trial of essential fatty acid supplementation in atopic dermatitis. Lancet 341, 1557–1560.

Buckle, 1997. Clinical aromatherapy in nursing. Arnold, London.

Casley-Smith, J.R., Casley-Smith, J.R., 1983. The effect of *Unguentum lymphaticum* on acute experimental lymphedema and other high-protein edemas. Lymphology 16, 150–156.

Chaitow, L., 2000. Field, T. (Ed.), Touch therapy. Churchill Livingstone, Edinburgh, p. vii.

Collins, A., Coleman, G., Landgren, B. M., 1993. Essential fatty acids in the treatment of premenstrual syndrome. Obstet. Gynaecol. 81, 93–98.

Culpeper, undated. Culpeper's complete herbal. Foulsham, Exeter, p. 262.

Emly, M., 1993. Abdominal massage. Nurs. Times 89 (3), 34–36.

Expert Panel, 1983. Cosmetic ingredient review: 4: Final report on the safety of sweet almond oil and almond meal. J. Am. Coll. Toxicol. 2 (5), 85–99.

Fern, E., 1992. Directorate of Maternity and Gynaecology. Practice Group (Midwifery, Gynaecology and Neonatal Care) Aromatherapy. Midwifery Procedure no. 23, Ipswich Hospital.

Ferrando, J., 1986. Clinical trial of topical preparation containing urea, sunflower oil, evening primrose oil, wheatgerm oil and sodium pyruvate in several hyperkeratotic skin conditions. Med. Cutan. Ibero Lat. Am. 14 (2), 132–137.

Field, T., 2000. Touch therapy. Churchill Livingstone, Edinburgh.

Field, T., Scafidi, F., Schanberg, S., 1987. Massage of preterm newborns to improve growth and development. Paediatr. Nurs. 13, 385–387.

Fleischner, A.M., 1985. Plant extracts: to accelerate healing and reduce inflammation. Cosmetics and Toiletries 100, 45.

Hertz, A.F., 1909. Constipation and internal disorders. Oxford University Press, Oxford.

Horrigan, C., 1991. Complementing cancer care. Int. J. Aromather. 3 (4), 15–17.

Horrobin, D.F., 1983. The role of essential fatty acids and prostaglandins in the premenstrual syndrome. J. Reprod. Med. 28, 465–468.

Kerscher, M.J., Korting, H.C., 1992. Treatment of atopic eeczema with evening primrose oil. Lancet 1 (8214), 278.

Leung, A.Y., Foster, S., 1996. Encyclopedia of common natural ingredients. Wiley, New York.

Lovell, C.R., 1981. Plants and the skin. In: Blackwell, London, p. 255.

Martindale, 1993. The extra pharmacopoeia. In: thirtieth ed Pharmaceutical Press, London, p. 1378.3.

Maxwell-Hudson, C., 1999. Aromatherapy massage. In: Dorling Kindersley, New York, p. 41.

Mennell, J.B., 1945. Physical treatment, fifth ed Blakiston, Philadelphia.

Millar, J.H.D., Zilkha, K.J., Langman, M. J.S., Payling Wright, H., Smith, A.D., Belin, J., et al., 1973. Double blind trial of linoleate supplementation of the diet in multiple sclerosis. Br. Med. J. 1 (5856), 765–768.

Newall, C.A., Anderson, L.A., Phillipson, J.D., 1996. Herbal medicines. In: The Pharmaceutical Press, London, p. 251.

Price, S., 1999. Practical aromatherapy, How to use essential oils to restore health and vitality, fourth ed Thorsons, London.

Price, S., 2000. The aromatherapy workbook, second ed Thorsons, London.

Price, S., Price, P., 2004. Aromatherapy for babies and children, second ed Riverhead, Stratford upon Avon.

Price, L., Price, S., 2008. Carrier oils for aromatherapy and massage, fourth ed Riverhead, Stratford upon Avon.

Sanderson, H., Harrison, J., Price, S., 1991. Aromatherapy and massage for people with learning difficulties. Hands On, Birmingham.

Scott, M.J., Scott Jr., M.J., 1982. Jojoba oil (Letter). J. Am. Acad. Dermatol. .

Shaparenko, B.A., Slivko, B.A., Bazarova, O.V., Vishnevetskaya, E.N., Selesneva, G.T., Berezhnala, L.P., 1979. On the use of medicinal plants for treatment of patients with chronic suppurative otitis. Zh. Ushn. Nos. Gorl. Bolezn. 39 (3), 48–51.

Stier, B., 1990. Secrets des huiles de première pression à froid. Self published, Quebec.

Swank, R.L., Dugan, B.B., 1990. Effect of low saturated fat diet in early and late cases of multiple sclerosis. Lancet 336, 37–39.

Tattam, A., 1992. The gentle touch. Nurs. Times 88 (32), 16–17.

Vickers, A., 1996. Aromatherapy and massage. A guide for Health Professionals. In: Chapman & Hall, London, p. 6.

Wilkinson, S., 1995. Aromatherapy and massage in palliative care. Int. J. Palliat. Nurs. 1 (1), 21–30.

Winter, R., 1999. A consumer's dictionary of cosmetic ingredients, fifth ed Crown, New York.

Worrell, J., 1997. Touch: attitudes and practice. Nurs. Forum. 18 (1), 1–17.

Wren, R.W., 1975. Potter's new cyclopaedia of botanical drugs and preparations. In: Health Science Press, Bradford nr. Holsworthy, p. 23.

Aromatic medicine

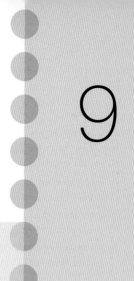

Robert Stephen

CHAPTER CONTENTS

Introduction

The practice of aromatic medicine has undergone something of a revolution in recent times. It has its origins in France, where essential oils are used internally and externally in larger dosages – and prescribed by those who are trained as medical practitioners. Unfortunately, in the UK there is a great suspicion of those who advocate internal use of essential oils. The fear is based on current legislation, which allows aromatherapy under a single exemption (Section 12 (1) of the Medicines Act 1968), effectively treating the use of essential oils as a cosmetic. To advance to claims for therapeutic use would necessitate new legislation, with the fear that current aromatherapeutic uses would be endangered by such revision. The exception permissible at the moment is that trained and qualified herbalists (who are not specifically qualified in the administration of essential oils) may prescribe them for internal use. However, there are aromatherapists who want to hold on to a distinct, yet related, aromatic practice that has little or no association with massage. Given that there are some clients who for various reasons may be

unable – or do not wish – to receive massage, the acceptance of aromatic medicine may be an equal opportunities issue, in that it allows access to the use of essential oils for those who, limited by movement, use of limbs or weight, cannot receive what would in the UK be regarded as a 'normal' aromatherapy treatment.

Aromatic medicine explained

Aromatic medicine has a number of distinctive elements that distinguish it from aromatherapy as it is practised in the UK:

- It is a therapy in which essential oils are used confidently and efficaciously in the most appropriate way for any presenting condition. The therapy is aromatic because it uses the aromatic, volatile molecules that constitute essential oils.
- It moves beyond the near-homoeopathic normal doses associated with aromatherapy massage and involves a considered response to a particular situation, balancing the presenting condition with a detailed knowledge of essential oils.
- It is built on knowledge of the therapeutic actions of the chemical components that make up essential oils, plus an understanding of the synergy within a single oil and the synergistic potential of blended oils.

It may well be that practitioners of aromatic medicine may have to train to the same level of recognition as herbalists before they will be permitted to prescribe for internal use, but as this is not the entire therapy one should look to building both understanding and confidence in what is a very precise and exacting branch of aromatherapy. There certainly should be no restriction in the intensive topical use. The intensive and specific use of essential oils is a valid expression of aromatherapy and is:

- intensive because of the higher dosage than that used in massage
- intensive because it is more focused on a particular presenting condition
- intensive because of the application of chemistry as the principal tool used in oil selection
- specific because essential oils are engaged for a particular health improvement rather than general wellbeing
- specific because whole-body massage is not always needed or wanted, a more focused application being more necessary.

Those who teach aromatherapy tend to attribute the advent of contemporary aromatherapy to the rediscovery made by **Gattefossé** of the healing properties of *Lavandula angustifolia* following a burn. Certainly this was an epiphany, supporting the intensive use of essential oils rather than the English-style aromatherapy, which owes as much to massage (a separate and independent therapy) and the use of carrier oils as it does to essential oils. It is this intensive use that will now be explored.

Beginning with essential oils

Any credible course in aromatherapy has an element of training in the chemistry of essential oils. This provides a foundation on which aromatic medicine is built. A much more detailed knowledge of the chemistry of essential oils and the therapeutic action of the various chemical components gives the use of essential oils in aromatic medicine its distinctiveness.

It is easy to read books on aromatherapy and to have claims for the various benefits from essential oils delineated. Many of these claims are based on traditional use (which is not to be disparaged, in that it has been tested through time – as valid a form of research as any), and without these uses practitioners may not be aware of how a benefit is to be achieved.

In aromatic medicine, treatment is based on the known and verifiable therapeutic effects of the chemical components found within the oils (Table 9.1), which means that practitioners need a

sound working knowledge of the constituent parts of the oils to be used. They also need to be competent enough to work out what the components in the synergy of an essential oil mix will achieve – this can only be understood by detailed training in the chemistry of essential oils.

Perhaps this approach is best illustrated with a recent example that caused a great deal of anxiety. Avian flu was followed by swine flu as a threatened pandemic. The few fatalities that ensued fuelled the hysteria that grew – disproportionately to the risk. The author, when taking a long-haul flight to China for a punishing teaching schedule of 7 days (including 10 flights), responded to the situation by researching the possible aromatic responses, the development in approaches 1–4 below showing the difference between the populist aromatherapy approach and that used in aromatic medicine (see Case 4.4 for the antiviral recipe used).

The available literature indicates that there are some essential oils and related products that are helpful in the treatment of viral conditions.

1. The general aromatherapy literature states that some essential oils are powerfully antiviral. Davis (2000 p. 308), for instance, suggests that bergamot, eucalyptus and tea tree may be used, but does not specify the oils, giving only the common names. These may indeed be effective, but there is no explanation as to how or why they work.

2. There is much more precision in the work of Pénoël and Franchomme. Franchomme (Franchomme & Pénoël 1990 p, 190) suggests that enveloped viruses respond to essential oils having a predominance of terpene-alcohols and phenols, whereas naked viruses respond to oils rich in terpenoid ketones. Pénoël is even more specific, suggesting that α-terpineol and the oxide 1,8-cineole should be administered. The oils suggested, in which these constituents are found, are *Laurus nobilis* [bay leaf], *Eucalyptus radiata* [narrow leaf peppermint] and *Melaleuca viridiflora* [niaouli].

3. Schnaubelt (1997 p. 98) states that terpenes enhance the immune system and metabolic activity by changing the receptors present on cell surfaces, and that new work is being undertaken on the reaction between sesquiterpenes and cell penetration.

4. Price and Price (2007 p.106) suggest that the effectiveness of essential oils may not be dependent upon any specific molecule, but rather

Table 9.1 Essential Oil Component Reference Chart Diagram (simplified) By kind permission of Penny Price Aromatherapy Ltd (www.penny-price.com)

Aromatic Medicine Essential Oil Component Reference Chart

Group	Monoterpenes	Sesquiterpenes	Alcohols gentle	Phenols can irritate	Aldehydes can irritate	Ketones use with care neurotoxic	Esters hydrophilic	Oxides can irritate
Properties	Mildly therapeutic Bulk of oil Hydrophobic Antiseptic	Mildly therapeutic Slightly hypotensive Anti-inflammatory	Analgesic Antiseptic Antiviral Stimulating	Antiseptic Anti-infectious Immunostimulant Nervine	Calming Hypotensive Anti-infectious Anti-inflammatory Nervine	Cicatrizant Lipolytic Mucolytic Sedative	Antifungal Anti-inflammatory Antispasmodic Cell regenerating	Mucolytic Expectorant Bronchodilators
Molecular structure	Two isoprene units joined head to tail	Three isoprene units joined head to tail	Hydroxyl radical (-oh) attached to a carbon chain	Hydroxyl radical (-oh) attached to a carbon in a benzene ring	Carbonyl radical (=o) and extra hydrogen (-h) attached to carbon chain or ring	Carbonyl radical (=o) attached to carbon chain or ring	Based on carboxyl group (-oh and =o together).	Rare in eos Except eucalyptol (1.8-cineole)
Component names	End in ene	End in ene	End in ol	End in ol	End in al or aldehyde	End in one	End in ate or acetate	End in oxide or ol
Comments				Short-term use	Short-term use	Short-term use		Medium-term use Used as excipient

on a property common to essential oils, perhaps lipid solubility.

5. The hypericin in *Hypericum perforatum* [St. John's wort] has been indicated as inhibiting the development of a virus within an infected cell (Miller 1998). Hypericin is active against several viruses, including cytomegalovirus, the human papilloma virus, hepatitis B and herpes virus. This antiviral activity has been shown in the laboratory and animal studies, but not in human studies. The herb seems to work against viruses by oxidation and its antiviral effect is stronger when exposed to light (as when animals eat the herb). St. John's Wort was studied in 1991 in people with HIV disease (Freeman & Lawlis, 2001, 415), where the doses were much higher than for treating depression. Patients were given intravenous doses of purified hypericin, but the study was stopped when every white-skinned patient in the trial became very sensitive to light. They developed skin rashes and some could not go outside until after they stopped taking hypericin. The one black-skinned patient did not have this reaction.

It is clear that essential oils are useful in the prevention of viral infection and in its treatment. Reflecting on the research, it appears as if essential oils are able to inhibit the absorption of a virus into a cell, and also to inhibit the reproduction of a virus once it has taken over a cell. On balance, the essential oils most useful are those with a predominance of 1,8-cineole and a significant presence of α-terpineol (although as has been seen, opinion varies and some viruses respond better to some oils than others – see Table 4.5 Ch. 4):

- *Eucalyptus radiata* [narrow-leaved peppermint]
- *Melaleuca viridiflora* [niaouli]
- *Ravensara aromatica* [ravensara]

One further essential which should be on this list, effective largely because of the powerful phenol eugenol, is *Syzygium aromaticum* (flos,) [clove bud].

It would be both possible and fitting to use the essential oil *Illicium verum* [star anise] as a preventative: the chemistry of the oil reveals that both 1,8-cineole and α-terpineol are present.

Given that viruses are contagious and very inventive in finding hosts, every care must be taken to prevent airborne infection and infection from contact. Diffusing an oil blend using a vaporizer is the best form of prevention. A blend of these oils added to a hand-wash would give further protection. If a viral infection has become established there are many proven and efficacious responses using essential oils, particularly to herpes simplex 1 and to the influenza viruses (Stephen 2010).

As aromatic medicine is a holistic therapy – a treatment tailored to an individual situation; it is a bespoke response in a therapeutic relationship.

Case study 9.1

Eye virus infection

Shirley Price – Aromatherapist

Assessment:

The editor (S Price) has suffered with a recurring herpes simplex virus in her left eye since it first appeared as a dendritic ulcer, necessitating an operation.

The prescription drops had to be collected each time from the hospital 15 miles away, which involved a day away from work (it included a test – and long wait), so she formulated what was to become her Chamomile Eye Drops (CED), a blend of orange flower water, distilled water and essential oil of *Chamaemelum nobile* (1 drop in 30 mL liquid). The virus disappeared as quickly with this as with the prescribed drops, and was used whenever it recurred (usually after a cold sore) until she retired in 1998.

Ten years later the virus appeared in a stronger form, necessitating a visit to the eye hospital, which prescribed a cream and two lots of drops to be put in separately several times of the day – a veritable nightmare! Hospital visits for check-ups went on for 2 years till the virus eventually 'went to sleep' again.

A year later it reappeared after a cold sore while in France, and as the nearest eye hospital was 2 hours away, S decided to try essential oils first – stronger than CED, as her eye was completely cloudy .

Intervention

- 1 drop of *Melissa officinalis* was added to 30 mL CED and 1 drop put into her eye each night.
- 3 drops of *Melissa* was put into 100 mL of *Thymus vulgaris* population hydrolat left from distilling the thyme in their field the previous year, and was used to bathe the eye three times daily.

Outcome

After a week the eye was less cloudy and after 3 weeks it was back to normal. Since then, S has put the drops in her eye once a week and applied one drop of *Melissa* around her lower lip as a preventative against the reappearance of a cold sore.

A practitioner need not be able to read a GC (gas chromatography) analysis, but should be aware of the principal components of the oils to be used (which should be obtained from a reputable supplier) and not just how an oil is generally made up. The prescription is used uniquely for the therapeutic action of chemical components in a properly calculated synergistic blend, to accomplish a specific objective. It is the whole oil that is used and not an isolate, which is why knowledge of the chemistry leads to awareness of the internal synergy of any resultant blend – as far as this is possible.

Matters of training and safety

Safety when using essential oils remains at the heart of practice; it is also at the heart of the debate between practitioners of aromatherapy and aromatic medicine. Aromatherapists – who may not always be aware of the full extent and possibilities of aromatherapy – will usually concede that intensive topical use of essential oils is sustainable as a practice, while rejecting any form of internal use, even though some schools teach the use of suppositories/pessaries and every aromatherapist uses and advocates gargling. It has been the author's contention for some time that topical use of essential oils (even in the quantities used in aromatherapy) becomes internal use, insofar as an essential oil is absorbed through the skin into the bloodstream and thence to the rest of the body. In 1877, Fleischer stated that the human skin was totally impermeable to all substances, including gases (Scheuplein et al., 1971 p. 703), but by 1945, Valette was able to demonstrate that essential oils penetrate the skin and goes on to say:

> Molecules which have passed through the skin's epidermis are carried away by capillary blood circulating in the dermis below. This tends to happen easily because the dermis is more or less freely permeable and the capillaries let small molecules pass through their walls. The most permeable regions of the skin to small molecules, including essential oils and vegetable oils, appear to be the palms of the hands and the soles of the feet, forehead, armpits and scalp (cited in Balacs, 1993c: 13)

Each time essential oils are applied to the skin there is a demonstrable presence of the chemical components in the blood. Essential oils molecules are carried into the cardiovascular lymphatic networks and thence diffused into all the organs. Hepatic sulfo- or glycurocombination then takes pace and renal elimination occurs (Byrne 1997: 35).

It is most unlikely that any essential oils fail to reach the bloodstream entirely when administered on to the skin; the factors that determine in what quantities they do, and how quickly and in what form, are many and complex (Balacs 1992a: 25).

Delieghere (1996) put up a strong defence for the internal use of essential oils at the first Australasian Aromatherapy Conference. He stated that anxiety about internal use of essential oils is due solely to a lack of knowledge. It is his contention that ingestion of essential oils may be safer than topical application for two reasons:

1. **Phototoxicity:** several essential oils (e.g. bergamot, lime etc.) contain furanocoumarins. There is a phototoxic effect if essential oils are used topically in combination with UV light. This does not happen when an essential oil is ingested.
2. **Allergic reactions:** the risk of allergic reactions is much reduced in ingestion compared to dermal administration.

Oral toxicity versus dermal toxicity

Table 9.2 (Devlieghere 1996: 17) is based on the work of Dr Maria Lis-Balchin (1997) and demonstrates that the LD50 (the median lethal dose applicable to 50% of the population) is sometimes safer in internal (oral) administration than when topically applied (dermal).

It is impossible to replicate naturally the chemical make-up of essential oils year after year, hence the importance of using the best-quality essential oils from trusted suppliers who have reliable sources.

Schnaubelt (1997 p. 128) responds adequately to questions of safety (particularly with reference to intensive use) when he says:

> A reasonable discussion of the safety of essential oils is distorted by the demand for "absolute safety" by consumers and practitioners. These demands are usually entertained by commercial interest looking for a way to sell to a public perceived as underinformed. The real intent of these demands is to ensure safety for the business venture. Alarmist attempts to discontinue completely the use of certain essential oils are a result of this. These warnings are made because there is a fear that accidents with essential oils could be used by government organizations to prohibit trade and thus hurt business. In light of the potential benefits, a modality as safe as aromatherapy should continue to be accessible despite the fact that minor accidents may occur, especially because the probability is much lower than for any other form of self-medication.

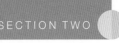

Table 9.2 Oral toxicity versus dermal toxicity

LD$_{50}$ – value in g/kg		
Essential oil	Oral LD50	Dermal LD50
Ocimum basilicum ct. linalool	1.4	0.5
Citrus basilicum ssp bergamia	>10	>20
Melaleuca leucadendron	4	>5
Cinnamomum camphora (white)	>5	>5
Cinnamomum camphora (yellow)	4	>5
Cedrus atlantica	>5	>5
Juniperus mexicana	>5	>5
Juniperus virginiana	>5	>5
Matricaria recutita	>5	>5
Chamaemelum nobile	>5	>5
Cinamomum zeylanicum ex foliae	2.7	>5
Cinamomum zeylanicum ex cotex	3.4	0.7
Cymbopogon nardus	>5	4.7
Salvia sclarea	5	>2
Eugenia caryophyllata ex flores	2.7–3.7	>5
Eugenia caryophyllata ex foliae	1.4	1.2
Anethum graveolens	4	>5
Eucalyptus citriodora	>5	2.5
Eucalyptus globules	4.4	>5
Foeniculum vulgaris var. dulce	4.5	>5
Foeniculum vulgaris var. vulgare	3.8	>5
Boswellia carterii	>5	>5
Zingiber officinale	>5	>5
Cinnamomum camphora var. hosho	3.8	>5
Jasminum grandiflorum	>5	>5
Juniperus communis ex fructus	8	>5
Lavandula angustifolia	>5	>5
Lavandula x burnatii	>5	>5
Lavandula latifolia	4	2

Table 9.2 Oral toxicity versus dermal toxicity—cont'd

LD$_{50}$ – value in g/kg		
Essential oil	Oral LD50	Dermal LD50
Citrus limonum	>5	>5
Citrus aurantium ssp amara ex flores	4.5	>5
Citrus aurantium ssp amara ex pericarpium	>5	>10
Citrus sinesis	>5	>5
Rosa damascene	>5	2.5
Salvia officinalis	2.6	>5
Salvia lavandulaefolia	>5	>5
Melaluca alternifolia	1.9	>5
Cananga odorata forma genuina	>5	>5
Citrus aurantium ssp amara ex pericarpium	>5	>10
Citrus sinesis	>5	>5
Rosa damascene	>5	2.5
Salvia officinalis	2.6	>5
Salvia lavandulaefolia	>5	>5
Melaluca alternifolia	1.9	>5
Cananga odorata forma genuina	>5	>5

Training

Training is essential for any complementary therapy and is vital if the intensive therapeutic use of essential oils is to be developed. It is extremely distressing to see advertisements for training in aromatology or aromatic medicine lasting but one or two days, after which a certificate in competence is issued. A course of such length, however well intentioned, lacks credibility and is a waste of money; a suitable course would be delivered at around Master's degree level in the UK.

An aspiring practitioner should have experience in using essential oils with a good grounding in theory and practice. Built onto this (or other related experience) should be an in-depth course in the chemistry of essential oils, followed by theoretical and practical knowledge of the specific techniques for intensive application or other appropriate use. Alongside this the specific philosophical theory of diagnostic triptychs, used to understand the development and progression of disease, was first suggested by Pénoël in 1988 and significantly developed by Gascoigne (1994).

It is essential that a period of supervised practice is undertaken, supported by case studies showing an understanding of reflective practice. Competence must be demonstrated by successfully completing an examination in both theory and practice, with regular study and engagement to sustain continuing professional development. This academic and technical rigour is necessary to ensure the wellbeing of clients.

Such a strict training regime is regarded as being elitist and unnecessarily academic, and beyond the intellectual reach of some. Quite so! By comparison, those who wish to practise aromatic medicine in France are expected to qualify as medical doctors before they begin their studies in aromatic medicine. An accredited course gives confidence to both clients and practitioners.

Treating clients

The potential of aromatic medicine is best seen in a case study, showing in one client both acute and chronic symptoms.

A full consultation leads to decisions being made about the priority of treatment needs. It would be accurate to state that, unlike aromatherapy, which anticipates an improvement and maintenance of general wellbeing and homoeostasis, aromatic medicine seeks to see specific and measurable responses to a targeted treatment.

Case study 9.2

MRSA

Debbie Moore – Aromatherapist and Penny Price – Aromatologist

Client assessment

Jim had had to have an amputation just above his ankle 3 years prior to his visit to the Penny Price Academy. The wound contracted MRSA. After the hospital had tried to cure the infection without success, Jim had to have another piece taken from his leg. This happened a further twice and Jim still had MRSA – he had become depressed and tired. His prosthetic leg could not be fitted until the infection had been cured and the skin over the wound had toughened enough not to break down when it came into contact with it.

Intervention

After a holistic assessment confirming both infection and depression, the following essential oils were selected:

- *Thymus vulgaris* ct. *thymol* [phenolic thyme] – powerful antiseptic, antidepressant, immunostimulant
- *Ravansara aromaticum* [ravensara] – antimicrobial, antiseptic, immunostimulant
- *Aniba rosaeodora* [rosewood] – analgesic, anti-inflammatory, neurotonic

The following were also used in the treatment:

- *Hypericum perforatum* [hypericum] macerated oil – antidepressant
- *Lavandula angustifolia* hydrolat [lavender] – anti-inflammatory, cell regenerating

The thyme, ravansara and rosewood oils were blended together in a 10 mL bottle for Jim to apply 4 drops three times a day to his wound, using a pipette to ensure that the oils went as deeply as possible into the infection.

He was given lavender hydrolat to spray on the stump regularly to help improve skin health.

He was also given a month's supply of capsules using hypericum as the base, with 1 drop each of thyme and rosewood per capsule – Jim took three capsules a day. The hypericum was chosen to help relieve the depression and strengthen the nervous system. The capsules were stopped after 1 month, but Jim continued with the drenches on the wound for 3 months.

Outcome

When Jim returned to the clinic after 3½ months, he walked through the door using his newly fitted prosthetic leg. The MRSA was no longer present, the wound had completely healed and the skin on the stump was strong and healthy. He was bright and cheerful and 'over the moon' that he had his independence back, no pain and no depression. Jim's wife was so impressed by the change in Jim that she has begun a training course in aromatology. Jim is using his prosthetic leg and is now well enough holistically to engage with life again – he says 'MRSA is not just about wounds – energy, appetite and will have all returned and everyone says how well I look'.

Conclusion

Aromatic medicine is a natural treatment using organic, unadulterated, whole plant volatile oils, hydrolats and fixed carrier oils, creating the most appropriate chemical synergy via the most effective interface as a targeted response to a presenting symptom or symptoms. It is often regarded as a development of aromatherapy, but should properly be understood as part of *complete* aromatherapy. As such, it is an exciting and safe therapy, using the same tools as in current aromatherapy practice but applied in distinct ways for specific outcomes.

References

Balacs, T., 1992a. Dermal crossing. Int. J. Aromather. 4 (2), 23–26.

Balacs, T., 1993c. Essential oils in the body: their absorption, distribution, metabolism and excretion. In: Proceedings of the AROMA 93 Conference.

Byrne, K., 1997. Ingestion of essential oils: food for thought. Simply Essential 26, 34–36.

Davis, P., 2000. Aromatherapy: an A-Z. Vermilion, London.

Devleighere, G., 1996. Oral use of essential oils. In: Proceedings of the Australasian Aromatherapy Conference.

Franchomme, P., Pénoël, D., 1990. L'Aromathérapie Exactement Roger Jollois Editeur.

Freeman, L.W., Lawlis, G.L., 2001. Complementary and Alternative Medicine: a researched based approach. Mosby, St Louis.

Gascoigne, S., 1994. The Manual of Conventional Medicine for Alternative Practitioners. Jigme Press, Dorking.

Lis-Balchin, M., Deans, S., Hart, S., 1997. A study of the changes in bioactivity of essential oils used singly and as mixtures in aromatherapy. Journal of Alternative and Complementary Medicine 3 (3), 249–256.

Miller, A.L., 1998. St. John's Wort (Hypericum perforatum): Clinical Effects on Depression and Other Conditions. Altern. Med. Rev. 3 (1), 18–26.

Price, L., Price, S., 2007. Aromatherapy for Health Professionals, third ed. Churchill-Livingstone, Edinburgh.

Scheuplein, R.J., Blank, I.H., 1971. Permeability of the skin. Psychol. Rev. 51 (4), 702–747.

Schnaubelt, K., 1996. Advanced Aromatherapy. Healing Arts Press, Vermont.

Schnaubelt, K., 1997. Medical Aromatherapy. Frog, Berkeley.

Stephen, R., 2010. Essential oils and viral illness. Aromatopia 19 (1), 9–13.

Sources

Balacs, T., 1993a. Hormones and health. Int. J. Aromather. 5 (1), 18–20.

Schnaubelt, K., 1989. Friendly molecules: aspects of essential oil constituents and their pharmacology. Int. J. Aromather. 2 (2), 20–22 and 2 (3), 16–17.

Valette, G., Sobrin, E., 1962. Absorption percutanée de diverses huiles animals ou végétales. Pharmaceutia acta Helvetiae 38, 710–716.

Valnet, C., 1945. Comptes Rendus. Société de Biologie (13th October).

Webster, R.C., Maibach, H.I., 1983. Cutaneous pharmacokinetics: 10 steps to percutaneous absorption. Drug Metab. Rev. 14 (2), 169–205.

Weyers, W., Brodbeck, R., 1989. Skin absorption of essential oils. Pharm. Unserer Zeit 18 (3), 82–86.

Williams, D.G., 1996. The chemistry of essential oils. Mycelle Press, Weymouth.

Zatz, J.L., 1993. Scratching the surface: rationale and approach to skin permeation. In: Zatz, J.L. (Ed.), Skin Permeation: fundamentals and applications. Allured, Wheaton.

Section 3

Aromatherapy in context

Section contents

Wound care

10

Denise Raines with contributions by Rhiannon Harris

Introduction

Of all the body's organs none is more exposed to infection, disease and injury than the skin, and wound healing is a prime example of how the body can maintain homoeostasis. This process often needs assistance to prevent the formation of chronic and sometimes fatal wounds. In this chapter we explore evidence to show how efficient aromatherapy and natural base products can be when used in the process of wound healing. The chapter also covers the stages of wound healing, previous research, the pros and cons of aromatic wound healing, pressure sores, burns and positive case studies.

The stages of wound healing

Wounds can be healed by primary intention, when the edges are brought together by stitches, staples or adhesive tape, e.g. following surgery or repaired lacerations; or by secondary intention, where the wound is left open and allowed to granulate. Very occasionally, owing to infection, wounds that are meant to heal by primary intention can break down and end up healing by secondary intention.

The classic model of wound healing is divided into several overlapping stages which normally progress in a predictable manner. If they do not, healing may not progress well, leading to a chronic wound. A good understanding of these stages is helpful in being able to provide effective aromatic treatment of wounds.

Inflammatory phase

Following injury a plug is formed to prevent further bleeding and becomes the main support for the wound until it is replaced with granulatory tissue and then collagen. Inflammation at the wound site causes an increase in circulation, resulting in tissue swelling and the release of factors involved in the next (proliferative) stage.

Inflammation facilitates the entry of white cells into the wound site, clearing it of debris and bacteria, the damaged tissue being removed after a couple of days. This debridement or cleaning of the wound

Case study 10.1

Penetrating wound with infection risk

Rhiannon Harris – Clinical aromatherapist

Assessment

Marcel (49) had just sustained a penetrating, ragged wound, approximately 3.5 cm deep, 1.5 cm to the left of the anal margin, after accidentally sitting on a blunt-ended rusty metal spike while gardening.

Intervention

First-aid intervention involved bathing and flushing the wound copiously with approximately 5 drops each of *Lavandula latifolia* [spike lavender] and *Melaleuca alternifolia* [tea tree] added to cool water. A tetanus booster was administered, but owing to the proximity of the wound to the anus and the consequent high infection risk, a decision was made not to suture. Instead, the wound was treated with essential oils and monitored closely.

The following wound care blend was chosen for anti-inflammatory, wound healing, analgesic and antimicrobial effects, the concentration being deliberately elevated because of the nature of the wound:

25% of the essential oil mix below in *Hypericum perforatum* macerated oil base:

- 40% *Thymus vulgaris* ct. *thujanol*
- 30% *Lavandula latifolia* [spike lavender]
- 10% *Matricaria recutita* [German chamomile]
- 10% *Cistus ladaniferus* [labdanum]
- 10% *Helichrysum italicum*.

The wound was irrigated daily (using a small syringe) with the above for 1 week, to ensure rapid healing of the deeper tissues and to prevent pockets of infection forming, which

might occur if epithelialization took place too swiftly. A gauze pad was soaked in the same mixture to form a compress over the wound, being changed twice daily. The same blend was used also to lubricate the anus prior to a bowel movement (to avoid over-stretching and straining), followed by careful washing of the area afterwards. A high-fibre diet and increased fluids were taken to reduce the risk of constipation.

One week after the injury irrigation was no longer required as the wound was closed and looking healthy. Two formulations were prepared for ongoing treatment until the new skin over the wound was fully stable.

Daytime use: the same blend of oils but at a concentration of 5% in *Aloe vera* gel. This was easy to apply during the day.

Night-time application: the same blend of essential oils in *Hypericum perforatum* at a 10% concentration.

Outcome

The immediate and lasting analgesic/local anaesthetic effect permitted Marcel to sit from the first day without discomfort. The speed of healing was equally remarkable, the wound diameter reducing by half in 3 days. There was also very little inflammation. On the first day the area was swollen and had a purplish appearance, and by day 2 it looked pink and healthy. At no point was there evidence of infection.

Two weeks after injury Marcel no longer needed aromatic intervention. All that remains is a small white scar that bears witness to a potentially serious penetrating wound of high infection risk.

(Taken from the *International Journal of Clinical Aromatherapy* 3 (2b): 14–15)

---

stimulates the cells that create granulation tissue and inflammation plays an important role during the initial stages; while there is debris in the wound (dirt or other objects) the inflammatory stage can become extended, leading to a chronic wound.

Proliferative (reconstructive) phase

After 2 or 3 days new blood vessels are formed within the wound. Special fibroblast cells grow, forming a new extracellular matrix (ECM) and granulation tissue. This activity requires oxygen and nutrients from the blood vessels, causing a typical red appearance of the tissue which is essential for further stages of healing to occur. The granulation tissue functions as rudimentary tissue, continuing to grow until the wound

bed is covered. At the end of granulation, fibroblasts begin converting granulating tissue into collagen – important because it increases the strength of the wound. Too little oxygen will inhibit the growth of fibroblasts and the deposition of ECM, which can lead to excessive, fibrotic scarring. Thus the therapist needs to be aware that smokers and people with poor circulation can have reduced oxygen flow to the wound site, which may slow the healing process.

Epithelialization

Once the wound is filled with granulation tissue, epithelial (skin) cells begin to advance across the wound until they meet in the middle. Epithelial cells only occur at the wound edges and require healthy tissue to migrate across, so if the wound is deep it must first be filled with granulation tissue. If this new membrane becomes damaged, re-epithelialization has to occur again from the wound margins. Therefore care must be taken during dressing changes not to destroy any part of the wound membrane; the more quickly migration of skin cells occurs, the less obvious the scar will be.

Contraction

Contraction can last for several weeks and is a key stage of wound healing; if it continues too long, disfigurement and loss of function can occur. Special cells, similar to smooth muscle cells, pull the extracellular matrix within the body of the wound when they contract, reducing the wound size, whilst fibroblasts lay down the collagen to reinforce the wound.

Maturation and remodelling phase

This can last a year or longer, depending on the size of the wound and how it was left to heal. During maturation, type III collagen is replaced by type I collagen and slowly the strength of the wound increases.

Unfortunately, the process of wound healing is complex and fragile and many factors can interrupt its progress, leading to the formation of chronic non-healing wounds (see Box 10.1).

The presence of a slow-healing wound has significant physical, psychological, psychosocial and financial impact. The psychosocial impact is even greater if the wound is malodorous or on a visible part of the body. The longer a wound takes to heal, the greater the microbial load, with further risk of complications and delayed healing (Bowler et al. 2001). Thus the challenge is to find interventions that promote and accelerate normal wound healing without complications, as outlined in Box 10.1.

The role of essential oils

The choice and specification of dressing is very important to achieve the above objectives and wound healing agents should adhere to certain specifications (Leach 2008). Natural bases and essential oils can play numerous roles in promoting wound healing, providing a range of treatment options (Box 10.2).

Few dressings satisfy all the criteria in Box 10.2, but it could be said that many plant extracts come close to being ideal wound-healing agents, e.g. aloe, calendula, hypericum and comfrey (Leach 2004), which leads to the question why are natural remedies, including aromatherapy, not used more widely in hospitals, hospices and the community? In 2002, John Kerr listed the following reasons:

Box 10.1

Factors inhibiting wound healing

- Infection
- Pre-existing disease, e.g. diabetes, cancer, venous or arterial disease, AIDS
- Immobility
- Advancing age
- Certain medications that cause immune suppression, e.g. cortisone
- Location of wound, e.g. areas of pressure, friction, in flexures etc.
- Poor tissue perfusion in area of wound
- Poor nutrition
- Smoking
- Obesity
- Psychological stress
- Social isolation

(adapted from Harris 2006)

Box 10.2

The roles of essential oils in wound healing

- Prevent and treat microbial contamination
- Reduce inflammation
- Debride the wound of slough and necrotic tissue
- Facilitate granulation and collagen formation
- Facilitate angiogenesis and tissue perfusion
- Increase the rate of wound contraction
- Alleviate pain
- Reduce odour
- Reduce scarring
- Cost effective
- Easily applied and removed

(adapted from Harris 2006)

- the current medical system is seen as effective, despite its shortcomings
- lack of scientific evidence
- limited anecdotal evidence, although there has been more in recent years
- a reluctance by aromatherapists to innovate
- administrative problems (e.g. patient liability issues, insurance, medical codes of ethics etc.)
- lack of education due to intensive use of essential oils not being taught by the majority of aromatherapy schools.

Famous pioneer aromatherapists such as Gattefosse and Valnet were well aware of the healing effects of essential oils, but the first report in the aromatherapy literature of using essential oils for wound healing in hospital was by clinical aromatologist Alan Barker (1994). He explored the aromatic treatment of pressure sores based on his experience of working in the English National Health Service, suggesting the following:

- application of undiluted essential oils in the presence of large amounts of pus and the need for debridement
- use of diluted oils in either honey or macerated vegetable oils
- use of sprays of distilled water with added essential oils.

NB Now that hydrolats are available, these would be preferable to water with essential oils.

Later, Ron Guba (1998/1999) used 10% of CO_2 extracts and essential oils in a cream containing a range of fixed oils on a number of wound types (venous ulcers, pressure sores, skin tears and abrasions) in nursing homes in Australia. The essential oils used were *Lavandula angustifolia* [lavender], *Artemisia vulgaris* [mugwort] and *Salvia officinalis* [sage], plus CO_2 extracts of *Matricaria recutita* [German chamomile] and *Calendula officinalis* [calendula]. The most significant results were obtained with chronic wounds.

Kerr (2002) reported the results of three years' work using essential oils for a range of wounds in Australian nursing homes. The main finding was that a 9–12% concentration of essential oils yielded better results than much weaker doses, with no side effects. The essential oils used included *Lavandula angustifolia*, *Matricaria recutita* [German chamomile], *Pogostemon patchouli*, *Commiphora myrrha* [myrrh] and *Melaleuca alternifolia* [tea tree] in *Aloe vera* gel.

Two American practitioners (Hartman & Coetzee 2002) conducted a study using *Lavandula angustifolia* and *Matricaria recutita* essential oils diluted in grapeseed fixed oil for the treatment of chronic ulcers of several months' duration and resistant to conventional treatments (the experimental group), comparing them with a control group who continued to receive conventional wound care. The results confirmed improved healing times in the experimental group. An important observation was that all wounds in the experimental group appeared to worsen initially for up to 2 weeks, with increased exudate and erythema, after which they showed signs of healing. A possible reason for this may be the increase in circulation and vascular permeability encouraged by the essential oil application – thereby accelerating angiogenesis. This observation has been confirmed in the author's own practice.

Primmer (2002) successfully treated a skin tear in an elderly patient using a mix of *Lavandula angustifolia*, *Eucalyptus radiata* [narrow-leaved peppermint], *Matricaria recutita* and *Boswellia carteri* [frankincense] at 3% dilution in sweet almond oil. When applied to the wound twice daily, a significant improvement was seen within 24 hours and the wound healed totally in 4 weeks with very little scarring, the therapist using this blend successfully several times with other patients.

Diane Ames (a family nurse practitioner and clinical aromatherapist) is endeavouring to integrate the use of essential oils into the healthcare system in Milwaukee. The cases dealt with were numerous – deep-seated infections, boils and abscesses, venous ulcers, several grades of pressure sore and fungating tumours, and all had good results (Ames 2006).

The author has found the following oils to be successful:

- *Melaleuca alternifolia* [tea tree] both neat and diluted for infected wounds, including those with methicillin-resistant *Staphylococcus aureus* (MRSA)
- *Matricaria recutita* and *Lavandula angustifolia* 50/50 at 10% dilution in macerated calendula oil for deep pressure sores.

In 2004, a team from Manchester Metropolitan University developed a dressing model for wounds to decolonize them from MRSA by vapour contact. This led to a phase 1 clinical trial on the effects of diffusion of essential oils to reduce infection risks. The study was carried out in the Burns Unit of

Wythenshawe Hospital (Edwards-Jones et al. 2004) (see also Case 9.2 MRSA).

Commonly used essential oils in wound healing

Concentrations of essential oil for wound healing formulas range from 1.5% to 25%, depending on each individual case and the expertise of the therapist. Always take an in-depth history and do a patch test. For direct application essential oils should be diluted in a suitable base or used on a dressing pad rather than straight on the wound.

With regard to the use of essential oils in wound healing, several are constantly mentioned in the research literature. What has not been properly researched is whether particular constituents are responsible for specific healing results – hence the use of the word 'may' when discussing this in the text.

Commiphora myrrha [myrrh]

Many aromatherapy texts cite myrrh as an effective wound healer from ancient times to the present (Price & Price 1999, Battaglia 1997, Kerr 2002), being specifically healing to bedsores, as it is highly antibacterial. It has an ability to increase the number of leukocytes in the blood (Bartram 1995) and is especially bacteriostatic against *Staphylococcus aureus* (one of the biggest bacterial wound invaders) and other Gram-positive bacteria (Price & Price 1999). The main constituents are sesquiterpenes, which may help decongest the wound and reduce inflammation (Price 1995). Myrrh can be bought as a resin but this should not be used for wounds – only distilled essential oil is safe for this purpose.

Abies balsamea [Canadian balsam/ balsam fir]

Canadian balsam is antiseptic against staphylococcus spp. and *E. coli* (Price & Price 2007), anti-inflammatory and cicatrizant, and is used by Native Americans for the treatment of burns, sores and cuts. It is high in monoterpenes (75–90%, mostly β-pinene), which may be why it is good for healing skin lesions and ulcerations. It is helpful for

depression, nervous tension and stress-related conditions, all of which add healing properties on a different level. Non-toxic and non-irritating, it may be chosen instead of myrrh for its ease of use, being a much thinner solution (Fact sheet, Penny Price Aromatherapy (2010).

Citrus limon [lemon]

Lemon has been found to be the most effective oil for debriding and desloughing wounds (Penny Price 2003 personal communication). This may be due to the high monoterpene content (90–95%), which can be aggressive to skin and mucous surfaces (Price L 2003 personal communication). It has exceptional antibacterial qualities, having the ability to stimulate the body's own white blood cells (Battaglia 1997). Lemon is useful in reducing wound odours and is both mentally and spiritually uplifting.

Lavandula angustifolia [lavender]

Lavender is highly cicatrizant, being an effective cell regenerator, which may be due to its high ester content (40–55%). It is especially good for all types of burn as well as skin problems and wounds (Price & Price 2007), providing also strong bactericidal and decongestant properties.

Melaleuca alternifolia [tea tree]

Tea tree is a proven antibacterial agent, active against a wide range of bacteria and fungi, including *Staphylococcus aureus* (Price & Price 2007), which makes it invaluable when treating infected wounds. Its high alcohol content (28–57%) may be responsible for its first-class desloughing and cleansing properties. Interestingly, Kerr (2002) mentions the possibility of *Backhousia citriodora* [lemon myrtle] being more antibacterial than tea tree.

Matricaria recutita [German chamomile]

German chamomile is invaluable in wound healing because of its excellent anti-inflammatory, antimicrobial and cicatrizant properties; the content of the sesquiterpene chamazulene is sometimes as high as 35%. The high oxide content (20–55%) may make it a good bactericide – also active against MRSA; oxides are also believed to have the ability to reduce inflammation and pain (ACS 2004, Price & Price 2007). German chamomile has been used successfully by Ames (2006) on leg ulcers and pressure sores.

Helichrysum angustifolium, H. italicum [everlasting, immortelle]

Helichrysum may be hailed as liquid stitching because of its remarkable healing properties on the skin's surface. The main constituent of helichrysum is the ester neryl acetate, which is reputed to be rejuvenating to the skin, as it is a cell regenerator with antimicrobial and anti-inflammatory properties (Price & Price 2007, Price L 2003 personal communication). Helichrysum has exceptional cicatrizant properties, speeding cellular growth and assisting in wound healing of all types (Guba 1997). Guba suggests that the ketones (italidiones) are responsible for this, owing to their power to regenerate and heal cutaneous tissue. Eileen Cristina (2006) successfully used helichrysum in reducing a scar following a burn and topical infection. Further, the author used helichrysum for three pressure sores to encourage final epithelial growth over the wounds, which proved positive.

Melaleuca viridiflora [niaouli]

Niaouli complements lemon in the action of initial cleansing and debridement of a wound (Price P 2003, personal communication). The synergy of its constituents helps deslough the wound, reduce bacteria, pain and inflammation and encourage cell regeneration.

Because of its antibacterial and antiseptic properties, niaouli is suitable for washing infected wounds. The high oxide content may cause worries about skin irritation.

Boswellia carteri [frankincense]

Esters are a predominant feature of this oil, including octyl acetate, which is cell regenerating (Price & Price 2007). Frankincense was used successfully on a skin tear as part of a 3% mix with lavender and German chamomile by Primmer (2002), and on a fungating tumour by Ames (2006). It is a good choice for people with wounds in a hospice setting because of its spiritual and uplifting properties (Price S 1995).

How can aromatherapy be beneficial?

According to Harris (2006), for the aromatherapist who is unable to treat a wound because of procedural protocols or resistance from medical staff, all is not lost. The impact of psychological stress and social isolation on delayed wound healing is well established (Detillon et al. 2004, Vurnek et al. 2006). Any aromatic intervention that reduces stress or provides positive social interaction can potentially speed healing times. Other interventions that improve quality of life, such as pain relief or removal of wound odours, are also extremely important and can be tackled by the aromatherapist without infringing the treatment 'rules'.

For simple or minor wounds the aromatherapist can usually intervene early and achieve swift and effective results; the implementation of aromatic interventions in more serious and chronic wounds may be dependent on the nurse practitioner or wound care specialist.

Safety/hazards

Hazards when applying essential oil-based products to areas of broken skin are irritation, allergy and wound contamination.

Leg ulcers are particularly susceptible to allergic contact dermatitis (Capriata et al. 2006), as happened to a woman using a leg ulcer cream containing geraniol (Guerra et al. 1987). The aromatherapist needs to be conscious of risks in patients with a perfume or cosmetic allergy, and patch testing before treatment is recommended. Allergy risk also arises when essential oils oxidize, as with *Melaleuca alternifolia* and *Lavandula angustifolia* (Hausen et al. 1999, Skold et al. 2002), those most often employed in wound care.

Irritation may be caused by high concentrations of essential oils, especially those rich in phenols and aldehydes. If used inappropriately these are capable of aggravating the wound by causing significant damage and cell death.

Maudsley and Kerr (1999) examined the viability and proliferation of microbes in essential oils and three fixed oils and concluded that using these oils in wound care constitutes safe practice, provided the essential oils are stored correctly and aseptic practices are followed. As indicated previously, even at concentrations of 25% no adverse reactions were noted; this may be partly due to the aromatherapist concerned selecting the appropriate oils.

Table 10.1 list those oils most commonly used in wound care based on case reports and the author's experience.

Natural base products

Essential oils are normally diluted in or administered in association with bases, which can bring additional wound healing. The following bases are commonly employed and have been successfully used for years by the author:

- Fixed oils
- Macerated/infused oils
- Honey
- Clay
- Aloe vera

Table 10.1 Properties of essential oils							
	Analgesic	Antibacterial	Anti-inflammatory	Antiseptic	Cicatrizant cell regenerating	Desloughing/debriding	Deodorizing
Abies balsamea Canadian balsam		X		X	X		
Achillea millefolium Yarrow	X		X	X	X		
Boswellia carteri Frankincense		X	X		X		
Cistus ladaniferus Cistus		X	X		X		
Citrus limon Lemon		X				X	X
Commiphora myrrha var. *molmol* Myrrh			X	X	X		
Helichrysum angustifolium (=*H. Italicum*) Everlasting or immo*rtelle*			X		X		
Lavandula angustifolia Lavender	X	X	X	X	X		X
Lavandula latifolia Spike lavender	X	X	X		X		X
Matricaria recutita German chamomile			X		X		
Melaleuca alternifolia Tea tree	X	X	X	X		X	
Melaleuca viridiflora Niaouli	X	X	X	X		X	
Pogostemon cablin Patchouli		X	X	X	X		
Thymus vulgaris ct. *thymol* Thyme		X		X			X

Case study 10.2

Bike accident wound

Penny Price – Clinical aromatherapist/aromatologist

Assessment

VP, 17 years old, had been knocked off his bike by a hit-and-run driver. He managed to get home and we looked at his wounds to assess treatment. His whole right side was grazed from the ankle to the hip, with two deep cuts in the thigh where the car's bumper had caught him. There were also abrasions to the right arm, hand and side of the face. When the blood had been cleaned away it was obvious that the amount of trauma caused was going to lead to deep bruising and possible scarring.

Intervention

It was decided that we would treat VP for four reasons:
1. To help heal with minimal bruising
2. To reduce pain and inflammation
3. To prevent infection from getting into the cuts and grazes
4. To help prevent scar formation.

The following treatment plan was put together:
- *Lavandula angustifolia* [lavender fine] – cicatrizant, cell-regenerating, pain-relieving, antiseptic, anti-inflammatory
- *Zingiber montana* [plai] – pain-relieving, muscle tonic, warming, antiseptic, circulatory
- *Origanum majorana* [sweet marjoram] – antiseptic, warming, muscular tonic, circulatory, phlebotonic
- *Thymus vulgaris* ct. *thymol* [thyme] – very antiseptic, immune-stimulant, nerve tonic, circulatory and vulnerary.

- *Hypericum perforatum* [St. John's Wort] – nervine, phlebotonic
- *Rosa canina* [rosehip seed] – regenerating, phlebotonic
- *Lavandula angustifolia* [lavender] hydrolat – soothing and healing

Application

After all areas had been washed and carefully dried, lavender hydrolat was sprayed onto the body and left to dry naturally. It was reapplied three more times and left to dry in the same manner. A 5% blend was made using 50/50 of each carrier oil and an equal blend of each essential oil. This was applied to all areas and reapplied after 2 hours. After a further 2 hours the whole treatment plan was repeated, starting with the hydrolat spray, before the client went to bed.

Outcome

The following morning there was one small bruise on the right knee. The grazes and cuts had covered over and looked healthy and infection free. The skin surrounding the grazes and cuts was soft and pink. There was a little pain, but it had improved dramatically.

After 6 days of treatment the grazes had healed over and the cuts were just visible. There was no pain and VP was able to resume normal life.

- Hydrolats (although essential oils do not dissolve in hydrolats, they are useful for administering them).

Fixed oils

Fixed oils have a role to play in assisting uncomplicated wounds to heal. Those indicated for wound repair include *Oenethera biennis* [evening primrose], *Borago officinalis* [borage], *Rosa rubiginosa*, [rosehip seed], *Calophyllum inophyllum* [tamanu] and *Azadirachta indica* [neem].

These fixed oils can produce an anti-inflammatory effect when applied topically, as they are rich in polyunsaturated fatty acids (PUFAs). These are crucial to cellular repair mechanisms, and so oral doses are also indicated.

Evening primrose and *borage* are high in PUFAs and borage has been studied for its beneficial wound healing effects (Marchini et al. 1998).

Neem oil has both traditional and research evidence (Biswas et al. 2002). It is antimicrobial, although its powerful odour may be offputting to some.

Rosehip seed's properties for skin regeneration are due to the presence of small amounts of *trans*-retinoic acid (Price & Price 2008).

Tamanu is traditionally used for promoting cellular regeneration (Guba 1997) because of its confirmed cicatrizant, anti-inflammatory, antioxidant, analgesic and antimicrobial properties (Kilham 2004). In the experience of Harris (2006), its analgesic activity is particularly useful for painful wounds and other lesions, such as blistering in shingles/zoster.

Macerated oils

The most popular macerated oils used in skin and wound care are *Calendula officinalis* [calendula] and *Hypericum perforatum* [St John's wort].

Calendula has been well documented for its anti-inflammatory and wound healing activity (Zitterl-Eglseer et al. 1997), with evidence indicating it as being the most favourable wound healing extract (Leach 2008). Calendula flowers demonstrate strong anti-inflammatory and antioedematous properties, research proving it to be as effective in reducing dermal inflammation as indomethacin (a potent non-steroidal anti-inflammatory drug) (Guba 1997). Used alone, calendula may facilitate wound healing by improving both local circulation and granulation tissue formation (Leach 2008), as proved by the author, who has used it alone to protect and strengthen the skin during the initial stages after healing. Its properties are enhanced when mixed with wound-healing essential oils (Price & Price 2008). Topical applications of calendula are safe, and it has been approved by the German Health Commission for topical administration in oral and pharyngeal mucosal inflammation, poorly healing wounds and leg ulceration (Leach 2008). It is advised that individuals with a known sensitivity to other species of the Asteraceae family, e.g. chrysanthemum, daisy etc., avoid calendula because of the potential risk of allergic reaction.

Hypericum perforatum is beneficial on wounds where there is nerve tissue damage and inflammation, including sunburn (Price & Price 2008), thought to be mainly due to the hypericin (a flavonoid) content, and has been approved for the treatment of first-degree burns (Blumenthal et al. 2000). The leaf extract has also been used for its wound healing potential (Mukherjee et al. 2000), partly due owing to the flavonoid content. Price and Price (2008) point out that the properties of St John's wort may vary according to harvest and that the flavonoids and proanthocyanidins useful in wound healing are highest when the flowers are in bud.

NB Homemade macerated oils carry the risk of contamination with fungal and bacterial spores. Both fixed and macerated oils should always be obtained from a reliable source, as they are normally micro-filtered and often sterilized.

Hydrolats

According to Harris (2006) hydrolats and aqueous plant extracts are useful for wound care and may be applied:

Box 10.3

Benefits of hydrolats in wound care (Harris 2006)

- Soothing
- Cooling
- Anti-inflammatory
- Antimicrobial
- Maintaining moist wound environment
- Analgesic
- Reducing bleeding
- Promoting cellular repair
- Deodorizing

- directly to the wound during cleaning
- in irrigation if the wound is deep
- on compresses for superficial lesions
- as a spray if the wound is extremely painful.

Hydrolats are cooling to the skin and help maintain wound moisture. They have a range of possible activities, e.g. pain relief and anti-inflammatory, depending on the species (see Box 10.3). They are active agents used alone or in combination with essential oils (up to 10%): it may be advisable to use an emulsifying/surfactant agent such as Tweens to permit even distribution of the essential oil, although this may perhaps reduce their antimicrobial activity (Lund 1994).

NB Depending on the hydrolat, regular handling and the passage of time may present a risk of microbial contamination, especially with microbes such as *Pseudomonas aeruginosa*. If hydrolats are to be used in wound care they should first be tested to ensure they contain no more than the permissible microbial load. Sterile preparations of hydrolats in unidose packaging are now becoming available in Europe.

Honey

A variety of wound types have been studied using honey; it has been demonstrated (Molan 2006) to be beneficial in dressing models and would be enhanced by the addition of essential oils. The beneficial effects of honey include:

- rapid clearing of infection
- reduction of inflammation and hence swelling, exudate and pain
- suppression of malodour

- induction of sloughing of necrotic tissue
- easy removal of sloughs without trauma
- promotion of granulation and re-epithelialization
- healing with minimum scarring.

Essential oils can be added to honey to further enhance healing, the amount added being judged according to the particular situation.

According to Molan (2006) and Winter (1962), wounds heal 50% faster if kept moist, although fear of increased bacterial growth sometimes causes clinicians to try keeping wounds dry. Honey prevents the growth of bacteria in a moist healing environment, which allows rapid removal of pus, dead tissue and debris, thereby speeding up tissue growth to repair the wound (Molan 2006). Honey also reduces inflammation, preventing blood vessels opening up and thereby reducing exudate and swelling.

The anti-inflammatory action reduces pain, with the added benefit of a reduction in the amount of blisters and scarring due to the mopping-up of free radicals at the time of occurrence (Subrahmanyam 1991, Subrahmanyam et al. 2003). Honey has a nutrient effect and draws out lymph from the cells by osmosis; this creates a honey solution in contact with the wound surface which prevents the dressing from sticking (Molan 1998).

The antibacterial property of honey helps avoid infection, which prevents wound healing, and the debriding action is important as it removes substances that harbour bacteria, stopping the healing and causing malodour.

NB When too much exudate is present the action of honey may be diluted.

Clay

The most commonly used clay is bentonite. Although there is little scientific evidence for its healing benefits (absorptive and adsorptive qualities), it is particularly suited for deep wounds with exudate and necrotic tissue, is extremely soothing and accelerates healing times. It also has deodorizing ability.

There are three main methods of using clay in wound care:

1. sprinkled on to the lesion in powder form
2. compresses in liquid form
3. poultices in paste form.

NB Clay should be obtained from reputable sources – contaminated clay risks wound infection. Powdered clay should be prepared with the addition of hydrolat or distilled water just before each use; if 'ready to use' clay is to be employed, this needs to be in a sterilized form.

Aloe vera

Aloe vera is anti-inflammatory (Vazquez et al. 1996, Gallagher & Gray 2003) and is traditionally used on wounds and burns and other skin disorders, e.g. psoriasis (Akhtar & Hatwar 1996, Syed et al. 1997, Reynolds & Dweck 1999) and appears to work best in superficial and uncomplicated wound care. Its advantage when used with essential oils is linked to its hydrophilic qualities, allowing the transfer of essential oil onto the tissues. It is rarely possible to incorporate more than 5% essential oil into aloe gel without separation unless a surfactant is used.

NB Delayed healing may be experienced in infected wounds or those healing by secondary intention (Schmidt & Greenspoon 1991). Few sterile *Aloe vera* preparations exist, which poses a risk of microbial contamination, those available showing a degree of inconsistency (Reynolds & Dweck 1999), with some containing ingredients that could cause contact dermatitis (Reider et al. 2005).

Pressure sores (decubitus ulcers)

Traditional medicine has limited success here, but nurses have found essential oils to effect healing (Price & Price 2007). Pressure sores occur mainly over bony prominences and are areas of inflamed or even necrotic (dead) tissue. They develop as a result of sustained localized pressure which compresses blood vessels in the area, causing ischaemia to the skin and underlying tissues. Pressure sores generally happen in people with reduced neurological integrity and mobility, other contributing factors including reduced padding of fat and muscle, anaemia, poor nutritional status, incontinence and infection. Extrinsic factors include pressure, shearing forces, trauma, moisture and friction. Possible complications include infection in the blood, heart and bone, amputations and prolonged bed rest – which brings its own complications, including death.

The severity of a pressure sore is graded according to the depth of ulceration and involvement of underlying tissues, which also helps determine the required treatment (see Table 10.2).

Table 10.2 The pressure sore grading system (based on EPUAP 2010)

Grade 1 Non-blanchable erythema	Discoloration of intact skin not affected by light finger pressure (non-blanching erythema). This may be difficult to identify in darkly pigmented skin, where it is likely to appear red, blue or purple
Grade 2 Partial-thickness skin loss	Partial-thickness skin loss or damage involving epidermis and/or dermis. The pressure ulcer is superficial and presents clinically as an abrasion, blister or shallow crater
Grade 3 Full-thickness skin loss	Full-thickness skin loss involving damage to subcutaneous tissue but not extending to underlying fascia. The pressure ulcer presents clinically as a deep crater with or without undermining of adjacent tissue
Grade 4 Full-thickness tissue loss	Full-thickness tissue loss with extensive destruction and necrosis extending to underlying tissue or supporting structures (muscle, bone and/or tendon)

First, dead or sloughy tissue needs to be removed before healing can take place, which sometimes requires surgery. If infection is present antibiotics may be required, therefore collaboration with the patient's healthcare team may be necessary, depending on the severity of the situation.

Burns

Essential oils were used with success on severe burns in University College Hospital in 1988; a consultant tried the effectiveness of essential oils, saying 'what I have been offered has been researched – but does nothing; what you have given me has not been researched – yet it works. This is what interests me' (Parkhouse 1988 personal communication). Most critical care units would not allow this use without research evidence, of which there is still not much. The cicatrizant properties of certain essential oils are very powerful, especially when used with macerated oil of *Hypericum perforatum* [St John's wort], which is used for treatment of injuries and first-degree burns (Blumenthal et al 2000):

Case study 10.3

Two clients with pressure sores

Denise Raines RN – Clinical aromatherapist/aromatologist

Assessment

Lucy (48) is paraplegic from C5 and presented with a pressure sore 4 cm in diameter over her left shoulder blade, due to friction from her wheelchair. The sore contained sloughy tissue and the intact skin around it was red and inflamed from constant dressing changes. There was no evidence of infection in the wound.

Bill (52) has multiple sclerosis and had developed a large pressure sore over his sacrum due to a recent relapse. This measured 6.5 cm across by 3.5 cm and was 2 cm deep, with the presence of a substantial layer of infected necrotic tissue within the wound. Initially this pressure sore was ungradable. The skin around the sore was very red and purple, with several abrasions over the buttocks.

Intervention

All pressure was removed from the sores, Bill having to stay on bed rest on a special air mattress for the duration of healing. It was more difficult to remove the pressure from Lucy's sore at the back of her wheelchair.

Bill's large pressure sore was initially debrided using manuka honey inserted into the wound, which was then packed with sterile gauze soaked in the honey. The wound was then covered with gauze pads to absorb any excess moisture and changed twice daily to maintain efficacy of the honey, and he started taking antibiotics to combat the infection. After 13 days the sore was fully debrided but was now 4 cm deep. Luckily this was still only a grade 3 pressure sore because no underlying bone, muscle or tendons were involved. The wound was now oozing an excessive amount of exudate, which rendered the honey ineffective despite more frequent dressing changes. Therefore, the treatment regimen was changed to the same as used for Lucy:

Stage 1 wound healing formula, 10% dilution

To debride and clean the sores of slough, encourage perfusion, prevent infection and commence granulation. All the wounds were cleaned with sterile sodium chloride 0.9% (normal saline solution), packed with

Continued

Case study 10.3

Two clients with pressure sores—cont'd

gauze soaked in this formula and covered with a secondary gauze dressing. The dressings were changed twice daily.

- 30 mL *Calendula officinalis* [calendula]
- 10 drops *Commiphora myrhha* [myrrh]
- 25 drops *Citrus limon* [lemon]
- 25 drops *Melaleuca viridiflora* [niaouli]

For the surrounding inflamed skin of both Lucy and Bill, a formulation of 1.5% dilution of myrrh in calendula was applied regularly throughout the day.

Stage 2 formula, still at.10% dilution

Once the slough was removed and the wounds were clean and pink, the wound formula was changed to:

- 30 mL calendula
- 40 drops myrrh
- 10 drops lemon
- 10 drops niaouli

Stage 3 formula, 7.5% dilution

As the wounds filled with granulating tissue and became more shallow, the dilutions were reduced and the myrrh was further increased in relation to the lemon and niaouli.

Helichrysum was added to help the final stages of healing, because of its exceptional efficacy at the skin's surface. At one stage the shallower sores started to dry out, which caused some minor bleeding of the new tissue on removal of the dressings. Therefore, non-adherent dressings were applied over the packed wounds, which made all the difference. In the final stages the formula was placed on the dressing pad and applied over the wound:

- 50 mL calendula
- 70 drops myrrh
- 24 drops helichrysum
- 3 drops lemon
- 3 drops niaouli

Outcome

Lucy's sore healed in 40 days (despite some continued pressure from the wheelchair). Bill's large sore healed in 63 days. The surrounding skin of both Lucy and Bill improved, becoming pink and normal within a short space of time. Apart from Bill's initial infection, at no other time were there signs of infection in either of the wounds. Bill's case was a challenge because of the close proximity of his sore to the anal area.

- *Boswellia carteri* [frankincense] – scars, wounds
- *Helichrysum italicum* [everlasting] – burns, open wounds, scars, skin regeneration
- *Lavandula angustifolia* [lavender] – burns, scars, wounds
- *Pelargonium graveolens* [geranium] – burns, wounds.

To keep the air antiseptic in a burns ward the following can be vaporised:

- *Citrus limon* [lemon]
- *Pinus sylvestris* [pine]

Pinus sylvestris [pine]

Other burns units that incorporate aromatherapy are the children's burns unit in the Red Cross War Memorial Children's Hospital in South Africa.

Radiation burns

Melaleuca viridiflora [niaouli] can be used to lessen radiation burns in those receiving this treatment for cancer (see Ch. 15).

Summary

This chapter shows that there is much evidence to support the use of aromatic extracts and related bases in wound healing, wound management objectives generally being achieved. Even so, their use in hospices and hospitals, plus feedback from the author's clients, is usually a final option when orthodox methods have failed, resulting in an extremely poor wound healing prognosis. As a result, some of the research regarding the use of essential oils involves the added difficulty that the wounds have not previously responded to conventional treatment and are usually chronic. Despite this, the majority of results are positive, emphasizing the efficacy of aromatic wound healing.

Depending on the health authority involved, one issue appears to be the cost and availability of manpower: many pharmaceutical dressings only need reapplying once a day or less, as opposed to the possibility of more frequent changes for aromatic dressings – depending on the type of wound. This leads to increased costs in more home visits by nurses to change the dressing. In terms of long-term cost-effectiveness, essential oil interventions prove much cheaper than typical dressing models and generally do not need more frequent application – in fact, because they are effective and cheap, there is every reason why they should be used.

Further support for the use of essential oils, hydrolats and related bases is the issue of infection. MRSA is one of the biggest problems in hospitals today, especially for the weak and elderly. Most essential oils used in wound healing are active against this superbug – and many other bacteria. Research shows that wounds treated with aromatics rarely become infected, resulting in more rapid healing and less need for antibiotics.

With the advent of postgraduate training in aromatherapy and the possibility of taking a diploma in aromatic medicine/aromatology (see Useful addresses), it appears that the necessary change is slowly taking place. More research is being carried out to support the use of plant extracts (including essential oils) in the healing of wounds, although to be accepted by the medical and nursing profession it must be more than anecdotal: rigorous clinical trials are needed to establish confidence and a turnaround in professional opinion.

References

ACS (American Chemical Society), 2004. Molecule of the week. http://www.chemistry.org/portal/a/c/s/1/acsdisplay.html.

Akhtar, A.M., Hatwar, S.K., 1996. Efficacy of Aloe vera extract cream in management of burn wound. J. Clin. Epidemiol. 49 (1 Suppl. 1), 24S.

Ames, D., 2006. Aromatic wound care in a health care system: a report from the United States. International Journal of Clinical Aromatherapy 3 (2), 3–8.

Barker, A., 1994. Aromatherapy and Pressure Sores. Aromatherapy Quarterly 41, 5–7.

Bartram, T., 1995. Encyclopedia of herbal medicine. Grace, Christchurch, p. 304.

Battaglia, S., 1997. The Complete Guide to Aromatherapy, second print. The Perfect Potion, Australia.

Biswas, K., Chattopadhyay, I., Banerjee, R.K., Bandyopadhyay, U., 2002. Biological Activities and Medicinal Properties of Neem (Azadirachta indica). Curr. Sci. 82 (11), 1336–1345.

Blumenthal, M., et al., 2000. Herbal Medicine. Expanded Commission E Monographs. Integrative Medicine Communications, Newton, MA.

Bowler, P.G., Duerden, B.I., Armstrong, D.G., 2001. Wound Microbiology and Associated Approaches to Wound Management. Clin. Microbiol. Rev. 14 (2), 244–269.

Capriata, S., Legori, A., Motolese, A., 2006. Contact sensitivity in patients with leg ulcers. Annali Italiani di Derm. Aller. Clin. Esp. 60 (1), 15–21.

Cristina, E.D., 2006. Scar reduction following burn and tropical infection: a case study. International Journal of Clinical Aromatherapy 3 (2), 19–20.

Detillon, C.E., Craft, T.K.S., Glasper, E.R., Prendergast, B.J., DeVries, A.C., 2004. Social facilitation of wound healing. Psychoneuroendocrinology 29 (8), 1004–1011.

Edwards-Jones, V., Buck, R., Shawcross, S.G., Dawson, M.M., Dunn, K., 2004. The effect of essential oils on Methicillin-resistant Staphylococcus aureus using a dressing model. Burns 30, 772–777.

EPUAP (European Pressure Ulcer Advisory Panel), 2010. International Pressure Ulcer Guidelines. http://www.epuap.org/guidelines.html.

Gallagher, J., Gray, M., 2003. Is Aloe vera effective for healing wounds? J. Wound Ostomy Continence Service 30, 68–71.

Guba, R., 1997. Aromatic Extracts as Wound Healing Agents (Part 1). Aromatherapy Today 3, 21–25.

Guba, R., 1998. Wound healing. International Journal of Aromatherapy 9 (2), 67–74.

Guerra, P., Aguilar, A., Urbina, F., Cristobal, M.C., Garcia-Perez, A., 1987. Contact dermatitis to geraniol in a leg ulcer. Contact Dermatitis 16 (5), 298–299.

Harris, R., 2006. Aromatic approaches to wound care. International Journal of Clinical Aromatherapy 3 (2b), 9–18.

Hartman, D., Coetzee, J.C., 2002. Two US Practitioners experiences of using essential oils in wound care. J. Wound Care 11 (8), 317–320.

Hausen, B.M., Reichling, J., Harkenthal, M., 1999. Degradation products of monoterpenes are the sensitizing agents in tea tree oil. Am. J. Contact Dermat. 10 (2), 68–77.

Kerr, J., 2002. Research Project – using Essential Oils in Wound Care for the Elderly. Aromatherapy Today 23, 14–17.

Kerr, J., 2003. Using Essential Oils in Wound Care. In Essence 1 (4), 13–17.

Kilham, C., 2004. Tamanu Oil (Calophyllum inophyllum) A Tropical Treatment Remedy. http//medicinehunter.com/tamanu1.htm.

Leach, M.J., 2004. A critical review of natural therapies in wound management. Ostomy Wound Manage. 50 (2), 36–46.

Leach, M.J., 2008. Calendula Officinalis and Wound Healing: A Systematic Review. Wounds 20 (8)Research.com.

Lund, W., 1994. Principles and Practice of Pharmaceutics, twelvth ed. The pharmaceutical codex. The Pharmaceutical Press, London.

Marchini, F.B., Martins, D.M., de Teves, D.C., Simoes M de, J., 1998. Effect of Rosa Rubiginosa Oil on the Healing of Open Wounds (in Portuguese). Rev. Paul. Med. 106 (6), 356.

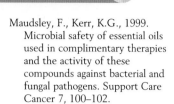
Maudsley, F., Kerr, K.G., 1999. Microbial safety of essential oils used in complimentary therapies and the activity of these compounds against bacterial and fungal pathogens. Support Care Cancer 7, 100–102.

Molan, P.C., 1998. A brief review of the use of honey as a clinical dressing. Primary Intention. The Australian Journal of Wound Management 6 (4), 148–158.

Molan, P.C., 2006. Using honey in wound care. International Journal of Clinical Aromatherapy 3 (2b), 21–24.

Mukherjee, P.K., Verpoorte, R., Suresh, B., 2000. Evaluation of in-vivo wound healing activity of Hypericum patulum (Family: Hypericaceae) leaf extract on different wound model in rats. J. Ethnopharmacol. 70, 315–321.

Price, P., 2003. Abies balsamea [Canadian balsam] Fact sheet. Penny Price Academy of Aromatherapy.

Price, L., Price, S., 2008. Carrier Oils for Aromatherapy and Massage, fourth ed. Riverhead, Stratford-upon-Avon.

Price, S., 1995. Aromatherapy Workbook. Thorsons, London.

Price, S., Price, L., 1999. Aromatherapy for Health Professionals, second ed. Churchill Livingstone, London.

Price, S., Price, L., 2007. Aromatherapy for Health Professionals, third ed. Churchill Livingstone, Elsevier, Philladelphia.

Primmer, J., 2002. Case study – healing a skin tear with essential oils. Aromatherapy Today 23, 20–21.

Reider, N., Issa, A., Hawranek, T., Schuster, C., Aberer, W., Kofler, H., et al., 2005. Absence of contact sensitization to Aloe vera. Contact Dermatitis 53, 332–334.

Reynolds, T., Dweck, A.C., 1999. Aloe vera leaf gel: a review update. J. Ethnopharmacol. 68, 3–37.

Schmidt, J.M., Greenspoon, J.S., 1991. Aloe vera dermal wound gel is associated with a delay in wound healing. J. Obstet. Gynaecol. 78, 115–117.

Skold, M., Borje, A., Matura, M., Karlberg, A.T., 2002. Studies on the autoxidation and sensitizing capacity of the fragrance chemical linalool, identifying a linalool hydroperoxide. Contact Dermatitis 46 (5), 267–272.

Subrahmanyam, M., 1991. Topical application of honey in treatment of burns. Br. J. Surg. 78, 497–498.

Subrahmanyam, M., Shahapure, A.G., Nagane, N.S., Bhagwat, V.R., Ganu, J.V., 2003. Free radical control – the main mechanism of the action of honey in burns. Annals of Burns and Fire Disasters 16 (3), 135–138.

Syed, T.A., Ali Ahmad, S., Ahmadpour, O.A., 1997. Management of psoriasis with Aloe vera extract in a hydrophilic cream – A placebo-controlled, double blind study. J. Eur. Acad. Dermatol. Venereol. 9 (Suppl. 1), S180.

Vazquez, B., Avila, G., Segura, D., Escalante, B., 1996. Anti-inflammatory activity of extracts from Aloe vera gel. J. Ethnopharmacol. 55 (1), 69–75.

Vurnek, M., Weinman, W., Whiting, J.C., Tarlton, J., 2006. Skin immune markers: Psychosocial determinants and the effect on wound healing. Brain Behav. Immun. 20 (3 Suppl. 1), 73–74.

Winter, G.D., 1962. Formation of the scab and the rate of epithelialization of superficial wounds in the skin of the young domestic pig. Nature (London) 193, 293–294.

Zitterl-Eglseer, K., et al., 1997. Anti-oedematous activities of the main triterpendiol esters of marigold (Calendula officinalis L.). J. Ethnopharmacol. 57 (2), 139–144.

Stress, depression and critical care

11

Penny Price   Shirley Price

CHAPTER CONTENTS

Introduction

A poster in the 1980s said, 'Don't ask me to relax – my stress holds me together!' This is important, as stress is not always negative and a certain amount of stress is needed in order to function efficiently.

Aromatherapy has been regarded by many as an effective means of reducing stress, and now some GPs recommend aromatherapy treatment for those who do not cope well with stress. This is because the use of essential oils is balancing and it is this balance – homoeostasis – that practitioners seek to establish and maintain. Aromatherapy is well established for reducing unwanted stress and is just beginning to be accepted in critical care.

What is stress?

There is no definitive, accepted definition of stress. One definition (Lazarus 1998) is that stress is any influence that disturbs the natural balance of a person's body or mind, including physical injury, disease, deprivation and emotional disturbance (Wingate & Wingate 1996). Anxiety (a state of apprehension) and worry (an over-anxious state of mind) are often the forerunners of both stressful and depressive states – in fact, the body has the same initial reaction as in the first stage of stress (see stress below). It can be due to:

a) a reaction to a potentially harmful situation; it is natural and healthy to experience anxiety when faced with danger or risk of some kind. Together with fear, it enables the body to deal with the situation by increasing the respiratory and heart rates, so that extra oxygen reaches the brain; it also releases energy and extra adrenaline (epinephrine) to help cope with the situation.

b) a reaction to an ongoing life event; here the anxious feeling or worry may be connected to work, a problematic marriage, illness, a son in the army who is sent into battle, etc. This sort of anxiety, if the situation becomes serious, usually develops into either stress or (and) depression, depending on the personality of the person.

Positive and negative stress

Stress is not necessarily something bad – it all depends
on how you take it. The stress of exhilarating, creative
successful work is beneficial, while that of failure,
humiliation or rejection is detrimental

(Selye 1956).

Stress need not be negative or even unwelcome –
indeed, a certain amount of stress can help our bodies to operate more successfully , i.e it uses stress as
a motivator and coping mechanism.

The production of adrenaline is one of the
positive side effects of stress which is needed to
motivate people and give the energy to do even
the simplest of tasks. Stress is therefore not
necessarily a problem – it only becomes one when
we have more stress than we can cope with in the
normal run of life; its depth is reflected by the rate
of wear and tear in the body caused by life. In the
introduction to his book on stress, Selye (1956) said
that stress, like the emotions, can be labelled
productive and unproductive, or positive and
negative. A sportsperson experiences pleasurable,
positive stress during a competitive game or when
climbing Mount Everest. Positive stress stimulates
us, giving us the energy to cope with challenging or
demanding tasks, after which both body and mind
return to their normal composure without any negative effect on health.

On the other hand, negative stress can cause
frustration and irritability to take hold – even
moodiness – and if not resolved, can weaken resistance
to ill-health. Some people may go through life suffering only mild stresses, with which they can cope,
having only minor disorders that do not seriously
affect their health.

Everyday stress can cause symptoms such as
headaches or tiredness. Some people tense areas
of their body, such as fists or shoulders; others
may suffer such severe stress that they become
physically and mentally ill, depending on the rate
of wear and tear the particular stress exerts on
their bodies and/or minds. The emotions associated
with stress can include deep anxiety, depression,
desolation, grief, heartache, pain and mental
torment.

Stress is accepted as a medical condition and is
generally viewed as a bad thing, with a range of harmful biochemical and long-term effects, but it is a
necessary part of being alive: the only unstressed
people are dead! Stress makes us competitive and
helps us to deal with unfamiliar situations.

Different people cope with different levels of stress
in different ways. What to one person is a normal and
motivating level of pressure is to another a debilitating
and disabling disturbance. Some experience stress
when too much is happening, whereas others cannot
cope when too little is happening – on the one hand
stress may be caused by over-stimulation, and on
the other by under-stimulation.

There are many types of stressors, which Lennard-Brown
(2001) has attempted to rank in a 'stress score' (p. 21)
(see Table 11.1).

The relationship between stress and depression

When stress is chronic, it can be a cause of depression.
Many depressive – and highly stressful – states are
brought about by a severe life event (such as the death
of a loved one) or a long-lasting bad situation (e.g. living with an incompatible partner) – in other words, a
provoking factor; whether or not this turns to depression depends on the vulnerability of the person concerned and the number of difficulties arising
together at any one time. In severe cases of stress
and/or depression, mental exhaustion or fatigue can
set in. Long-term stress can raise blood pressure and
damage the body's immune system, and it is linked
to problems such as heart disorders, stomach ulcers
and cancer. Highly stressed people are also more likely
to have accidents (Haughton 1995 p. 6).

Aromatherapy is particularly beneficial to both
stress and depression, as one of its main aims is to
bring balance and harmony to the mind; essential
oils generally are balancing substances (especially those
containing esters) and can, as such, help the *whole* person to adjust to their particular situation in life.

In the tradition of aromatherapy, specific essential oils are stress reducing, whereas others are
energizing, and still others can have either effect,
depending on the user's state of mind/body interaction (Warren & Warrenburg 1993).

Response to stress

The body deals with all stress (positive or negative)
by releasing extra energy from its nutritional 'store';
at the same time, extra oxygen is transported to the

Table 11.1 Stressful life events

Event	Score/100	Event	Score/100
Death of spouse	100	Son or daughter leaving home	29
Divorce	73	Trouble with in-laws	29
Separation	65	Outstanding persona achievement	28
Jail term	63	Spouse begins or stops work	26
Death of a close family member	63	Beginning or end of school or college	26
Personal injury or illness	53	Change in living conditions	25
Marriage	50	Change in personal habits	24
Fired from work	47	Trouble with boss	23
Marital reconciliation	45	Change in work hours or conditions	20
Retirement	45	Change in residence	20
Change in health of a family member	44	Change in school or college	20
Pregnancy	40	Change in recreation	19
Sexual difficulties	39	Change in church activities	19
Gaining a new family member	39	Change in social activities	18
Business readjustment	38	A moderate loan or mortgage	17
Change in financial state	38	Change in sleeping habits	16
Death of a close friend	37	Change in the number of family	15
Change to a different line of work	36	gatherings	
Change in number of arguments with spouse	35	Change in eating habits	15
A large mortgage or loan	30	Holiday	13
Foreclosure of a mortgage or loan	30	Christmas	12
Change in responsibilities at work	29	Minor violation of the law	11

brain and extra adrenaline produced. These changes prepare us to cope with the situation causing stress. There are three stages in the development of the body's response to stress (Selye 1956):

1. The initial direct effect of the body exposed to a stressor, bringing about the alarm stage, where:

   - a temporary cessation of digestive juices occurs
   - the respiratory and heart rates increase
   - extra oxygen is transported to the brain and the muscles (in preparation for strenuous action or emotional strength)
   - energy is released quickly from stored fats and sugars
   - extra adrenaline is produced
   - the immune system shuts down.

2. The second, resistant stage is the action taken using these extra resources, where the extra oxygen, energy and adrenaline act to enable the body to cope with the unacceptable situation. Lacking relief from the situation, the responses in stage 1 continue as the body tries to adapt and reach a balanced state. If the level of stress becomes chronic and continues without help, the body reaches the third stage.

3. With excess build-up of stress stage three commences and true (clinical) stress is experienced. This can occur because of an emotional disturbance like the above, severe physical injury, illness or work overload. There is exhaustion, resulting eventually in health problems. These may manifest as headaches, insomnia, digestive problems, skin disorders and susceptibility to infection owing to the gradual closing down of immune responses (Price & Price 2007 p. 252).

Breakdown

Figure 11.1 illustrates the relationship of stress to performance: when stress goes beyond a certain level, fatigue sets in and the performance level drops.

In stage 3, people may become irritable, aggressive, critical, restless, inefficient, withdrawn, moody. They may find that coffee, cigarettes or alcohol give

Table 11.2 Stress-associated problems

Physical problems	Psychological problems	Social problems
Tiredness during the day	Vivid dreams	Increased arguments at home
Difficulty going to sleep	Lack of interest in the world	Tendency to avoid people
Frequent waking at night	Lack of motivation	Abuse of alcohol, tobacco or other drugs
Aches and pains	Listlessness	Increased aggression – particularly in young men
Increased number of infections	Irritability	Inappropriate behaviour
Palpitations	Tearfulness	Over-reaction to problems
High blood pressure	Anxiety	Ignoring problems
Heart attacks	Poor performance at work	Loss of libido
Stroke	Eating problems – too much or too little	
Diarrhoea	Poor self image	
Constipation	Lack of patience	
Irritable bowel syndrome	Depression	
Stomach cramps		
Dental problems (often due to teeth grinding)		
Mouth ulcers		
Skin problems		
Menstrual problems		
Hormone imbalances		

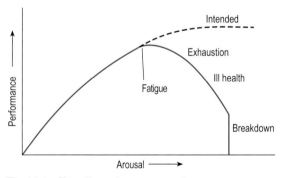

Fig 11.1 • The effect of stress on performance.

temporary relief to the mental stress or they may resort to tranquillizers, any of which may eventually add to their discomfort.

The combination of several ongoing stressors can result in a nervous breakdown, or what is sometimes termed 'burnout'. The nervous system, influenced so strongly by the mind, is unable to cope, and lethargy, inactivity, apathy and indifference set in. It is important to be able to recognize the danger signals and find a natural method of combating them, so that severe consequences can be avoided.

Mental and emotional health go hand in hand with certain attitudes to life. People who are happy-go-lucky remain mentally and physically fitter than those who are negative or who have too much stress in their lives to cope with rationally.

Modern life

O'Hanlon (1998) estimated that 40 million working days were lost each year in the UK as a result of stress; related problems account for more than six out of ten visits to doctors' surgeries.

Health professionals should recognize stress, both within themselves and in their patients/clients, as the commonly held belief is that emotional and physical stress eventually leads to emotional and physical dysfunction (disease).

It is possible to suffer from an acute stress reaction:

> [These] occur in individuals without any other apparent psychiatric disorder, in response to exceptional physical or psychological stress. While severe, such reactions usually subside within hours or days. The stress may be an overwhelming traumatic experience or an unusually sudden change in social circumstances.
>
> (Kumar & Clark 2000 p.1134)

In an attempt to identify and treat stress, healthcare practitioners need to be able to recognize the symptoms. Since almost everyone suffers from some sort of stress discretion is needed; most people do not discuss medical stress comfortably, as stress is essentially being out of control of your own personal situation, relationships and work environments. During periods of stress, emotions are out of proportion to what situations warrant.

Left untreated, stress can lead to self-destructive or harmful behaviour towards others. Stress-related disease is not only on the increase (Seaward 2000), but has a pathogenic effect on the immune function (Hori et al. 2003), appearing to exert an effect on the immune system similar to ageing (Hawkley & Capioppo 2004).

Fight or flight – good or bad?

When an organism experiences a shock or perceives a threat, hormones are released which help cope with the situation. In times past this reaction was valuable in protecting life and limb, but today it is experienced frequently in a modern civilization, and it is not only life-threatening events that trigger this reaction.

Case study 11.1

Stress and depression

Penny Price – Clinical aromatherapist/aromatologist

Assessment

Mr M was so emotionally pressured that on his first visit he had difficulty in articulating his condition. His speech was stilted and often the words were confused and incorrectly pronounced. He had been made redundant 2 years previously and had suffered from cystitis periodically during that time. The antibiotics had lowered his resistance and the cystitis had taken self-confidence away from him. He was difficult to talk to and the taking of his case history was prolonged and uncomfortable.

Mr M felt depressed, tired, listless, apathetic, and did not want to face the world. He suffered from dizziness and disorientation, which was believed to be related to his stress condition and to fear of going out and meeting people.

Intervention

A fresh, natural diet was discussed, moderate exercise and limiting of alcoholic beverages. Mr M seemed happy with our joint plan and signed an agreement to say he would put it into action.

Massage was not an option as Mr M felt too embarrassed to be touched, so a blend of essential oils in a vitamin E base was made for him to apply every day, together with the same essential oils in a bath foam. The aim was to strengthen the immune system and to bring the stress under control.

Equal proportions of the following essential oils were selected for both prescriptions.

- *Eucalyptus staigeriana* [lemon-scented Eucalyptus] – antiseptic, calming
- *Nepeta cataria* [catnip] – anti-infectious (urinary). antiseptic, calming, neurotonic
- *Citrus aurantium* var. *amara* por (bitter orange) antiseptic, calming, sedative
- *Pinus sylvestris* [pine] – antiseptic (particularly to the urinary system), uplifting, energizing.

The above essential oils were blended in a 5% dilution in organic vitamin E cream, which Mr M was to apply to his feet and legs (his choice) twice a day.

The same essential oils were blended 3% in an organic bath foam base for use in the bath (1 dessertspoonful). Mr M had a bath every evening before bed and was encouraged to spend 20 minutes in it so that the oils could penetrate effectively.

Outcome

With the self-help treatments and the essential oils, Mr M began to improve. Progress was slow, as his confidence also had to be rebuilt, and he was referred to a local self-help group near his home. However, within 2 months his speech had improved and he had experienced no further infections. Over the following 3 months Mr M continued to improve and has now reduced his treatments to a 1% blend in the bath foam in the evenings.

When the threat is small, the response is small and can pass unnoticed among the many other distractions of a stressful situation. This mobilization of the body for survival has negative consequences: people are excitable, anxious and irritable, less able to work effectively, more accident prone and less able to make good decisions (http://www.mindtools.com/pages/article). The fight-or-flight response is discussed in Ch 7.

Dealing with stress

Advice commonly given for dealing with stress includes:

- healthy eating – vital to maintaining homoeostasis (fresh fruit and vegetables, complex carbohydrates combined, moderate amounts of protein-rich foods, some fats (in small amounts)
- rest and relaxation techniques, particularly those that focus on controlling the breathing
- aromas with or without massage help relaxation
- counselling or the more short-term cognitive behaviour therapy can change patterns of response and teach ways to deal with change.

Prescription medication, usually tricyclics and SSRI antidepressants, may be given by a medical practitioner. Such a course of action is to be avoided if possible because the side effects can outweigh any benefits and may present difficulties at first when discontinued.

Hospitalization

For many, hospitalization is the most stressful thing that could happen (Jamison, Parris & Maxon 1987). Patients lose their identity and become a number, exchanging their daily attire for nightwear and taking on a new role as a 'condition' in a bed (Buckle 1997 p. 165). However, despite being intimidated by the high-tech environment, the state of mind can be calmed by the use of essential oils (Mullen 2005 personal communication). Stress connected with hospitals is not confined to patients – they are tended by nurses and doctors who are also under stress.

Aromatherapists working in hospitals often have to treat the staff to help relieve the pressures they are under. Tysoe (2000) conducted a study to discover the effect on staff of essential oil vaporizers

Case study 11.2

Severe emotional distress – aromatology class

Jane Guscott – Aromatherapist/aromatologist

Assessment

Sue, a care worker, was experiencing extreme pain in her jaw. When presented to the class as a potential case study she was tense, having just returned with a diagnosis from the GP that she had severe emotional stress. Her jaw was clenched and her teeth were aching. Her blood pressure was slightly raised, her skin was sallow and she was losing more hair than normal from her head.

Intervention

After a holistic assessment, the following essential oils were chosen:

- *Chamaemelum nobile* [Roman chamomile] – antispasmodic, calming and sedative, digestive
- *Melissa officinalis* [Melissa] – uplifting, calming, neurotonic, hypotensor
- *Cymbopogon citratus* [lemongrass] – analgesic, hypotensor, relaxing
- *Lavandula angustifolia* [lavender] – analgesic, antispasmodic, hypotensor, neurotonic, relaxing
- *Origanum majorana* [sweet marjoram] – analgesic, antispasmodic calming, hypotensor 5 drops of each oil

were added to 80 mL sunflower oil and 20 mL mustard oil (for warmth).

The oils were applied initially with a deep facial massage and treatment by self-application was to be continued at home between weekly clinic appointments.

For home treatment 50 mL of an organic moisture cream base was blended with 2 drops of the same oils for morning and evening application. These were also used in an undiluted blend for Sue to use in her aromatizer every day, and also in the bath.

Outcome

This was a difficult case study, as when the massage was applied to the tense facial muscles, Sue began to release her emotions. Perhaps more time was spent letting her cry than treating her, but this was felt to be a positive release that would help the outcome of the treatment and shorten her recovery time. She returned every week to the classroom clinic and in 10 weeks was showing a remarkable improvement. Her hair had stopped shedding and the tension in her jaw was 90% less. Sue continues with the treatments.

in extended care settings using lavender oil in burners. A significant number (88%) indicated that the use of essential oil had a positive effect in the workplace.

Complementary treatment

Of the numerous ways of reducing stress by employing complementary techniques, the following are the most frequently practised in hospitals in the UK and USA:

- **Relaxation**.
- **Counselling**.
- **Reflexology** and/or Swiss reflex massage.
- **Massage** (without essential oils).
- **Therapeutic touch**. This is massage by another name to circumvent some State regulations in the USA, used by nurses belonging to the American Holistic Nurses Association (Krieger 1979).
- **Hydrotherapy** (often followed by massage).

- **Laughter**. Boosts endorphin levels and gives a good feeling. Michigan psychologist Zajonc maintains that even fake smiling triggers a reaction in the brain, making a patient feel better (cited in Price 2000).
- **Essential oils**. A large number of essential oils are stress reducing when inhaled, and to this end can be used independently on a paper tissue, in the bath and in a vaporizer.

Aromatherapeutic treatment

The main function of aromatherapy as introduced in the 1960s (always with massage in the UK) was to relieve stress. Aromatherapists were initially taught to concentrate only on stress relief, so that the body's own healing mechanism would be enabled to alleviate symptoms brought on by the stress, such as migraines, menstrual problems, eczema etc. The effects of massage are enhanced when essential oils

Case study 11.3

Glandular fever and stress

Penny Price – Clinical aromatherapist/aromatologist

Assessment

Ms R (53) has two grown-up children. She had been off work for 9 weeks, initially due to glandular fever diagnosed by her GP through blood tests.

For several years Ms R had been going to her GP for various complaints, mainly muscular aches and pains, which her GP has now diagnosed as fibromyalgia. It was decided that she was also suffering from adrenal fatigue.

After going through a full medical history and consultation for nutritional therapy, it appeared that Ms R has been suffering from long-term stress due to her work and personal life. She has had to raise her children on her own and work long hours in a very demanding and stressful job.

Intervention

The essential oils were selected for her adrenal fatigue and anxiety, and also those that would boost the immune system:

- *Litsea cubeba* (may chang) – anti-infectious, calming, nervine
- *Cinnamomum verum* (cinnamon) – analgesic, anti-infectious, nervine, stimulating, uplifting
- *Aniba rosaeodora* (rosewood) – anti-infectious, stimulating (overwork), tonic
- *Eucalyptus smithii* (gully gum) – analgesic, anti-infectious, balancing, warming.

A blend was made up with 1 mL of each oil. Her feet were warmed, then 30 drops were applied carefully to the soles of both feet (15 drops to each) and covered in plastic film to ensure maximum penetration of the essential oils. After the third visit Ms R was given *Rosa damascena* [rose] hydrolat to ease her mouth ulcers, with instructions to swill and gargle with 10 mL each day (or as needed) and swallow. As well as dealing with the mouth ulcers this was also to help with mental strain, as it is calming and sedative.

Outcome

Ms R shows improvement at each visit and is still taking the rose hydrolat internally. She is happy with the skin drenches and has had no adverse reaction. Her hands and feet are warmer and her skin is pinker. She is going to require further treatments which will include balancing her adrenal glands and help with the pain caused by the fibromyalgia. However, she is improving and becoming stronger, with reduced stress. Oils to be considered for adrenal support once the initial stress is completely under control will be *Picea mariana* [black spruce] combined with *Pinus sylvestris* [pine needle] for application to the kidney area. They contain the monoterpens α-pinene, β-pinene and δ_3 carene, which mimic the action of cortisone and have a modulating effect on the activity of the adrenal cortex.

are added to the basic massage oil (Passant 1990). Patients who experienced aromatherapy reported its beneficial effects in aiding relaxation and reducing stress and anxiety. Sleep patterns improved dramatically for those patients who had previously experienced sleep difficulties, as Cannard (1994) found in his trial on elderly people in hospital.

Childhood stress

Ill effects from stress can begin in early childhood, and Price and Price (2005) give the uses of essential oils for childhood depression and distress, highlighting the fact that the sense of smell has always played an important part in the emotional development of human beings. When trying to calm a child at night, if a parent's garment is put in the cot, the child will snuggle into the garment and feel the closeness of the parent. Essential oils can also be used on a tissue to help to put the child at ease with babysitters, childminders, or in unfamiliar surroundings (Price & Price 2005 p. 12). The familiar smell of security objects apparently serves as a substitute odour when a loved one is not present (Schleidt 1992 p. 43).

A study in 2003 showed that aromas could influence children in the learning environment. This study took place in a special needs classroom, which was apart from the main school. Although the children felt safe in their own area, they became disruptive and unruly when moved into the main school for science lessons. A subtle aroma was established in the special needs rooms using *Eucalyptus staigeriana* and *Aniba roseaodora* in an aromatizer. After establishing the effects of the aroma, the same aroma was placed in the science rooms in the main school for up to 1 hour before the class started. The behaviour of the children was shown to improve dramatically in that they became calmer, less disruptive and quieter (Price 2001).

Essential oils and mood changes

After 7 years' experience of psychological measurement of mood in relation to aroma, Warren and Warrenburg (1993 p. 12) made the following observations:

- Fragrance-evoked mood changes are small, but beneficial to our wellbeing.
- Fragrance can be used to reduce the stress response in humans, but its physiological effects on a non-stressed subject are minimal.

- Measurement of fragrance-evoked mood changes by psychological methods is feasible and yields intriguing results.

Stress can be dissipated by an aroma:

> Fragrances may be used to cope with stressful situations throughout a person's lifespan. Clinical and laboratory studies have shown that certain smells enhance relaxation and reduce stress (Schiffman 1992 p. 57).

Conditioning

Personal experience shows that many people experience stress relief when they inhale, or apply the same blend of oils over a period of time. This is partly due to the creation of a conditioned response – repeated use of a particular aroma for a particular condition will produce the required response; this is known as 'conditioned reflex'. Parents use this technique every day when putting their children to bed: the same bath routine, a story, a drink, then sleep!

Stress can be a learned behavioural pattern, but aromatic treatments can break into that circle to create learned patterns of calm.

Betts (1994) used olfaction to control arousal symptoms in epileptic seizures, not only in those who experienced olfactory auras, but in any patient who had an aura long enough to give them time to apply a countermeasure before a major seizure started. Betts says that using the autohypnotic technique it is possible to train the patient to associate intense relaxation with the smell of the oil (see Ch. 7).

Depression

Depression seems to affect women more than men. Like stress, it is a much abused word, many people saying they are depressed when in reality they are simply feeling temporarily sad or low-spirited; fortunately, after a relatively short period of several days at most, most of us 'snap out' of a temporary dejected state and are able to resume our normal 'emotional' lives.

Depression takes in a whole range of melancholic dispositions, not least those connected with moodiness and apathy, as sufferers can feel lethargic, bored, suffer mood swings and often show little interest in anything at all. Other emotions can also play a part in the whole depressed state, for example sadness, grief, remorse, shame etc. Carter (1998) says that depression is more than just a mood – because the brains of people who are depressed are less active than normal, this probably accounts for physical symptoms such as fatigue and lethargy.

There can be pain and disturbance of sleep and appetite, the memory is affected and thinking is slowed. Anxiety, irrational fear and agitation may be present, and a depressed person typically feels guilty, worthless and unloved. Life seems pointless – the 'meaning' is missing from things (Carter 1998 p. 100).

Before a person can be clinically diagnosed as depressed, two factors have to be confirmed:

- that the social life of the person is interfered with
- that the condition has been going on for more than 2 weeks – some clinicians say a month.

The symptoms a clinician looks for are

- lack of energy – a feeling of being 'washed out' all the time
- sleep problems: difficulty in getting to sleep or waking early and unable to get back to sleep
- slowing down in everything they do
- irritation and inability to concentrate on things (Wood 1990 p. 64)

When depression becomes chronic, people feel that their situation is going to continue interminably; they feel helpless to do anything about it and can become mentally exhausted, as well as often being pessimistic and withdrawing into themselves (Wood 1990 p. 63–65).

Causes of depression can be:

- lack of sunshine in winter
- a feeling of inadequacy
- inability to cope – as in postnatal depression
- rejection – at work, in sport, drama group etc.
- illness – even if minor
- frustration at missing an important social function
- not being able to finish an urgent task.

If the illness is chronic or hopeless or due to immobility, fear, despair and even anger can be experienced. Even minor illnesses such as coughs, colds and flu or general aches and pains can trigger feelings of despondency which can lead to depression; if someone does not make a full recovery after a viral illness such as flu, for example, they are left feeling drained and without energy, which can change despondency into full-blown depression, called postviral fatigue syndrome. When depressed people think about themselves in a negative way, remembering mistakes more easily than successes, unhappy memories return more easily than happy ones.

Drug alternatives

In conventional treatment, patients with anxiety who visit their GPs are often prescribed tranquillizers. The effects of these drugs are to repress the individual because the drugs are designed to slow down the body. Gascoigne (1994 p. 360) quotes the figure of 8.5 million prescriptions for stress/depression in the UK in 1989. The prescriptions given are based on the belief that stress and/or depressive illness is caused by a chemical imbalance in the brain (thyroxin level is now a standard test).

The rationale seems to be that if the thought processes are slowed down then life is easier to cope with. From observation of those who have been treated in this way it seems that this leads to further depression born out of the inability to live life from day to day because they lack motivation. Therefore, rather than use essential oils to depress the system, it is better to use oils known to be stimulating and invigorating.

Aromatherapy provides a harmless alternative to psychotropic drugs and muscle relaxants commonly used to treat anxiety allopathically. See Essential oils for stress and depression below.

Essential oil choices

The underlying anxiety and all the accompanying states of mind can be treated effectively with essential oils, either with or without massage. As each essential oil is capable of a variety of health effects, both mental and physical, there is quite a long list of those that could be beneficial, therefore the final choice depends on which emotional and physical symptoms are being experienced.

When treating a client holistically, a list should first be made of all essential oils that will benefit anxiety or depression (see Appendix A (II) on the CD-ROM) – whichever is the client's basic problem. Should any other physical or emotional states also need to be addressed, check whether they match any already on the list.

Essential oils for treating stress

Schnaubelt (1998 p. 103) says that nervousness, tension and stress call for the sedative qualities of aldehydes, the diverse action of ester compounds on the nervous system and the sympatholytic (calming, dilation of blood vessels) effects of some phenyl-propanes (found in oils such as aniseed and fennel). This may mean that essential oils such as *Citrus aurantium* var. *amara* per. [petitgrain], *Citrus bergamia* [bergamot], *Litsea cubeba* [may chang] and *Melissa officinalis* [melissa] (among others rich in at least two of these chemical groups) would suffice to relieve tension, and he advocates the application of these oils neat to the temples every day.

Ocimum basilicum [basil], because of its methyl ether content, soothes, calms and relaxes, and is recommended for people with schizoid tendencies.

A blend of up to four different essential oils could be required to treat stress holistically, and the synergy between them will enhance the total effect.

Essential oils for lifting depression

Some essential oils have been singled out empirically for their effects on the human psyche, such as *Boswellia carteri* [frankincense], which has been recognized as being good for nervous depression (see Appendix A (II) on the CD-ROM).

Traditionally, *Melissa officinalis* [melissa] has been used as a treatment for depression – Paracelsus called it the 'elixir of life'. Culpeper said that it 'driveth away all troublesome cares and thoughts out of the mind'. Since melissa oil contains around 70% aldehydes (mainly citral), this fits Schnaubelt's theory that aldehydes are essential for psychological health and wellbeing.

Eucalyptus staigeriana [lemon-scented iron bark]. Of all the eucalyptus family, *E. staigeriana* appears to have an effect at the emotional level. It is uplifting, antidepressive, and has been used in the treatment of ME. The aldehyde content (21–37%) means that it may be a mild skin irritant, especially if used neat (however, there are no reported incidents of such).

Ocimum basilicum var. *album* [European basil] has been used widely in many healing traditions since antiquity. The phenol content of the oil (eugenol 1–19%) is reputed to kick-start the nervous system, but there is no published research for this.

Thymus vulgaris ct. *thymol*. Thyme helps to revive and strengthen both body and mind. The phenol (thymol) content is 60–80%; when blended with *Ocimum basilicum* [European basil], whose uplifting alcohols complement the stimulating phenols, the resulting blend is effective for depression.

Neurotonic and energizing essential oils to relieve depression and stimulate the mind are:

aniseed, basil, bergamot, **Roman chamomile**, **clary sage, cypress**, frankincense, **geranium**, ginger, juniper, **lavender, marjoram, neroli, bitter orange**, peppermint, petitgrain, pine, rosemary, **rose otto**, sage, sandalwood, sweet thyme.

Balancing oils – calming and uplifting

Many essential oils which help depression can also relieve stress (these are in **bold** above)because many have a balancing effect, probably due to the ester content. Essential oils have many properties: those needed to lift someone out of a depressive state can not only target the depression but also maintain equilibrium and (if selected carefully and knowledgeably help to heal) other physical or mental problems.

The following are taken from Price (2000) and Franchomme and Pénoël (2001):

- *Chamaemelum nobile* [Roman chamomile] – headaches, insomnia, indigestion, irritability, muscle tension
- *Citrus aurantium* var. *amara* (flos) [neroli bigarade] – agitation, insomnia
- *Citrus bergamia* (per.) [bergamot] – agitation, insomnia, indigestion, irritability
- *Lavandula angustifolia* [lavender] – agitation, headaches, hypertension, insomnia, irritability, muscle tension
- *Lavandula* x *intermedia* 'Super' [lavandin] – agitation, headaches, hypertension, muscle tension
- *Origanum majorana* [sweet marjoram] – agitation, headaches, hypertension, insomnia, indigestion, irritability, muscle tension
- *Pelargonium graveolens* [geranium] – agitation, headaches, irritability, low immunity.

Gatti and Cayola (1923) researched the psychotherapeutic effects of essential oils, attempting to identify sedative and stimulating essences by measuring pulse rate and cardiovascular and respiratory activity. Recommended oils for anxiety were neroli, petitgrain, cedarwood, chamomile, melissa and valerian (Damien & Damien 1995 p. 150). As is the case with much research, no Latin names are mentioned and assumptions have to be made regarding the identity of the essential oils mentioned.

Paolo Rovesti, in the 1970s, practised aromatherapy to treat stress and psychological distress using inhalation techniques, preferring to use blends rather than single essential oils, thereby introducing many variables into his research. For anxiety Rovesti listed petitgrain and neroli, bergamot, cypress, lavender, lime, marjoram, rose and violet leaf (Damien & Damien 1995 p.151).

Selecting a blend

The method of selecting and combining essential oils described above is illustrated by the following examples:

- Depression, with headaches and insomnia: *Chamaemelum nobile, Lavandula angustifolia* and *Origanum majorana*. If the immune system is felt to be low, *O. majorana* should be present in the highest proportion in the mix. Should the aroma need adjusting for the client, select any other essential oil from the antidepressive range above or the fuller list in Appendix A (II) on the CD-ROM.
- Anxiety with agitation, and high blood pressure: *L. angustifolia* and *O. majorana*.
- Anxiety with agitation, indigestion and muscle tension: *L. angustifolia* and *O. majorana*.

Should a third oil be desired, one may be selected for whichever symptom is strongest. Consult Appendix A (II) for other symptoms which can be helped with the same oils as those helping to reduce stress or lift depression.

Having selected the essential oil(s), it is advisable and time-saving to make up the blend in a dropper bottle, which must be labelled with instructions for use. For stress, the relative proportions of essential oils should be influenced by the aroma preferences of the patient concerned.

Stress in critical care

Many factors need to be addressed when looking after a patient in critical care, including the severe stress experienced by patients and relatives, to say nothing of the possibility of further invasive infections, both of which will respond to essential oils, with or without aromatherapy massage.

It is difficult to talk generally about the use of aromatherapy in critical care, simply because the reasons for needing it are many and often sudden, e.g. breathing difficulties, lung viruses, strokes, heart attacks, heart surgery, road accidents etc.

Critical care is concerned predominantly with the management of patients with acute life-threatening conditions in a specialized unit. Teamwork and a multidisciplinary approach is central to the provision of intensive care and is most effective when directed and coordinated by a committed specialist. In the UK, about 1–2% of the beds in the hospital are usually allocated to intensive care. In critically ill patients, the immediate objective is to preserve life and prevent, reverse or minimize damage to vital organs such as the brain.

(Kumar & Clark 2000 p. 829–830)

The acute emotional and psychological trauma that patients endure in a strange and unfamiliar place (often without their loved ones beside them) can leave them with an intense feeling of loneliness and isolation. The CCU can be a hostile environment to patients who are surrounded by a bewildering array of monitoring and support equipment and subjected to a variety of invasive therapeutic techniques (Waldman et al. 1993).

Touch is a very important part of care for any patient, particularly those in critical care. It has been found that a nurse who is able to take the time to touch patients in critical care – holding their hand, even without talking – could establish in a relatively short time an empathetic relationship with them (McCorkle 1974). Essential oils with and without massage are used generally in critical care units throughout the UK for relaxation, comfort and well-being: massage of even just the feet has been shown to have beneficial effects (Hayes & Cox 2000); but massage with essential oils needs careful consideration for those patients needing a high level of intensive care, as it could be damaging (Shepherd 2005 personal communication).

Use of aromatherapy

Most recorded uses of aromatherapy in critical care are concerned with heart surgery, where the overriding concern of the aromatherapist is patient stress. Anxiety can precipitate life-threatening arrhythmia and extend infarction areas, if not allayed quickly enough (Harris 1993). Although frequent nursing reassurances may prevent intimidation by the high-tech environment, patients' anxieties have been found to be centred on their personal illness rather than on the hospital surroundings (Herxheimer et al. 2000); essential oils can calm their state of mind still further.

Critical care is considered a stressful environment at both physiological and psychological levels for patients. A research study in which a five-minute foot massage was offered to 25 patients (68 sessions in total) as a stress-reduction intervention. Physiological data (heart rate, mean arterial blood pressure, respirations and peripheral oxygen saturation) were collected before, during and after the intervention. There was no significant effect on peripheral oxygen saturation, but a significant decrease in heart rate, blood pressure and respiration was observed during the foot massage using jasmine. Results indicated foot massage had the potential effect of increasing relaxation, as evidenced by physiological changes during the brief intervention administered to critically ill patients in intensive care.

(Hayes & Cox 2000 p. 77–82)

Inhalation

Inhalation is a non-intrusive way of using essential oils in critical care, where the interaction between the molecules and the receptors in the central nervous system is responsible for the sedation caused by inhaling the fragrant molecules (Buchbauer & Jirovetz 1994) and there is no need for physical contact with the patient. The higher the level of intensive care needed, the more should inhalation be the method chosen for aromatherapy care – if intervention is permitted at all.

The sedative influence of lavender has been shown by many early research works and was confirmed by Karamat et al. in 1992; similarly, anxiety and fear can be masked by orange (Lehrner et al. 2000). Miyake, Nakagawa and Asakura (1991) found that inhalation of bitter orange oil increased sleeping time significantly under conditions of mental stress. Sugano and Sato (1991) discovered that lavender, orange and rose countered the effects of stress. There is concern that only common names are given for the oils used in many research studies, especially when there are so many varieties of, for instance, 'chamomile', 'eucalyptus' and 'lavender'. Full botanical and analytical identification is essential if such trials are to be of practical use.

Massage

Massage should not be given to patients requiring a high level of care, as it could possibly endanger those under heavy sedation or on ventilators. Massage of the hands or feet is the least intrusive if wishing to use this method when helping to wean people off a ventilator.

Essential oil choice

The following essential oils contain sedative properties suitable for use in critical or coronary care:

- Citrus oils – *Citrus aurantium* var. *amara* flos, fol., per. [neroli, petitgrain, bitter orange], *Citrus bergamia* [bergamot], *Citrus limon* [lemon], *Citrus reticulata* [mandarin] – calming and/or sedative to various degrees
- *Chamaemelum nobile* [Roman chamomile] – sedative
- *Melissa officinalis* [melissa] – sedative
- *Commiphora myrrha* [myrrh] – sedative, cardiotonic
- *Lavandula angustifolia* [lavender] – calming and sedative.

Research trials and studies

Several trials and studies have been carried out to evaluate the effectiveness of essential oils and massage in the nursing care of patients in critical care units:

- Royal Sussex County Hospital (Woolfson & Hewitt 1992) – massage of the feet – (Box 11.1)
- Middlesex Hospital, London (Stevensen 1994) – massage of the feet – (Box 11.2)
- Battle Hospital, Reading (Dunn, Sleep & Collett 1995) – massage on various parts of the body (back, outside of limbs, scalp) – (Box 11.3).

There may be a role for relatives of critically ill patients to use essential oils to help them cope with their stress, as this is a huge crisis in their lives (Green 2005 personal communication) although this, albeit effective, is limited.

There is widespread belief that the use of aromatherapy and massage in an intensive care environment offers a means of increasing the quality of sensory input that patients receive, in addition to reducing stress and anxiety. Despite a wealth of anecdotal evidence in support of these claims, there have been few objective studies to evaluate the effects of these therapies. In a study by Dunn, Sleep and Collett (1995 p. 34–40) 22 patients admitted to a general intensive care unit were randomly allocated to receive either massage, aromatherapy using lavender essential oil, or a period of rest. Both pre- and

Box 11.1

Royal Sussex County Hospital – foot massage

Intervention

Lavender (botanical name not given) was used. Two treatments a week were given to three groups of 12 patients each for 5 weeks, observations being recorded at the beginning, end and 30 minutes after each session:

- Group 1: 20 minute massage using lavender in a vegetable oil
- Group 2: 20 minute massage using only vegetable oil
- Group 3: 20 minute undisturbed rest period only

Results

The results showed a consistent decrease in blood pressure, heart rate, pain, respiratory rate and wakefulness in all three groups, the greatest benefits being experienced by group 1, especially in the reduction of the heart and respiratory rates:

- Heart rate: group 1 – 11/12 (91.6%); group 2 – 7/12 (58.3%); group 3 – 5/12 (41.6%)
- Respiratory rate: group 1 – 9/12 (75%); group 2 – 5/12 (41.6%); group 3 – 16.6% (Woolfson & Hewitt 1992).

Box 11.2

Middlesex Hospital, London – foot massage

Intervention

Each of the four groups of cardiac patients in critical care was assessed physiologically for heart rate, respiratory rate and blood pressure, and psychologically for pain, anxiety and tension before the intervention and 5 days afterwards. Assessments were made of all patients both before and after each session:

- Group 1: 20 minute standardized foot massage
- Group 2: as above, using only apricot oil
- Group 3: 20 minute conversation with a nurse – no tactile input or formal counselling
- Group 4: 20 minute period with routine care – no intervention of any kind

The feet of patients in groups 1 and 2 were massaged once a day, using 2.5% *Citrus aurantium* var. *aurantium* (flos) [neroli bigarade], chosen for its calming, antispasmodic, antidepressant and gentle sedative actions, in apricot kernel vegetable oil.

Results

Immediately after the intervention, both the respiratory rate and the psychological (pain and anxiety) results showed statistically significant reduction differences between groups 1 and 2 and the control groups 3 and 4.

Even though no difference was seen physiologically at the next measurement period, groups 1 and 2 had statistically significantly better psychological results than the control groups, 3 and 4 at the end of day 5. (Stevensen 1994)

Box 11.3

Battle Hospital, Reading — massage of parts of the body

The following study was carried out to evaluate the effectiveness of aromatherapy and massage in the nursing care of patients in critical care, the protocol being approved by the Research and Ethics Committee for the West Berkshire Health District.

Intervention

Three groups were each given a different treatment: Group 1 received a light massage on areas of the body available to the therapist – back, outside of limbs, scalp – using grapeseed oil alone; the same carrier but with the addition of 1% of *Lavandula vera* [lavender] essential oil was used on Group 2, and Group 3 were left to rest

for half a hour, with no massage being given. Areas assessed were:

- Behavioural – categorized into a four-point scale
- Physiological – systolic and diastolic blood pressure, heart rate and rhythm, respiratory rates
- Psychological – also using a four-point scale for patients to self-assess their level of anxiety, mood and ability to cope with the present situation.

Results

These showed that the use of essential oils with massage proved to be more effective than massage and rest alone in reducing anxiety. (Dunn, Sleep & Collett 1995) post-therapy assessments included physiological stress indicators and patients' evaluation of their anxiety levels, mood and ability to cope with their intensive care experience. Ninety-three patients (77%) were able to complete subjective assessments. There were no statistically significant differences in the physiological stress indicators or observed or reported behaviour of patients' ability to cope following any of the three interventions. Those patients who received aromatherapy reported significantly greater improvement in their mood and perceived levels of anxiety, and felt less anxious and more positive immediately following the therapy, although this effect was not sustained or cumulative.

Another study points out the beneficial effects of essential oils in reducing anxiety in a dentist's waiting room (Lehrner et al. 2000 p. 83–6), which may also be of use in critical care.

Summary

This chapter has examined stress in modern life and the role essential oils can play in reducing its effects. A trial project (Gonella 1993 unpublished) clearly demonstrates that massage with essential oils can significantly reduce stress levels in GPs' patients. The guide to the selection of stress-reducing oils presented here is intended to enable readers to choose and administer essential oils for their patients to achieve beneficial results. Nurses currently using aromatherapy in critical care units will have little doubt that it can help relieve some of the stress related to the intensive treatments and procedures. The fact that carers are actively helping their patients may also reduce their stress. The case studies and trials presented in this chapter demonstrate the efficacy of essential oils in reducing stress levels both in and out of hospital, for both carers and patients.

References

Betts, T., 1994. Sniffing the breeze. Aromatherapy Quarterly 40 (spring), 19–22.

Buchbauer, G., Jirovetz, L., 1994. Aromatherapy – use of fragrances and essential oils as medicaments. Flavour and Fragrance Journal 9, 217–222.

Buckle, J., 1997. Clinical aromatherapy in nursing. Arnold, London.

Cannard, S., 1994. On the scent of a good night's sleep. Trial project. Midland Health Board News January, 3.

Carter, R., 1998. Mapping the mind. In: Weidenfeld & Nicholson, London, pp. 99–100.

Damien, P., Damien, K., 1995. Aromatherapy scent and psyche: using essential oils for physical and emotional well-being. Healing Arts Press, Rochester, Vermont.

Dunn, C., Sleep, J., Collett, D., 1995. Sensing an improvement: an experimental study to evaluate the use of aromatherapy, massage and periods of rest in an intensive care unit. J. Adv. Nurs. 21, 34–40.

Franchomme, P., Pénoël, D., 2001. L'aromathérapie exactement, second ed Jollois, Limoges.

Gascoigne, S., 1994. The manual of conventional medicine for alternative

practitioners, vol. II. Jigme Press, Surrey.

Gatti, G., Cayola, R., 1923. Azione terapeutica degli olii essenzioli. Rivista Italiana delle Essenze e Profume 5 (12), 133–135.

Gonella, 1993. Unpublished work.

Harris, C.M., 1993. Is there a benefit to patients in using aromatherapy oils in a coronary care unit? Pilot study results. (copies available from The Royal Shrewsbury Hospital).

Haughton, E., 1995. Dealing with Stress. Wayland, Hove.

Hawkley, L.C., Capioppo, T.J., 2004. Stress and the aging immune system. Brain Behav. Immun. 18, 114–118.

Hayes, J.A., Cox, C.L., 2000. Immediate effects of a foot massage in intensive care. Complement. Ther. Nurs. Midwifery 6 (1), 9.

Herxheimer, A., et al., 2000. Database of patients' experiences (DIPEx): a multi-media approach to sharing experiences and information. Lancet 355, 1540–1543.

Hori, Y., Ibuki, T., Hosokawa, T., Tanaka, Y., 2003. The effects of neurosurgical stress on peripheral lymphocyte subpopulations. J. Clin. Anaesth. 15, 1–8.

Jamison, R.N., Parris, W.C.V., Maxon, W.S., 1987. Psychological factors influencing recovery from outpatient surgery. Behav. Res. Ther. 25, 31–37.

Karamat, E., Ilmberger, J., Buchbauer, G., Roblhuber, K., Rupp, C., 1992. Excitatory and sedative effects of essential oils on human reaction time performance. Chem. Senses 17.

Krieger, D., 1979. The therapeutic touch. Simon & Schuster, New York.

Kumar, P., Clark, M., 2000. Clinical Medicine, fourth ed Harcourt Brace and Co, London.

Lazarus, R.S., 1998. Stress and emotion. Springer, New York.

Lehrner, J., Eckersberger, C., Walla, P., Potsch, G., Deecke, L., 2000. Ambient odour of orange in a dental office reduces anxiety and improves mood in female patients. Physiol. Behav. 71, 83–86.

Lennard-Brown, S., 2001. Stress and Depression. White-Thomson, Lewes.

McCorkle, R., 1974. Effects of touch on seriously ill people. Nurs. Res. 23 (2), 125.

Miyake, Y., Nakagawa, M., Asakura, Y., 1991. Effects of odours on humans 1.

Effects on sleep latency. Chem. Senses 16, 183.

O'Hanlon, B., 1998. Stress – the common sense approach. Newleaf, New York.

Passant, H., 1990. A holistic approach in the ward. Nurs. Times 86 (4), 26–28.

Price, S., 2000. Aromatherapy and your emotions. Thorsons, London.

Price, P., 2001. Managing School Environments: Children's Responses to Changes in the Aromatic Environment. An Action Research. Oxford University Masters Dissertation.

Price, P., Price, S., 2005. Aromatherapy for babies and children, second ed Riverhead, Stratford on Avon.

Price, S., Price, L., 2007. Aromatherapy for Health Professionals, third ed Churchill Livingstone, Edinburgh.

Schleidt, M., 1992. The semiotic relevance of human olfaction: a biological approach, chapter 4. In: Van Toller, S., Dodd, G. (Eds.), Fragrance: the psychology and biology of perfume. Elsevier Science, Essex.

Schnaubelt, K., 1998. Advanced aromatherapy: the science of essential oil therapy. Healing Arts Press, Rochester, Vermont.

Seaward, B.L., 2000. Stress and human spirituality 2000: at the crossroads of physics and metaphysics. Appl. Psychophysiol. Biofeedback 25 (4), 241–246.

Selye, H., 1956. The stress of life. McGraw Hill, New York.

Stevensen, C.J., 1994. Psychophysical effects of aromatherapy massage following cardiac surgery. Complement. Ther. Med. 2, 27–35.

Sugano, H., Sato, N., 1991. Psychophysiological studies of fragrance. Chem. Senses 16, 183–184.

Tysoe, P., 2000. The effects on staff of emotional oil burners in extended care settings. Int. J. Nurs. Pract. (April), 110–112.

Waldman, C.S., Tseng, P., Meulman, P., Whitter, H.B., 1993. Aromatherapy in the intensive care unit. Care of the Critically Ill 9 (4), 170–174.

Warren, C., Warrenburg, S., 1993. Mood benefits of fragrance. The International Journal of Aromatherapy 12 (2), 12–16.

Wingate, P., Wingate, R., 1996. Medical encyclopaedia. Penguin, London.

Wood, C., 1990. Say yes to life. Dent, London.

Woolfson, A., Hewitt, D., 1992. Intensive aroma care. Int. J. Aromather. 4 (2), 12–13.

www.mindtools.com/pages/article.

Pregnancy and childbirth

Penny Price   Shirley Price   Jo Kellett

Introduction

Aromatherapy and massage on expectant mothers have proved to be effective throughout their pregnancy, especially where some allopathic medications are contraindicated because of possible adverse effects on the fetus. Aromatherapy can offer a gentler means of achieving optimum wellbeing during the antenatal period and labour, as essential oils can help combat many of the physical and emotional symptoms. This chapter seeks to advise the professional in their safe and effective use, while stressing that aromatherapy is not an alternative to the orthodox care of a pregnant woman, but a complementary aid.

Ethical, legal and safety aspects in pregnancy

Aromatherapy during pregnancy and childbirth has gained enormous popularity in the last decade; many midwives were already using it at the turn of the century (Ager 2002, Reed & Norfolk 1993), as it blends in easily with the one-to-one situation of labour and delivery care and enables both midwives and aromatherapists to provide more holistic care.

> Aromatherapy offers a wonderful means of helping women to cope with the physiological symptoms of pregnancy and early parenthood and to ease discomfort and pain in labour.
>
> (Tiran 2000)

However, UK law states that only a midwife or doctor can take sole responsibility for the care of an expectant or labouring mother, except in an emergency. Treatment with essential oils is complementary to normal antenatal, intrapartum or postnatal care, from confirmation of conception until 28 days after delivery, when the legal period of midwifery care comes to an end.

Only aromatherapists with specialized training in the changing anatomy and physiology of pregnant women should administer essential oils, always liaising with the maternity care team. On the other hand, it is not appropriate for midwives to advise women on the use of aromatherapy unless they have undertaken accredited training, to ensure that the information and care given is accurate, safe and up-to-date (NMC 2002a, b). A cooperative team of experienced professional midwives and aromatherapists can enhance the wellbeing of the mother and add to her overall pleasure and sense of achievement. Protocols may be devised not only to ensure best midwifery practice but also to include the protection of mothers and midwives. Although not actually a safety issue, cigarettes and alcohol are best avoided during pregnancy.

Insurance

Aromatherapists should be well insured for their work, and nurse-aromatherapists should have personal professional indemnity insurance cover in addition to their nursing insurance, which does not cover them for essential oil use. If permission to use aromatherapy within their midwifery practice has been obtained from the employing authority, the Trust's liability insurance cover will usually apply. Midwives having a private aromatherapy practice should notify the Local Supervising Authority if intending to use essential oils on a pregnant client.

Keeping records

Most women keep their pregnancy notes with them and have access to midwife or consultant comments. The Congenital Disabilities Act 1976 says that notes must be kept for a period of 25 years after the baby is born, in case of any legal claims for error at birth. With this in mind, it would be prudent for a therapist also to keep their consultation and follow-up notes for this same period, giving the expectant mother a copy to keep with her maternity notes.

Safety issues

There is little scientific evidence for or against the safety of essential oils in pregnancy, as it is impossible and unethical to conduct randomized controlled studies on pregnant women; most available evidence comes from anecdotal and empirical knowledge accumulated by practitioners. Antenatal

application of a limited number of essential oils is assumed to be safe, based on anecdotal evidence from years of use by pregnant women, currently available knowledge, and the increasing number of research findings (these have been carried out on animals, however, and so are not necessarily relevant to humans). Lists of essential oils contraindicated in pregnancy differ from one authority to the next, emphasizing the need for continual training to ensure that therapists are practising according to current information, whether based on experience or research.

It is standard practice for aromatherapist-midwives or aromatherapists administering essential oils to pregnant and labouring women to use only those that are considered to be safe. They should apply both knowledge of essential oil chemistry and common sense to the physiology and potential pathological complications of pregnancy.

Some aromatherapists, who have taken only a short course or one not recognized by a leading aromatherapy organization, feel they should not treat pregnant women: considering their lack of knowledge and experience, such people should not even be calling themselves aromatherapists (O'Hara 2002).

Emmenagogues and abortifacients

Although some aromatherapists prefer not to use essential oils with emmenagogic or abortive properties on pregnant women, there is only real danger if these oils are used in excess (i.e. 5–10 mL) and/or internally, neither of which a proficient aromatherapist would do. During the first 3 months of pregnancy the developing child is particularly sensitive to chemicals, and remains vulnerable throughout. There is good evidence that different fetal systems are sensitive to different chemicals at specific times (Tisserand & Balacs 1995 p. 110).

Where oils have been reported to cause spontaneous abortion, it has been as a result of ingesting quantities more than 20 times the amount that would normally be used – even in therapeutic aromatherapy, when maternal hepato- or renal toxicity is a far more likely primary outcome (Balacs 1992). Essential oils considered to be abortifacient (such as pennyroyal) are not used during pregnancy (see Ch. 3 Pt II and Appendices B2 and B3 on the CD-ROM).

Emmenagogues

An emmenagogue is a substance that promotes and regulates menstruation, and it is therefore understandable that oils with this property are usually avoided until the end of the first trimester once a woman realizes she is pregnant. Although essential oils with emmenagogic properties are used extensively in aromatherapy for conditions such as polycystic ovaries, dysmenorrhoea, amenorrhea and PMT, such oils should be avoided during pregnancy. There is no conclusive evidence that essential oils can cause a miscarriage, but women experiencing such a loss may look to the oils as a reason and may blame their aromatherapy treatment for their loss, even though the overall risk from essential oils is very small indeed.

Certain individual constituents, e.g. ketones, are claimed to stimulate uterine contractions, although this may depend on the isomer present in the particular oil; it may be wise to refrain from using oils containing ketones, particularly for women with a history of preterm labour. On the other hand, ketones can be useful at the end of pregnancy as they stimulate contractions and so reduce the time spent in labour.

Abortifacients

An abortifacient is a substance which can provoke an abortion (Collin 1993 p. 2). It is necessarily powerful as it has to *fight* nature, not help it. Essential oils known to be abortifacient should not normally be used in general practice – savin, tansy, juniper and pennyroyal have all been considered abortifacient. However, work using the isolated human uterus shows that the essential oils of these plants have no direct action on uterine muscles (Gunn 1921). There appears to be no clear evidence that any essential oils present an abortifacient risk, as far as external use in aromatherapy is concerned (Tisserand & Balacs 1995 p. 112).

Most abortion cases reported have been due to oral ingestion of a large quantity of an essential oil. Rather than advising oils for different stages of pregnancy, the wisest course is to avoid potentially hazardous oils throughout.

A note on photosensitivity

Although photosensitizing oils are not a major problem in aromatherapy because possible ill effects are ineffective within 2 hours of administration (see Ch. 3), pregnant women should take extra care as they have an increased production of melanocytic hormone, which may make them more prone to being affected if the minimum waiting period of 2 hours is not observed before going into direct sunlight. Citrus oils, expressed or distilled, contain furanocoumarins, which trigger phototoxicity (Naganuma et al. 1985). Women who develop chloasma (the butterfly-shaped facial pigmentation of pregnancy) have higher circulating levels of melanocytic hormone and should not apply such oils on parts of the body most likely to be exposed to the sun. However, citrus essences and essential oils are otherwise considered relatively safe during pregnancy (see also Ch. 3 Pt II).

Aromatherapy and massage during pregnancy

Choice of oils and methods of use

The selection of essential oils can only be made in conjunction with the mother, following assessment of her condition at the time of the treatment. The oils suggested below are given as a general guide. Aromatherapy used to relieve specific physiological disorders in pregnancy offers mothers, midwives and aromatherapists additional tools to treat the unwanted symptoms which can present during the 9 months, as well as making the birth itself much easier. Most methods of use can be employed, although oral use (see Ch. 9) is the most effective way of treating digestive disorders, should the mother request it: it should not be used for any other problem. Not enough schools teach this aspect, so it is best used on the prescription of an aromatologist working with a medical practitioner. Regular antenatal aromatherapy, whether by massage, inhalation or self-application, is a pleasant way of enhancing the mother's wellbeing by aiding relaxation, sleep, and easing physiological discomforts.

Massage during pregnancy reduces stress hormones such as cortisol and may contribute to a lower incidence of antenatal, intranatal and postpartum complications (Field et al. 1999), as well as being invaluable for treating oedematous ankles, constipation, backache and headaches etc.

See Ch. 8 for help in positioning a woman advanced in pregnancy for massage, in order to avoid supine hypotension, especially in later pregnancy, and to prevent discomfort.

Firm sacral massage on a woman with a history of preterm labour must be avoided, as inadvertent stimulation of the acupuncture points in the intravertebral foramen may trigger uterine contractions. Additionally, there are certain points on the feet that should be avoided, for example massage of the area

Case Study 12.1

Massage throughout pregnancy treatments

Jo Kellett – Aromatherapist

Assessment

Ms E, age 38 – pregnant with non-identical twins (her first baby had died at 11 months old 7 years previously).

Recent diagnosis of gestational diabetes – under control. A history of polycystic ovaries was diagnosed in her early 20s, she experienced bad PMT, mood swings and had a 45-day cycle. She is emotionally tender over losing her first baby and is feeling tired, often aching.

Intervention

1st treatment – at 26 weeks

(1% blend in sweet almond oil used for all treatments)

Aim: to help Mrs E to feel relaxed, more confident about pregnancy and help dispel feelings of fear. Full body massage was given and the following oils selected:
- *Citrus sinensis* – calming, sedative, aids sleep
- *Santalum album* – cardiotonic, general tonic
- *Citrus aurantium* var. *amara* flos – calming, neurotonic, aids sleep

The same blend of essential oils given in a lotion to apply on shoulders each night.

2nd treatment – 3 weeks later – Mrs E had been sleeping better

Assessment: her sacroiliac area was painful and she was congested, with excess mucus.

Aim: To decongest system and relieve muscular aches and pains
- *Boswellia carteri* – analgesic, anticatarrhal, anti-inflammatory, energizing, expectorant, immunostimulant
- *Pelargonium graveolens* – analgesic, anti-inflammatory, relaxant
- *Myrtus communis* – anticatarrhal, expectorant, decongestant

The same blend was given for local application morning and night at home.

3rd treatment – 2 weeks later

Assessment

Having frequent Braxton–Hicks contractions; was told not to overdo it, to drink more water and to rest. Mrs E was not sleeping well again, this time because it was difficult to get comfortable; her feet were swollen and tight. Heartburn was a regular occurrence. Scan showed twins gaining weight, so no worries. The oils selected were:
- *Chamaemelum nobile* [Roman chamomile] – calming, sedative (aids sleep), carminative, digestive
- *Citrus paradisi* [grapefruit] – digestive (indigestion), diuretic
- *Citrus limon* [lemon] – calming, carminative, digestive, diuretic (oedema)
- *Lavandula angustifolia* [lavender] – balancing, calming, cardiotonic, carminative

The blend was given for home application twice a day

Last treatment – before caesarean section booked for 2 weeks' time

Assessment

Babies have dropped so heartburn has eased. Mrs E excited but nervous. Has had medication altered to combat insulin dropping sharply after meal times. Feeling fed up and very tired!

Aim: To energize Mrs E and relieve her anxiety
- *Boswellia carteri* – energizing, immunostimulant
- *Citrus limon* [lemon] – calming, diuretic, pancreatic stimulant
- *Pelargonium graveolens* – antidiabetic, relaxant
- *Thymus vulgaris* ct. *thujanol* [sweet thyme] – hormone-like (diabetes), immunostimulant, neurotonic

Blend of essential oils alone given for inhalation at home

Final outcome – after birth

Both babies well, each being a good weight (one boy, one girl). Still in hospital, having had some trouble establishing feeding, but expressing well – and babies taking a bottle. Mrs E continues with regular treatment and also brought her babies for infant massage.

between the heel and the inner ankle is contraindicated in early pregnancy as this is the reflexology zone for the uterus (Price 1999 p. 55).

Essential oil use

A 1% dilution is recommended during all stages of pregnancy – for application, compresses and baths; it is advisable not to use the oils neat during this time, except in an emergency, such as a burn. As a woman's sense of smell can change dramatically during pregnancy (see morning sickness and Box 12.1), always involve the client in the choice of oils and blends. It would perhaps be prudent to use a seed oil such as sunflower or grapeseed in case the client has a nut allergy.

Common problems in pregnancy

Blood pressure

Blood pressure is monitored closely in pregnancy and is checked at each antenatal visit – some women may suffer from hypertension throughout their pregnancy. If pre-eclampsia (a serious condition involving oedema, high blood pressure and protein in the urine (Collin 1993 p. 278)) is present, or if the mother-to-be is already on medication for high blood

---

Box 12.1

Taste and smell in pregnancy

A report by Nordin et al. (2004) showed that abnormal taste and smell was reported by 76% of 187 pregnant women tested, typically believed to be caused by their pregnancy. Increased smell sensitivity was common during the early stages of pregnancy (67%), occasionally accompanied by qualitative smell distortions (17%) and phantom smells (14%). Smell abnormalities occurred less in the later periods of pregnancy and were virtually absent postpartum. Abnormal taste sensitivity was fairly commonly reported (26%), often described as an increase in bitter and a decrease in salt taste. The authors conclude that pregnancy smell and taste disorders relate to fetal protection mechanisms to avoid poisons and increase salt levels for the expanded fluid levels.

---

pressure, the authors do not advocate the use of aromatherapy; however, elevated blood pressure in the parameters of what is considered normal can be treated effectively with massage using hypotensive essential oils. Those reputed to lower blood pressure include: *Cananga odorata* [ylang ylang], *Citrus aurantium* var. *amara* (flos) [neroli], *Citrus limon* [lemon], *Lavandula angustifolia* [lavender] and *Melissa officinalis* [melissa].

Digestive disorders

Digestive disorders such as constipation, diarrhoea and indigestion, even if not directly connected with pregnancy, are likely to occur at some stage (see Table 4.6, which gives essential oils for all types of digestive disorder.

As massage is not appropriate for digestive problems, they are most easily relieved by taking essential oils orally – but only when prescribed by an aromatologist! Using 3 drops maximum in total, 1 drop each of two or three of the oils below should be blended with a little honey, followed by a teaspoonful of boiling water; the cup should then be half-filled with cold water; 10–15 drops each of two or more of the oils can be put into a dropper bottle for easy use.

Alternatively, should internal use not be considered advisable, 15 drops of the blended essential oils should be added to 50 mL lotion for self-application. Aromatherapists familiar with Swiss reflex treatment (see Ch. 8) can massage the whole area of the arches of the soles of the feet with the relevant oils, in a clockwise direction, to stimulate the digestive system reflex zones, especially those of the large intestine.

Constipation

The hormonal action of progesterone relaxes the digestive system, which can result in the slowing down of peristalsis. It is often made worse by high doses of iron supplements to alleviate anaemia symptoms. A diet rich in fruit and vegetables and at least 2 litres of water a day will assist defecation. Essential oils which can help constipation include *Citrus aurantium* var. *amara* per. [bitter orange], *Citrus reticulata* [mandarin], *Piper nigrum* [black pepper], *Rosmarinus officinalis* [rosemary] and *Zingiber officinale* [ginger]. *Coriandrum sativum* [coriander seed] and *Elettaria cardamomum* [cardamon] aid a sluggish digestion, which may in turn aid constipation.

Clockwise massage over the abdomen can bring relief, but would have to be very light to be comfortable in later pregnancy (see above).

Diarrhoea

Diarrhoea can be helped by the following oils (see also Table 4.6): *Citrus limon* [lemon], *Cupressus sempervirens* [cypress], *Melaleuca viridiflora* [niaouli] and *Pelargonium graveolens* [geranium].

Treatment is as above for constipation.

Heartburn

Heartburn can be relieved by inhalation, ingestion or applying a blend of oils in a carrier firmly on to the chest area. Suggested oils are *Carum carvi* [caraway], *Citrus aurantium* var. *amara* fol. [petitgrain], *Citrus aurantium* var. *amara* per. [bitter orange], *Citrus limon* [lemon], *Citrus reticulata* [mandarin], *Mentha x piperita* [peppermint] and *Origanum majorana* [marjoram].

Haemorrhoids and varicose veins

Although very different, these two conditions have been grouped together as they can be alleviated using the same essential oils. Haemorrhoids, which are sometimes protruding, often occur in pregnancy due to weight gain and/or a sluggish digestion. The changing levels of oestrogen and progesterone cause the smooth muscles of the body to soften, leading to changes in the digestive and circulatory systems, when the increase in blood volume sometimes results in varicose veins.

The client needs to reduce the amount of time spent standing and the legs should be elevated for 10 minutes every hour – or, if there is another child, for half an hour twice a day, when the child is resting or while reading a story. Exercising the feet several times a day is also beneficial.

When treating haemorrhoids, aloe vera gel makes a good base for the essential oils, which can be self-administered. Spending 10 minutes in a sitz bath with essential oils (blended first in a little honey and hot water or an emulsifier) is also useful, as is a compress. There is a wide choice of phlebotonic oils, some of which are also astringent, such as *Cupressus sempervirens* [cypress]; two or three oils together always gives an enhanced result.

Phlebotonic essential oils which help to relieve haemorrhoids and varicose veins are: *Citrus aurantium* var. *amara* flos. [neroli], *Citrus limon* [lemon] *Citrus paradisi* [grapefruit], *Cupressus sempervirens* [cypress], *Pelargonium graveolens* [geranium], *Helichrysum angustifolium* [everlasting], *Melaleuca alternifolia* [tea tree], *Melaleuca leucadendron* [cajuput], *Melaleuca viridiflora* [niaouli], *Nardostachys jatamansi* [spikenard] and *Pogostemon patchouli* [patchouli].

When treating varicose veins there are rules to follow for massage or self-application: this must always start above the affected vein in order to help clear the blood from this area up towards the heart, before encouraging the upward flow of blood from below – direct pressure over the vein itself must be avoided.

Headaches

Some women suffer from headaches in early pregnancy, sometimes due to increased blood flow leading to vasodilatation; nausea can also bring on a headache, as can stress when pregnancy nears termination and as the breasts become heavier. If severe headaches are reported in the final trimester and are accompanied by oedema and sickness, this may be an indication of hypertension or pre-eclampsia. If so, it should be reported to the midwife or consultant.

Several methods of using decongestant and relaxing essential oils can be employed to relieve headaches:

Inhalation – tipping the bottle against a finger, then rubbing this on the forehead, behind the ears or at the hairline of the back of the neck is an effective and easy method. *Mentha x piperita* [peppermint] has been shown to be effective (Göbel et al. 1994).

Massage – head, back of neck and shoulders with essential oils in a carrier.

Compress – a small compress on the places mentioned above can be a helpful addition to inhalation.

Essential oils effective for headaches are *Chamaemelum nobile* [Roman chamomile] (antispasmodic, sedative), *Eucalyptus smithii* [gully gum] (decongestant), *Lavandula angustifolia* [lavender] (calming, sedative), *Mentha x piperita* [peppermint] (analgesic, decongestant) and *Rosmarinus officinale* [rosemary] (analgesic, decongestant).

Morning sickness

Nausea and vomiting are two of the earliest symptoms of pregnancy, the degree differing from woman to woman. Some sail though pregnancy without any concerns, but approximately 50% are adversely affected, resulting in time off work, feelings of despondency, and in severe cases the need for medical intervention. The medical term for this degree of severity is hyperemesis gravidarum; it affects less than 3% of women, requiring hospital admission and intravenous fluid replacement.

Studies have shown that women who have morning sickness tend to have healthier and easier pregnancies, with lower rates of miscarriages and stillbirths, than women who have nausea-free pregnancies (Flaxman & Sherman 2000). It is not fully understood why morning sickness occurs, but there is a change in a woman's sense of smell, which pregnancy is known to heighten; feelings of nausea will exaggerate this (see Box 12.1).

The best method to combat nausea is to place 2–3 drops of the favoured oil on a tissue or cotton wool ball and inhale deeply three times. A light massage can also help, as can a bath containing 6–8 drops – swished well before entering.

Melissa officinalis [lemon balm] and *Matricaria recutita* [German chamomile] are especially effective for morning sickness.

Other digestive oils which help to combat nausea and morning sickness include *Citrus limon* (lemon), *Mentha* x *piperita* (peppermint), *Mentha spicata* (spearmint) and *Zingiber officinale* (ginger).

Ginger tea may also be helpful, as the whole herb has been shown to be statistically significant in its effectiveness in trials on expectant mothers (Bartram 1995 p.198–199).

Muscular aches and pains (e.g. backache and sciatica)

As the fetus grows the mother's body changes, causing postural changes that lead to muscular aches and pains. Often expectant mothers will have increased lumbar lordosis due to their increasing size and change in centre of gravity, which may lead to lower back pain and sometimes sciatic pain from trapped

---

Case Study 12.2

Morning sickness

Penny Price – Aromatherapist

Client assessment

Lesley suffered from nausea and sickness from very early stages of pregnancy and was offered orthodox medication in the form of antacids by her GP. These helped for only a few minutes before the feeling returned, and she was often sick afterwards. When I talked to Lesley, I found that she had a very sensitive sense of smell and so it was necessary to find aromatherapy treatments that worked but were not overly invasive in aroma.

Intervention

The following essential oils and hydrolats were chosen:
- *Citrus aurantium amara* fol [petitgrain] – uplifting, refreshing, digestive
- *Coriandrum sativum* [coriander] – digestive, anti-nausea, stomach relaxant
- *Santalum austrocaledonicum* [sandalwood] – digestive, heartburn, sedative
- *Mentha* x *piperita* [peppermint] hydrolat – digestive, antispasmodic

Petitgrain, coriander and sandalwood were blended 1% in two different bases, first, at 5%, in a heavy massage cream that was applied to the soles of Lesley's feet during a Swiss reflex treatment that her husband was going to carry on at home. After the treatment she was given a peppermint hydrolat drink.

Second, for home use, a white lotion, at 1%, was given to Lesley to apply to her solar plexus and chest as many times a day as she needed (recommended up to four times). This was to calm the stomach area and also to give a slight ongoing aroma during the day.

Finally, it was suggested that Lesley used 10 mL of peppermint hydrolat in a glass of warm water to drink 20 minutes before taking food – and if she felt sick, with a maximum of five drinks a day.

Outcome

Lesley began to improve during the first treatment, and particularly so when she took the hydrolat drink before leaving the couch to return home. Lesley reported that although she did still feel slightly nauseous during the next few days, she was able to control it and keep it minimal. She much preferred the natural approach and continued to improve. After the first 10 days of treatment the nausea had gone, although Lesley continued using the same blends throughout the pregnancy as she found they relaxed and comforted her.

nerves. Sciatica is difficult to treat, although many have benefited from applying a lotion (50 mL containing 3 drops each of the following analgesic or/ and anti-inflammatory oils) which is known to relieve muscular aches and pains: *Chamaemelum nobile* [Roman chamomile], *Mentha x piperita* [peppermint], *Myristica fragrans* [nutmeg], *Ocimum basilicum* [basil], *Pelargonium graveolens* [geranium], *Piper nigrum* [black pepper], *Zingiber officinalis* [ginger].

The same oils can be used also in a bath (6–8 drops) or in a compress.

Massage of the head, neck, shoulders, arms, hands and upper back can be helpful: back massage in particular is both psychologically and physically relaxing by altering the sense and perception of pain, thus bringing relief. (See Ch. 8 for massage positioning during pregnancy).

Analgesic and anti-inflammatory oils which help to relieve muscular aches and pains include: *Chamaemelum nobile* [Roman chamomile], *Boswellia carteri* [frankincense], *Elettaria cardamomum* [cardamom], *Matricaria recutita* [German chamomile], *Origanum majorana* [sweet marjoram], *Piper cubeba*, [cubeb] and *Zingiber officinale* [ginger].

Symphysis pubis dysfunction (SPD)

This is when the symphysis pubis, the cartilage that joins the two sections of the pubic bone, separates slightly from the bone owing to increased levels of the hormone relaxin, resulting in mild to severe pain. Some women describe the experience as their 'pelvis coming apart'. Pain is felt on making certain movements, such as turning in bed, climbing stairs etc. The pain radiates anywhere from the pubis, into the groin, the inner side of the thighs, the hips and into the buttocks.

A client who is experiencing this condition may be unable to get on and off the couch for treatment (she should be advised to keep her thighs together rather than moving first one leg then the other, as this would exacerbate the diastasis (Tiran 2005). Essential oils with analgesic properties can be used effectively in local application (see Muscular aches and pains above).

Oedema

Oedema in pregnancy, particularly of the feet and ankles, results from weight gain and the general slowing down of the blood circulation. It can be worse in hot weather or if the client has spent a long time on her feet. If sudden or extreme it should be reported to the midwife or consultant, as it may be an early sign of hypertension and in severe cases pre-eclampsia (see Headaches above).

Massage is known to relieve fluid retention in the legs and ankles, particularly if performed with long, upward strokes, always moving away from the ankle. The condition can also be helped by raising the legs, taking regular gentle exercise and keeping up fluid intake. Essential oils with diuretic properties are useful and can be applied in treatment (should be offered for local application between treatments).

Diuretic essential oils which can reduce oedema include *Angelica archangelica* [angelica root], *Citrus paradisi* [grapefruit], *Cupressus sempervirens* [cypress], *Citrus limon* [lemon], *Cedrus atlantica* [Atlas cedarwood] and *Juniperus communis* fruct. [juniper berry].

Skin problems in pregnancy

Various skin changes may occur in pregnancy, such as the appearance of acne, dry or sweaty skin, stretch marks or even changes to moles, freckles and birth marks (the latter due to an increase in the production of melanin). Local application at home can bring relief to many skin complaints.

Extreme chloasma (darkened pigmentation to the face) can make a woman feel self-conscious. *Citrus limon* [lemon] undiluted is reputed to help such a condition; essential oils having euphoric, antidepressant or sedative properties may also be of help: Citrus aurantium var. amara flos [neroli], Pelargonium graveolens [geranium], Rosa damascena [rose otto].

Acne or oily skin: this may be hormonal and often leads to distress, in which case the essential oils above may be of benefit. A diet without fatty foods combined with the use of antiseptic, anti-infectious, anti-inflammatory and/or astringent oils such as the following can help to clear the skin: *Cedrus atlantica* [Atlas cedarwood], *Citrus aurantium* var. *amara* fol. [petitgrain], *Citrus limon* [lemon], *Eucalyptus radiata* [narrow-leaved peppermint], *Melaleuca alternifolia* [tea tree], *Myrtus communis* [myrtle], *Juniperus communis* ram. [juniper branch], *Pelargonium graveolens* [geranium], *Pogostemon patchouli* [patchouli].

Itchy skin: many women suffer skin irritation (often on the abdomen) during pregnancy. Severe itchy skin in the third trimester may indicate obstetric cholestasis; this is not common but is due to a build-up of bile acids in the bloodstream and must be reported to the primary carer. Oils for irritated skin include: *Angelica archangelica* rad. [angelica root], *Chamaemelum nobile* [Roman chamomile], *Mentha x piperita* [peppermint].

Stretch marks: women always fear they will develop stretch marks; although genetics can play a role in determining whether a woman will develop them, regular use of essential oils is a great preventative. Ethnicity is also a factor, women with darker skin being less likely to get stretch marks than those with fairer skin. Stretch marks are caused by a loss of elasticity in the deeper layers of the skin and the following cicatrizant, skin-softening, cytophylactic essential oils (32 drops in total) in 25% macerated carrot oil and 75% almond oil have been proved by the editor to be successful with all clients who used the blend twice a day from the fourth month: *Boswellia carteri* [frankincense], *Cymbopogon citratus* [lemongrass], *Lavandula angustifolia* [lavender], *Pogostemon patchouli* [patchouli].

Case Study 12.3

Stretch marks

Penny Price – Aromatherapist

Assessment

Fiona, a model, was expecting her first baby. She was in her fourth month and was very concerned about possible stretch marks – this was her biggest worry!

Intervention

Both carrier and the first four essential oils were chosen for their emollient, cicatrizant (scar reducing) and/or skin softening properties, the oil mix being as follows:

- 75 mL sweet almond oil – emollient (dry skin)
- 25 mL macerated carrot oil – cicatrizant, emollient
- 8 drops each of *Boswellia carteri* [frankincense], *Lavandula angustifolia* [lavender] and *Pogostemon patchouli* [patchouli]
- 8 drops *Cymbopogon citratus* [lemongrass] – chosen for its refreshing and toning properties

Fiona was told that she must apply the oil every night and every morning without fail if she wanted a good result, and to increase the area covered as her tummy increased in size, including the tops of her thighs during the last month.

Outcome

Fiona had a baby boy weighing 7 lb 4 oz – and was delighted to report that she had not a single stretch mark!

Emotional concerns

Owing to increased hormone levels, pregnant women are prone to a range of emotional symptoms such as tearfulness, anger, elation and depression. A study carried out by Field et al. (1999) concluded that massage given during pregnancy reduces anxiety by reducing cortisol (a stress hormone) and may contribute to a lower incidence of antenatal, intranatal and postpartum complications.

Society has changed dramatically; family members are not always close, leaving some women feeling isolated and anxious. Textbooks and the media present a rosy view of the experience to come, but many women feel a loss of their identity, are fearful of a change in their financial situation and have very little knowledge or experience of being around newborn infants. Aromatherapy and massage at this time can alleviate some of the anxieties and concerns that women go through in the lead-up to labour. Symptoms presented at treatment may be insomnia, mood swings or general fear of the unknown.

Essential oils which may help emotional symptoms are: *Mood swings*: Balancing essential oils and those which are uplifting and calming are a good choice: *Citrus aurantium* var. *amara* fol. [petitgrain], *Citrus aurantium* var. *amara* [bitter orange], *Citrus reticulata* [mandarin] *Commiphora myrrha* [myrrh] *Lavandula angustifolia* [lavender], *Lavandula x intermedia* [lavandin], *Pelargonium graveolens* [geranium], *Santalum album* [sandalwood].

Oils can also be chosen for the properties below:

Euphoric: *Citrus aurantium* var. *amara* (flos) [neroli], *Cedrus atlanticus* [Atlas cedarwood], *Rosa damascena* [rose otto].

Antidepressant: *Citrus aurantium* var. *amara* (flos) [neroli], *Citrus bergamia* [bergamot], *Citrus sinensis* [sweet orange], *Citrus reticulata* [mandarin], *Citrus aurantium* var. *amara* (fol) [petitgrain] *Pelargonium graveolens* [geranium], *Rosa damascena* [rose otto], *Santalum album* [sandalwood].

Refreshing/stimulating: *Citrus limon* [lemon], *Citrus paradise* [grapefruit], *Citrus bergamia* [bergamot], *Boswellia carteri* [frankincense].

Grounding/strengthening: *Boswellia carteri* [frankincense], *Cedrus atlantica* [Atlas cedarwood], *Cedrus deodar* [Deodar], *Santalum album* [sandalwood], *Zingiber cassumunar* [plai].

Sedative/calming: *Lavandula angustifolia* [lavender], *Nardostachys jatamansi* [spikenard], *Origanum majorana* [marjoram], *Vetiveria zizanioides* [vetiver].

Miscarriage and stillbirth

Only about a quarter of all conceptions culminate in the birth of a live child – obvious recognized miscarriages occur in approx 15% of all pregnancies. These statistics do not lessen the blow to the individual, but show how common miscarriages are.

- A pregnancy that ends spontaneously before the 28th week of pregnancy is termed a miscarriage or a spontaneous abortion.
- Stillbirth is the term used if a baby is born dead any time after the 28th week of pregnancy up to full term.
- Neonatal death is when the baby dies in the first 4 weeks of life.

These occurrences affect the mother and father in many ways and counselling is often offered. A client suffering any of the above may return to the aromatherapist for help to cope with the loss. Essential oils for grief and loss include: *Citrus aurantium var. amara* (fol) [petitgrain], *Citrus aurantium var. amara* (flos) [neroli], *Cupressus sempervirens* [cypress], *Melissa officinalis* [melissa], *Nardostachys jatamansi* [spikenard] and *Rosa damascena* [rose otto].

Massage at this time is most effective, but whether or not the treatment should include an abdominal massage depends on the client's individual feelings about touch on this area – a gentle placing of hands could bring some sense of comfort.

Aromatherapy for labour

Preparation for labour

Towards the end of pregnancy, during the last 6 weeks, essential oils can be used to prepare the uterus for labour. Adding 3 drops of *Rosa damascena* [rose otto] to the stretch mark mix helps the uterus to gain tone and strength.

Perineal management

Aromatherapy can be used to reduce the perineal trauma and discomfort that may result from childbirth. Perineal management is becoming part of the midwife's role; it is not uncommon for women to experience some extent of perineal trauma in childbirth, especially those having their first baby, a trial

Table 12.1 Essential oils to help with labour

Essential oil	Properties
Boswellia carteri [frankincense]	Circulatory stimulant, respiratory tonic, helpful for anxiety and nervous tension
Chamaemelum nobile [Roman chamomile]	Analgesic, antispasmodic, helpful for anxiety, shock and nervousness
Chamomilla recutita [German chamomile]	Analgesic, helpful for anxiety, fear and tension
Citrus aurantium var. *amara* (flos) [neroli]	Antispasmodic, helpful for anxiety, exhaustion, stress and shock
Citrus limon [lemon]	Refreshing, cleansing, helpful for anxiety and dark moods
Citrus sinensis [sweet orange]	Hypotensive, antispasmodic, helpful for anxiety, depression and has the ability to 'bring sunshine to a situation'
Commiphora myrrha [myrrh]	Uterine tonic, emotionally warming
Cymbopogen martinii [palmarosa]	Tonic, cooling and refreshing – helpful for a summer labour

having been carried out in 2000 (Labrecque et al. 2000). To help prepare the perineal muscles to expand, the mother-to-be can moisten two fingers with her stretch mark oil mix and place them inside the vulva to stretch the space by moving the fingers in a circular fashion; this should be done every day. Having an intact perineum and preventing tears and other damage saves the midwife from having to suture the perineum after the birth.(see Table 12.1).

Also during the last 6 weeks uterotonic essential oils such as aniseed and fennel are useful in order to facilitate delivery (Franchomme & Penoel 2001 p. 382, 416). Drinking sage tea during this time is also helpful; Bernadet (1983 p. 120) recommends a tea made with sage leaves, but an alternative is to make a tea by putting two drops of *Salvia officinalis* [sage] essential oil on a tea bag (preferably tannin free) and adding hot water.

Commencement of labour

As soon as the first signs of labour appear, the client's partner can apply the following blend to her back, in between contractions; the feet can also be massaged with the same blend: *Chamaemelum nobile* [Roman chamomile], *Citrus reticulata* [mandarin] and *Santalum album* [sandalwood] in a carrier oil.

A 'must' in the labour ward is a ball of cotton wool with several drops of *Salvia sclarea* [clary sage]; this should be kept in the palm of the hand and really deep breaths taken from it each time a contraction begins – the relaxing benefits are enormous.

A woman hoping to labour in a birthing pool will not be allowed to use essential oils in the water during the second stage because of the risk of the baby ingesting them, but a blend may be used in a bath prior to this, which is an effective way to reduce pain and worry. Most labours involve a certain degree of pain, and if the client wishes to take those essential oils into the labour suite it would be prudent to include some with analgesic properties.

If the therapist has permission to attend, blends can be administered at the client's request. Some women prefer to use the oils themselves and/or ask their birthing partner to administer them; either way, they can be of benefit.

Massage and touch can be very soothing for labouring women, and firm deep pressure is often requested by the women over the sacrum area, while lying on their side. Massage to certain areas may be restricted because of medical interventions, e.g. an epidural, or the fact that the woman may be supine on the bed.

Citrus oils are light and fresh and are beneficial in the labour suite, an effective method being to inhale the chosen oil or oils from a tissue or cotton wool ball as above. Essential oil burners with a naked flame are not allowed in hospitals for obvious reasons, and an

---

Box 12.2

Lavender baths during labour (Reed & Norfolk 1993)

This trial was carried out by Reed and Norfolk (1993), with the support of the Director of Midwifery Services at Ipswich Hospital – using her practical procedures.

Purpose of trial

19 primigravidae and 19 multigravidae clients took part in a trial to determine whether pain relief and relaxation could be achieved without adverse side effects, using 5 drops of lavender (unspecified) in the bath.

Results from questionnaires

Apgar scores

- 3 women scored 10
- 30 scored 8 or 9
- 2 scored 7 (pethidine given – 150 g and 250 g, respectively)
- 1 scored 6 (stale meconium present)
- 2 did not have their score recorded

Deliveries

- 34 of the 38 clients achieved a normal delivery
- 2 had forceps
- 1 LSCS (failure to progress)
- 1 had ventouse extraction

Additional pain relief given

- 18 out of the 19 primigravidae
- 12 out of the 19 multigravidae

Length of labour:

- 8 multigravidae: up to 8 hours
- 5 multigravidae: up to 5 hours
- 2 multigravidae and 8 primigravidae: up to 6 hours
- 4 primigravidae: under 10 hours
- 2 multigravidae: 7–13 hours
- 5 primigravidae: 14–22 hours

Perceived benefits

- 31 of the clients felt they had benefited from the relaxation effects (2 negative, 5 did not reply)
- 23 clients felt that the baths had given pain relief (7 negative, 8 did not reply)
- 30 clients had enjoyed the experience (1 negative, 7 did not reply)

Conclusion

The good Apgar scores would suggest that 5 drops of lavender in baths present no risks to the baby.

Although it was not possible to assess whether or not labour was shortened by the lavender baths, labour in some clients appeared to progress very rapidly. Progress was better in those clients who:

- used the lavender bath when a 2+ or more dilation was established
- spent more than 30 minutes in the bath.

Case Study 12.4

Postnatal treatment after stitches

Jo Kellett – Aromatherapist

Assessment

Ms K (33) had a long, slow first labour. The baby presented occipitoposterior (spine to spine) and pethidine was given, with eventual assisted delivery using episiotomy and ventouse. Stitches were administered.

Intervention

The treatment was by self-administered essential oils.

On postpartum day 2 Mrs K used the following essential oils in a sitz bath twice a day to assist healing from the episiotomy:

- 2 drops of *Lavandula angustifolia* – analgesic, antibacterial, anti-inflammatory, cicatrizant
- 2 drops of *Cupressus sempervirens* [cypress] – antibacterial, anti-infectious, phlebotonic

She continued to do this for approximately 5 days, after which she had one sitz bath daily until day 10.

Outcome

On day 3 Mrs Ks midwife commented on the extreme change to the whole genital area, noting how rapidly it was healing; there was also a huge reduction in discomfort. Mrs K was able to sit comfortably and was able to pass a stool by day 5 without anxiety or pain.

---

electric vaporizer must be checked by the hospital electrician. For essential oils and their properties useful for labour see Table 12.1.

Postnatal care

With the birth of a baby many physical and emotional changes can occur and aromatherapy can be of help.

As soon as possible after the birth, women who have suffered perineal tears may benefit from a sitz bath containing *Lavandula angustifolia* [lavender] and *Cupressus sempervirens* [cypress] to assist healing. Even without tearing the perineal and vulval areas will be bruised and stretched. Application can be repeated twice a day until healing has taken place (see Case Study 12.4). The blend will also benefit if haemorrhoids are present, when again they should be used in a sitz bath. Parents and babies are assisted in the early days of parenthood by midwives, GPs and health visitors, with various tests and aftercare advice

being given. At about 6 weeks postpartum mother and infant have a postnatal check, which includes physical examination and a chance to air any concerns.

Breast care

When essential oils are used for breast care whilst breastfeeding, they should only be applied *immediately after* feeding – never just before; this gives the oils time to be thoroughly absorbed, leaving none for the baby to ingest at feeding time.

Mastitis

Infection of the breast tissue is usually compounded by tiredness and the infant not latching on to the nipple efficiently; symptoms include tenderness, redness and occasionally lumpiness. Over 50% of mothers who have mastitis experience 'flu-like' symptoms, and if the mother is given a course of antibiotics, this may affect the composition of the milk. A compress using essential oils can be helpful alongside the orthodox treatment. The signs are often a tingly feeling in the breast and acute discomfort on feeding. Anti-inflammatory essential oils can be used as a preventative and applied via a compress at the initial sign of inflammation or infection.

The following oils can be applied as a blend alongside antibiotics to help the healing process: *Lavandula angustifolia* [lavender], *Pelargonium graveolens* [geranium], *Chamaemelum nobile* [Roman chamomile].

Lack or insufficiency of milk

A woman's ability to produce enough milk for her infant may be hindered by stress levels, her state of tiredness and her dietary intake. Assurance and the application of lactogenic essential oils can be beneficial. The safest essential oil to increase milk flow is: *Foeniculum vulgare var. dulce* [fennel].

Stimulating the pituitary gland reflex by massaging the centre of each big toe with Swiss reflex cream containing fennel oil could also be of help.

It was once thought that *Jasminum grandiflorum* [jasmine] (an absolute, not an essential oil) acted as a galactogogue until evidence showed the reverse – it actually works as a suppressant (Shrivastav et al. 1988).

Involution of the uterus – afterpains

As the uterus is returning to its original size, cramp can sometimes be felt in the lower abdomen; although breastfeeding encourages the uterus to shrink, the cramps are often stronger while the baby is at the breast. A blend containing the analgesic and antispasmodic essential oils below applied to the lower abdomen can help reduce the pain: *Zingiber cassumunar* [plai] – used traditionally in Thailand for many generations, massaged into the mother's abdomen directly after the birth *Matricaria recutita* [German chamomile] *Eucalyptus citriodora* [lemon-scented gum].

Confidence

Aromatherapy can offer valuable postnatal support to women who live at a distance from their immediate family and who feel isolated with the arrival of the baby. To encourage confidence and give support, the following essential oils have been chosen, as they are balancing, energizing, relaxing, tonic or/and uplifting: *Boswellia carteri* [frankincense], *Citrus aurantium* var. *amara* [neroli], *Citrus bergamia* [bergamot], *Cananga odorata* [ylang ylang], *Ocimum basilicum* [basil], *Pelargonium graveolens* [geranium], *Origanum majorana* [sweet marjoram], *Rosa damascena* [rose otto], *Thymus vulgaris* ct. geraniol, ct. linalool [sweet thyme].

Postnatal depression

After giving birth, approximately eight out of ten new mothers experience 'baby blues', which are different from postnatal depression. They usually occur 3–4 days after the birth, when the colostrum (the thin, yellow fluid that the mammary glands secrete before the normal breast milk) is changing to normal breast milk. There is a huge swing in hormone levels at this time and women may feel tearful, anxious or mildly depressed. Fortunately this usually lasts a few days only.

Postnatal depression may affect around one in every ten women and is much more serious. It usually occurs during the first 6 months, but can occur at any time during the first year. It generates a deep feeling of hopelessness and inability to perform even the simplest task, leaving women exhausted, angry and bewildered. It is only when they are obviously unable to cope that medical intervention occurs. The use of essential oils to treat depression is well known, and aromatherapists have a selection of euphoric, antidepressant, strengthening and uplifting oils to draw upon: *Boswellia carteri* [frankincense], *Cananga odorata* var. *genuina* [ylang ylang], *Citrus aurantium* var. *amara* [neroli] (aids fatigue, sleep and nervous system imbalance), *Citrus bergamia* [bergamot], *Citrus paradisi* [grapefruit] (relieves exhaustion), *Origanum majorana*, *Pelargonium graveolens* [geranium] (also relaxing, relieving anxiety and nervous fatigue), *Rosa damascena* [rose otto], *Thymus vulgaris* ct. geraniol, ct. linalool [sweet thyme] (also uterotonic).

Aromatherapy for infants

According to Field (1995), massage has been shown to have a variety of very positive effects on both full-term and preterm babies. Many societies use massage daily as part of a baby's routine, and the addition of essential oils can enhance this if used correctly. A blend of 0.25% is recommended for infants up to 1 year old, increasing to 0.5% for those between 1 and 2, after which a 1% blend is suitable.

Among the mild essential oils suitable for babies – and the favourites – are: *Chamaemelum nobile* [Roman chamomile] and *Lavandula angustifolia* [lavender]

as they can be used for a variety of infant complaints. Other oils may be added to help the following complaints:

Colic, fever or raised temperature, insomnia, nappy rash and undue crying (stress): *Citrus sinensis* per. [sweet orange] can be added for colic and insomnia.

Santalum album [sandalwood] is a helpful addition for undue crying and nappy rash. **Coughs/colds can be helped by two effective anti-infectious and expectorant oils:**

Eucalyptus smithii [gully gum] and *Myrtus communis* [myrtle].

Cradle cap is a type of seborrhoeic eczema and can be a worrying problem in small babies. A mild shampoo (very little!) should be used on the baby's scalp and hair then rinsed off thoroughly. It is easier to treat successfully as soon as the scaling is noticed. One drop each of the following essential oils should be blended into 10 mL grapeseed oil and massaged gently into the scalp at night after washing the hair. Leave overnight – the scales should be rubbed off gently the next morning while re-washing the baby's hair (Price & Price 2005 p. 96–97).

Cedrus atlantica [cedarwood], *Pogostemon patchouli* [patchouli], *Santalum album* [sandalwood].

Summary

Aromatherapy can be used safely to benefit and enhance a woman's health and wellbeing during the whole of her pregnancy and her early days as a mother. The transition from adult to parent is huge. In a society that often undervalues the importance of parenthood, massage and the application of essential oils can bring confidence, care and support to women and their partners at this critical and wonderful time.

References

Ager, C., 2002. A complementary therapy clinic: makin it work. RCM Midwives' J. 5 (6), 198–200.

Balacs, T., 1992. Safety in pregnancy. Int. J. Aromather. 4 (1), 12–15.

Bartram, T.H., 1995. Encyclopaedia of herbal medicine. Grace, Christchurch.

Bernadet, M., 1983. La phyto-aromathérapie pratique. Dangles, St-Jean-de-Braye, p. 120.

Collin, P.H., 1993. Dictionary of medicine. Peter Collins, Teddington.

Field, T., 1995. Massage Therapy for infants and children. J. Dev. Behav. Pediatr. 16 105–111.

Field, T., Hernandez-Reif, S., Hart, Theakston, H., 1999. Pregnant women benefit from massage therapy. J. Psychosom. Obstet. Gynaecol. 19.

Flaxman, S.M., Sherman, P.W., 2000. Morning sickness: a mechanism for protecting mother and embryo. Q. Rev. Biol. 75 (2), 113–148.

Franchomme, P., Pénoël, D., 2001. L'aromathérapie exactement. Jollois, Limoges.

Göbel, H., Schmidt, G., Soyka, D., 1994. Effect of peppermint and eucalyptus oil preparations on neurophysiological and experimental algesimetric headache parameters. Cephalalgia 14, 228–234.

Gunn, J.W.C., 1921. The action of the emmenagogue oils on the human uterus. J. Pharmacol. Exp. Ther. 16, 485–489.

Labrecque, M., Eason, E., Marcoux, S., 2000. Randomised trial of perineal massage during pregnancy. Am. J. Obstet. Gynaecol. 180 (3 Pt 1), 593–600.

Naganuma, M., Hirose, S., Nakayama, Y., et al., 1985. A study of the phototoxicity of lemon oil. Arch. Dermatol. Res. 278 (1) 31–36.

Nordin, S., et al., 2004. A longitudinal descriptive study of self-reported abnormal smell and taste perception in pregnant women. Chem. Senses 29 391–402.

Nursing & Midwifery Council, 2002a. Midwives' rules and code of practice. NMC, London.

Nursing & Midwifery Council, 2002b. Scope of professional practice. NMC, London.

O'Hara, C., 2002. Challenging the rules of reflexology. In: Mackereth, P., Tiran, D. (Eds.), Clinical reflexology: a guide for health professionals. Elsevier, Edinburgh, pp. 33–52.

Price, S., 1999. Practical aromatherapy, fourth ed. Thorsons, London.

Price, S., Price, P., 2005. Aromatherapy for babies and children. Riverhead, Stratford-on-Avon, p. 55.

Reed, L., Norfolk, L., 1993. Aromatherapy in midwifery. Aromatherapy World (Nurturing, Summer issue), 12–15.

Shrivastav, P., George, K., Balasubramaniam, N., Jasper, M.P., Thomas, M., Kanagasabhapathy, A.S., 1988. Suppression of puerperal lactation using jasmine flowers (Jasminum sambac). Aust. N. Z. J. Obstet. Gynaecol. 28 (1) 68–71.

Tiran, D., 2000. Clinical aromatherapy for pregnancy and childbirth. Churchill Livingstone, Edinburgh, p. 13.

Tiran, D., 2005. Using aromatherapy in pregnancy and labour. Expectancy, London, p. 275.

Tisserand, R., Balacs, T., 1995. Essential oil safety: a guide for health care professionals. Churchill Livingstone, Edinburgh.

Learning difficulties and autism

13

Julia Fearon   Louise Anderson

CHAPTER CONTENTS

Introduction

Although the term learning disability is widely used, people who are themselves affected prefer the term 'learning difficulty' (Northfield 2004, DoH 2001), but this change in terminology has yet to be widely adopted, as can be seen from the quotes and references used throughout this chapter.

Currently there are over 1.5 million people in the UK with diagnosis of a learning disability (Mencap 2010a). Statistically it is difficult to ascertain the number of people affected by autistic spectrum disorder (ASD) in the UK due to lack of data, but it is thought to be about 1% of the population, both children and adults (Brugha et al. 2009, Green et al. 2005). Comparable figures for the USA estimate that 1 in 110 children have a diagnosis of ASD, a prevalence of 1% (Centers for Disease Control Prevention, 2007).

Types of learning and behavioural disorder

Learning difficulties

Learning disability is not a mental illness (Mencap 2010b). This term can cover a broad range of disabilities or difficulties with which a person may present (BILD 2007). Founded on the belief that people with learning difficulties are people first, learning difficulty can be defined as a significantly reduced ability to understand new or complex information or to learn new skills (impaired intelligence), with a reduced ability to cope independently (impaired social functioning) and which started before adulthood with a lasting effect on development (Department of Health (DH) DoH 2001).

People with learning difficulties have poorer health and are more likely to die prematurely than the rest of the population (DH DoH 2008). Health-related conditions that may coexist with the diagnosis of learning disability include Down's syndrome (a lifelong genetic disorder that causes delays in development and learning (Mills 2007)), cerebral palsy, epilepsy, autism and Asperger syndrome (Mencap 2010c).

Asperger syndrome

The National Autistic Society (NAS) 2009a explains Asperger syndrome (AS) as a form of autism (see below). Although there are similarities with autism, people with Asperger syndrome have fewer problems with speaking and are often of average, or above average, intelligence. They do not usually have the accompanying learning disabilities associated with autism, but may have specific learning difficulties including dyslexia and dyspraxia, or other conditions such as attention deficit hyperactivity disorder (ADHD) and epilepsy. People with AS can find it harder to read signals such as facial expressions and body language which most of us take for granted. Thus they find it more difficult to communicate and interact with others, which can lead to high levels of anxiety and confusion, frustration, anger, depression and a lack of self-esteem.

Autism (ASD)

Autism is a lifelong developmental disorder characterized by impaired social interaction and communication, severely restricted interests and highly repetitive behaviour (Brugha et al. 2009). 'Spectrum disorders' is the collective term used, as the symptoms can present with varying degrees of severity (Autism Society of America 2006). Further classifications used are high-functioning autism, low-functioning autism, mild, moderate, severe and autistic traits or tendencies (Bogdashina 2006).

Autism can also occur in association with other conditions such as metabolic disturbances, epilepsy, visual or hearing impairments, Down's syndrome, dyslexia, cerebral palsy, attention deficient disorder and ADHD (Bogdashina 2006). Other health problems that may be experienced by children with autism include sleep problems, eating difficulties, bowel problems, and difficulties developing motor skills such as holding a pencil (NAS 2009b).

Some people with autism have severe learning disabilities, and some are non-verbal. They may also have abnormal sensory perceptions, for example being hypo- or hypersensitive to tastes, smells and sounds (NAS 2009c, Royal College of Psychiatrists 2004), each altered perception possibly fluctuating between hypo- and hypersensitivity (Autism & Practice Group (APG) 2007).

However, some people with autistic tendencies are very high achievers and their oddness may show up only in their preference for being alone, lack of empathy and single-minded pursuit of their

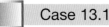

Case 13.1

Introducing touch

L Anderson – Aromatherapist

Assessment

Michael, aged 60, is non-verbal with mild to moderate learning difficulties and challenging behaviour which could involve attacking other people and throwing things and furniture. He was learning to adapt from having spent 30 years in an institution before coming to the group home.

Intervention

The first month of meeting was spent walking outside together for him to get used to the therapist. Initial sessions were only 15 minutes long, with limited eye contact, as he did not like this. Gentle, relaxing strokes were used on his feet, avoiding any sudden movements. Gradually his hands were touched to introduce closer contact. After another month, sessions up to 30 minutes and occasional eye contact were possible.

The following sedative essential oils were used one at a time in 1% dilution:
- *Boswellia carteri* [Frankincense], [Roman chamomile], *Citrus reticulate* [mandarin].
- Later, *Melaleuca alternifolia* [tea tree] and *Lavandula angustifolia* [lavender] (also sedative) were used, for their antiseptic and bactericide effects.

Outcome

By about the third month, Michael had started to smile and could take off his shoes and socks. He giggled and chattered, sometimes touching the therapist's hand spontaneously and occasionally vocalizing a hello-like sound.

own interests (Wing 1997). Many very successful academics are thought to fall into this category (Carter 1998).

Altered sensory perception in autism

Touching, tasting and smelling – everyday experiences – inform us about the world we live in, each experience leading on to the next, assisting in learning and development. Those with autism may not be able to process the information in the same way, leading to 'abnormal' behaviour as the affected individual struggles to cope with altered perceptions (Table 13.1).

People with autism might display what are known as autistic traits, e.g. rocking, flapping hands, or

Table 13.1 Examples of behaviours that might result from the altered sensory perception of autism

Hypersensitivity	Hyposensitivity
Dislikes dark and bright lights	Moves fingers or objects in front of the eyes
Looks at minute particles, picks up smallest pieces of dust	Fascinated with reflections, brightly coloured objects
Covers ears	Makes loud, rhythmic noises
Dislikes having hair cut	Likes vibration
Resists touch	
Avoids people	

(Autism and Practice Group 2007, Sensory Issues in Autism, p. 8)

pressing fists into their eyes when experiencing a hypersensitive reaction to a sensory stimulus. This is because they are trying to induce different sensations in an attempt to block out the pain or calm themselves down. When autism causes hyposensitive sensory perception, the affected individual might bang objects/doors, seek out noises such as the vacuum cleaner, prefer tight clothing or self-injure in an attempt to cause sensations to help their brain get more information from the outside world. Aromas can be overpowering, so can background noise, and touch can be excruciating;

> 'I was frightened of the vacuum cleaner, the food mixer and the liquidizer because they sounded about five times as loud as they actually were.'
>
> (White 2007, cited in APG 2007, p6.)

Contending with smell, noise and touch can cause a person to go into hypersensitive overload, leading to sensory shutdown (APG 2007). Although aromatherapy might not seem to be the obvious therapy choice for anyone with ASD, when used with discernment and care by a responsible, professional therapist, it can provide valuable support.

Consent

The Disability Discrimination Act (2005) and Mental Capacity Act (2005) highlighted the health requirements of people with a learning disability or autism. It should never be assumed that people cannot make their own decisions, simply because of their problem (DoH 2003), and consent – where the person is able to give it – should be sought before commencing an aromatherapy intervention.

Children 16 years or older and competent to do so, or under 16 years and deemed 'Gillick' competent, can legally consent to their own treatment (DoH 2009). Gillick competence is a term used in medical law to decide whether children under 16 are able to consent to their own medical treatment without parental permission or knowledge (Wikipedia 2010). Those with parental responsibility may consent to treatment for those under 16 (DoH 2009). Written consent is not always necessary, but the therapist should always record what consent was given and by whom.

Particular care should be taken to ensure that children and adults with learning difficulties or autism are given every opportunity to communicate their needs, wishes and feelings regarding care and treatment.

If an adult is not competent to consent, then the relatives/carer/key worker should be involved in the decision – when the treatment is in the client's best interest, it is lawfully possible to provide it (DoH 2009).

Validity of aromatherapy and essential oil use

Although there is little research evidence, there is a consensus of opinion that aromatherapy has a positive effect. The individual parts of an aromatherapy treatment – the relationship between client and therapist, touch/massage, essential/carrier oils and olfaction – can each provide support, and the synergistic effect of the whole package can produce significant physical and psychological benefits. Research has revealed that aromatherapy can have profound effects on the mind by affecting the autonomic level of the cognitive part of the brain (see Ch. 7); this can be seen in a study with older adults, linking postural stability to the olfactory system, where some changes in stability were noted (Freeman et al. 2009 (see Box 13.1, Broughan 2005; also Ch. 7).

Essential oils can have powerful effects on the body and the nervous system, evoking memories, changing human perception, altering behaviour, reducing aggression and agitation, improving communication and activating cognitive responses (Buck 2007, Cook 2008, Ouldred & Bryant 2008), and it is important that unadulterated essential oils are used for the best therapeutic effect and to avoid the risk of adverse reactions.

The choice of oils and their mode of use should be decided upon as for any other client, but with special attention to the complexity of the individual's

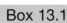

Box 13.1

Olfactory stimuli and enhanced postural stability in older adults (Freeman et al. 2009)

This study tested the effect of olfactory stimuli on the postural stability of 17 older adults. The subjects were randomly exposed to the odour of *Lavandula angustifolia* [lavender] or *Piper nigrum* [black pepper] or the sham (distilled water) while standing with feet slightly apart on a force plate which measured movement of the body's centre of pressure. The odour was presented to the subject on a spill which had been dipped in one of the oils or the water and held a few centimetres from, but not touching, the right nostril. They stood for 1 minute with eyes open, looking straight ahead with the odour stimulus, then a 2-minute break during which they sat and relaxed. The spill was re-dipped in the oil or water and presented again for 1 minute, during which time the subjects were asked to stand on the force plate with eyes closed. Subjects also underwent the same protocol with no odour exposure. The study found that with eyes closed, olfactory stimulation with either *Lavandula angustifolia* or *Piper nigrum* significantly reduced the velocity of postural adjustment, suggesting that olfactory stimulation may improve postural stability in older adults.

particular needs, bearing in mind known and potential medical conditions, including acknowledged contraindications to existing drug regimens and possible side effects.

Touch and communication

Touch is a vital sense and a valuable form of communication, and is a significant aspect of our daily lives. The deprivation of touch between parents/carers and the child/adult with learning difficulty/ASD can have dramatic impacts on the development of bonding and relationships.

Herbert (2002) states that touch is one of the first senses to develop – within the first 8 weeks of fetal life. It is related to both physiological and psychological development, and children who are deprived of loving touch can develop serious emotional and psychological disturbances (Blackwell 2000, Field 2002a, b). For people with learning difficulties and ASD experiences and perception of touch are often very different from those unaffected by these

disorders. Touch may frequently be functional rather than loving, e.g. the touch they feel is related to personal care: washing, dressing, being fed, being moved in and out of a wheelchair or bed.

Individuals with ASD often have a distorted perception of touch.

'Light touch feels like a cattle prod'

(Grandin 2007, cited in APG p7)

The impaired touch communication experienced by some can cause difficulties both for the affected individual and their relatives/carers. Parents of children with autism describe their distress and 'hurt' in response to the 'aloof' nature of the child, where natural parenting instincts such as spontaneous cuddling are limited (Cullen & Barlow 2002).

Where a person is not able to communicate verbally or to understand facial expressions or body language, it is clearly difficult to obtain an accurate understanding of his/her feelings or response to touch (Baron-Cohen, 2004). However, aromatherapy with massage has been said to promote more effective communication with this client group (Armstrong & Heidingsfeld 2000, Cullen & Barlow 2002, Thompson 2002 – see Case 13.2).

Case 13.2

Agitation (Armstrong and Heidingsfeld 2000)

Assessment

Kate is aged 35 with autism. She self-mutilates, rocks and head-bangs when unhappy or frustrated.

Intervention

Initially, gentle hand massage was given, avoiding eye contact. At the third visit, sedative essential oils – *Lavandula angustifolia* and *Citrus bergamia* [bergamot] – were introduced by holding each aroma to her nose on a spill, and Kate was encouraged to demonstrate a preference. She showed her choice by pointing with quick finger movements at one of the spills. Over several months, more oils were introduced – *Pelargonium graveolens* [geranium] (relaxing) and *Citrus aurantium var. sinensis* [sweet orange] (calming); up to three oils of her choice were included at each treatment.

Outcome

Gradually over several months Kate allowed more areas of her body to be massaged. She becomes calm and serene during treatments, but is agitated at the start and aromatherapy is viewed by her carers as a valuable support for Kate.

Some clients with autism may prefer deeper massage pressure, as this can help block out unwanted external stimuli that may cause a hypersensitivity overload (Ellwood 2002). Conversely, some clients with learning difficulties prefer simple effleurage and stroking techniques (Anderson 2008). Whichever form is preferred, careful use of touch and massage with essential oils can help develop trust and build up tolerance to touch (Armstrong & Heidingsfeld 2000, Cullen & Barlow 2002).

Developing the aromatherapy treatment

It may be inappropriate at first to treat a client with a full body aromatherapy massage; often this is unlikely ever to be suitable, but inhalation of essential oils can be beneficial. It is best to take a considered approach, introducing single components of aromatherapy one at a time to reduce the risk of inducing fear or over-sensitization.

Introducing essential oils

Initially spend time just getting to know each other. Each time you meet, offer a spill with a drop of essential oil on it, using the same oil for the first two or three visits – preferably one with a gentle aroma. Discover whether the client has any physical problems that might be helped by essential oils, and select your gentle oil from there – the aim is to find an aroma which is acceptable to the client. It is important to allow the client the opportunity to express a preference for one essential oil – or blend – over another, as it enables him/her to exercise personal choice and independence, thereby enhancing the end result. Having selected the essential oils most helpful to the person concerned, the way in which these are presented is of great importance. Always offer aromas one at a time – never more than three in one session, noting any reaction carefully. Those preferred by the client can also be vaporized. Armstrong and Heidingsfeld (2000) used aromatherapy bubble baths, flower waters and creams for many months with a deaf/blind client for her enjoyment and to enhance her femininity, before progressing onto any form of massage.

A blend can be used once each individual oil has been approved – it will be a new aroma to be experienced.

Possible reactions to note

- Did the client reach out for the hand holding the aroma?
- Did the client's hand push it away?
- Was his/her head averted?
- Did the client come closer?

Introducing touch and massage

These should be introduced gradually to accustom the client to the sensation of oil on skin. The client's favourite essential oil should be used in a carrier oil for the first contact. The hands are usually the best place to start, as these are easily accessible without causing a great deal of stress. To be able to hold and gently stroke a hand may take more than one visit, after which 5–10 minutes' massage of the hands may be as much as a client can tolerate at first. The treatment should not be lengthy, as it may be counterproductive if the client's attention starts to wander or he/she becomes frustrated. Once touch is accepted, a blend of two or three essential oils can be introduced, when the synergy enhances the treatment.

After a simple hand massage has been accepted, the lower arm could be included, but it is important not to force the pace, even if progress seems slow. Some clients will find the feet and lower legs less threatening than hands and arms, as the therapist will not be in such close proximity.

As one of the aims of treatment is to relax and calm the client, music could enhance the aromatherapy experience; singing nursery rhymes, especially with children, may help increase enjoyment of the session.

People with learning difficulties and autism often favour regular routines, so where possible, visits should be made at the same time and day of the week, in the same environment and with the same music (if enjoyed). Wearing the same clothes and having a drop of the client's favourite oil on your wrist is equally helpful.

The preferred essential oils and music can also be used by the client between sessions. Olfaction is powerfully linked to memory and can be really useful to help a client evoke memories of the calm experienced during a therapy session if they should become agitated, stressed or distressed between sessions.

Case 13.3

Social interaction and positive touch

Louise Anderson – Aromatherapist

Assessment

P. is a 60-year-old man who has Down's syndrome – a genetic abnormality that causes physical and intellectual impairments. He has good verbal communication and understanding; enjoys interacting with others but sometimes finds this difficult, isolating himself from others in the house. He lives in a housing association care home with five other individuals and various care staff who provide 24-hour care and support. He has his own room, in which he spends a lot of time on his own.

Intervention

P enjoys massage on his legs and feet using a base with 1% of *Lavandula angustifolia* [lavender] for its pleasant aroma and its antiseptic, antiviral, bactericide and carminative properties. He does not like other strong smells and asks only for this. The massage consists mainly of gentle effleurage and can last up to 30 minutes, on a

weekly basis. P likes the therapist to follow the same routine, finding it really difficult if something is changed. He does not like change – this can lead to him becoming upset, when he may challenge verbally and walk off. He likes to sit in the lounge with the other residents in the same place each week. He will engage with the therapist, talking and telling them about the activities he has done during the week.

Outcome

The treatment provides P with positive touch and one-to-one time; at the end of each session he will hug and thank the therapist. He appears to find this comforting and is very settled and relaxed after the session, staying with the rest of the residents for the remainder of the evening. Staff comment on how much more relaxed and calm he is after the sessions.

Disturbances during treatment should be kept to a minimum (sometimes difficult in a group setting), and staff and residents should be informed when therapy is about to take place.

Essential oil choice

As with any client, a full medical history must be obtained and recorded, including any medication used and any precautions or contraindications concerning current medications and treatments. Epilepsy (and therefore antiepileptic medication) is more common in people with a learning disability than among the general population (Searson 2008). Although there is little evidence to suggest that antipsychotic medication is effective for the challenging behaviour of people with learning difficulties (Benson & Brooks 2008), unfortunately many individuals will be receiving it. These medications have implications in the choice of essential oils – some antipsychotics may be photosensitizing and some medications to reduce anxiety may lower blood pressure; however, there is no evidence to demonstrate that any essential oil used in aromatherapy has ever induced a seizure. Hyssop may be the only oil prudent to avoid, although it would not in any case be used when treating people with autism or learning difficulties (see Table 13.2).

Table 13.2 Oils high in phenols, aldehydes and ketones – avoid or use with caution

Phenols	*Cinnamomum verum* fol. [cinnamon leaf] *Foeniculum vulgare* var. *dulce* [sweet fennel] *Ocimum basilicum* – ct. eugenol [basil] *Syzygium aromaticum* flos, per. [clove bud and leaf] *Thymus vulgaris* ct. thymol, ct. carvacrol [thyme]
Aldehydes	*Cympbopogon citratus* [lemongrass] *Cymbopogon nardus* [citronella] *Eucalyptus citriodora* [lemon scented eucalyptus] *Litsea cubeba* [litsea, may chang] *Melissa officinalis* [melissa]
Ketones	*Hyssopus officinalis* [hyssop] *Mentha spicata* [spearmint] *Salvia officinalis* [sage]

Because of the large range of essential oils available, it is not necessary to include any that might sensitize the skin or have a possible toxic effect on the nervous system. Photosensitizing essential oils pose no problem unless the client is going into direct sunlight within 2 hours of the treatment – a sunbed is definitely unwise for anyone. Generally, essential oils high in terpenes,

Case 13.4

Agitation and poor sleep

M Slaney – Aromatherapist

Assessment

H is a delightful 5-year-old who has leukodystrophy (Aicardi–Goutieves syndrome), a progressive neurological condition. She has globally delayed development, is unable to sit without support and gets frequent urine infections. Her limbs can become very stiff, her hips are painful as they are out of joint, and she is a poor sleeper.

Intervention

H has aromatherapy massage using grapeseed oil with 1% dilution of one of the essential oils below to her back, arms legs, tummy, neck and shoulders. Before starting the massage, the blend is wafted under her nose to see if there is a positive reaction – a smile. Her mother and the therapist sing nursery rhymes or play little games to keep her engaged during the massage. When she is enjoying the massage, she stays quite still and smiles a lot, but when she has had enough she starts to wriggle or moan. Massage time is between 20 and 40 minutes, depending on H's mood. Essential oils to induce sleep were used:

- *Citrus reticulata* [mandarin] – also gentle antispasmodic.
- *Citrus bergamia* [bergamot] – also antiinfectious (urinary)
- *Lavandula angustifolia* [lavender] – also calming/balancing when she is upset.

Outcome

Her mother and carer report that H is a happier, calmer and more relaxed little girl for the remainder of the day. The night after the treatment she always sleeps well.

---

alcohols and esters are suitable and will address both emotional and physical discomfort. Essential oils with a high oxide content can be useful (use with care if the client is asthmatic) – *Eucalyptus smithii* and *E. staigeriana* are the appropriate oils to use, as they are gentler in action and aroma than other eucalyptus oils.

Summary

For clients with learning disabilities and autism, the use of essential oils and massage can help build bridges of communication, add choice and have a positive and beneficial influence on an individual's life, providing relaxation where anxiety and agitation are often commonplace. There are now plans to reform the way care is provided for these people (NAS 2009d), which may result in complementary and alternative therapies bridging the gap often left when conventional interventions are used (DoH 2009).

In spite of the largely anecdotal nature of aromatherapy's reported successes on people with learning disabilities and autism, it is clear that it would be worth holding properly conducted trials, especially for adults, whose habits, obsessions and survival techniques have already been ingrained. Not only could more be discovered about the benefits of aromatherapy, but much could be learned about the nature of the disabilities themselves. Treating this client group with aromatherapy is a privilege and can be wonderfully rewarding – not only for the client but for the therapist and carers too.

References

Anderson, L., 2008. Making contact through loving touch. In Essence (Journal of the International Federation of Professional Aromatherapists) 7 (3), 9–12.

Armstrong, F., Heidingsfeld, V., 2000. Aromatherapy for deaf and deafblind people living in residential accommodation. Complement. Ther. Nurs. Midwifery 6, 180–188.

Autism and Practice Group (Learning Disability Services), 2007. Sensory issues in autism. East Sussex County Council. Available on: https://czone. eastsussex.gov.uk/specialneeds/autism/Documents/sensory%20issues%20in%20autism.pdf (accessed 07.06.10).

Autism Society of America (ASA), 2008. What is Autism. Available at: http://www.autism-society.org/site/PageServer?pagename=about_whatis (accessed 02.05.09).

Baron-Cohen, S., 2004. Theories of the autistic mind. The Psychologist 21 (2), 112–116.

Benson, B.A., Brooks, W.T., 2008. Aggressive challenging behavior and Intellectual Disability. Curr. Opin. Psychiatry 21 (5), 454–458.

Blackwell, L., 2000. The influence of touch on child development: Implications for intervention. Infants Young Child. 13 (1), 25–40.

Bogdashina, O., 2006. Theory of Mind and the Triad of Perspectives on Autism and Asperger Syndrome: A view from the Bridge. Jessica Kingsley Publishers, London & Philadelphia.

British Institute of Learning Disabilities (BILD), 2007. Factsheet–Learning Disabilities 2007. Available on: http://www.bild.org.uk/docs/05faqs/Factsheet%20Learning%20Disabilities.pdf (accessed 07.06.2010).

Broughan, C., 2005. The psychological aspects of aromatherapy. The International Journal of Aromatherapy 15, 3–6.

Brugha, T., McManus, S., Meltzer, H., et al., 2009. Autism Spectrum Disorders in adults living in households throughout England. Report from the Adult Psychiatric Morbidity Survey 2007. The Health and Social Care Information Centre, Social Care Statistics. Available on: http://www.ic.nhs.uk/webfiles/publications /mental%20health/mental%20health%20surveys/Autism_Spectrum_Disorders_in_adults_living_in_households_throughout_England_Report_from_the_Adult_Psychiatric_Morbidity_Survey_2007.pdf (accessed 07.06.10).

Buck, P., 2007. Childhood behavioural disorders. In Essence 6 (1), 9–12.

Carter, R., 1998. Mapping the mind. Weidenfeld & Nicolson, London, p. 145.

Centers for Disease Control Prevention Autism Spectrum Disorders Overview, 2007. Available on: http://www.cdc.gov/ncbddd/autism/addm.html (accessed 07.06.10).

Cook, N., 2008. Aromatherapy: reviewing evidence for its mechanisms of action and CNS effects. British Journal of Neuroscience Nursing 4 (12), 595–601.

Cullen, L., Barlow, J., 2002. Kiss cuddle and squeeze: the experiences and meaning of touch among parents of children with autism attending a Touch Therapy Programme. J. Child Health Care 6 (3), 171–180.

Department of Health, 2001. Valuing people: a new strategy for Learning Disability in the 21st Century. HMSO, London. Available on: http://www.archive.official-documents.co.uk/document/cm50/5086/5086.htm (accessed 07.06.10).

Department of Health, 2003. Seeking Consent: working with people with learning disabilities. Available on: http://www.dhsspsni.gov.uk/consent-guidepart4.pdf (accessed 07.06.10).

Department of Health, 2008. Healthcare for all. Report of the independent inquiry into access to healthcare for people with learning disabilities. Available on: http://www.dh.gov.uk/prod_consum_dh/groups/dh_digitalassets/@dh/@en/documents/digitalasset/dh_106126.pdf (accessed 07.06.10).

Department of Health, 2009. Reference guide to consent for examination or treatment, second ed. Available on: http://www.dh.gov.uk/prod_consum_dh/groups/dh_digitalassets/documents/digitalasset/dh_103653.pdf (accessed 07.06.10).

Disability Discrimination Act, 2005. HMSO, London. Available on: http://www.opsi.gov.uk/acts/acts2005/ukpga_20050013_en_1 (accessed 07.06.10).

Ellwood, J., 2002. Touching the spirit. In Essence 1 (3), 10–13.

Field, T., 2002a. Infants' need for touch. Hum. Dev. 45 (2), 100–104.

Field, T., 2002b. Violence and touch deprivation in adolescents. Adolescence 37 (148), 735–750.

Freeman, et al., 2009. Olfactory stimuli and enhanced postural stability in older adults. Gait and Posture 29, 658–660.

Grandin, T., 2007. My experience with visual thinking sensory problems and communication difficulties. Available on: http://www.autism.org.

Green, H., McGinnity, A., Meltzer, H., Goodman, R., 2005. Mental health of children and young people in Great Britain. 2004. Palgrave Macmillan, Basingstoke. Available on: http://www.statistics.gov.uk/downloads/theme_health/GB2004.pdf (accessed 07.06.10).

Herbert, M., 2002. Typical and Atypical Development: From Conception to Adolescence. BPS Blackwell.

Mencap, 2010a. About learning disability. http://www.mencap.org.uk/landing.asp?id=1683.

Mencap, 2010b. What is a learning disability? Available on: http://www.mencap.org.uk/page.asp?id=1684 (accessed 07.06.10).

Mencap, 2010c. Associated conditions. http://www.mencap.org.uk/page.asp?id=1702 (accessed 07.06.10).

Mental Capacity Act, 2005. HMSO, London. Available on: http://www.opsi.gov.uk/acts/acts2005/ukpga_20050009_en_1 (accessed 07.06.10).

Mills, S., 2007. Downs' Syndrome A New Parents Guide. Down's Syndrome Association, Middlesex.

National Autistic Society, 2009a. What is Asperger syndrome?. Available on: http://www.autism.org.uk/About-autism/Autism-and-Asperger-syndrome-an-introduction/What-is-Asperger-syndrome.aspx Updated 25/05/10 (accessed 07.06.10).

National Autistic Society, 2009b. Living with autism, understanding behaviour. Available on: http://www.autism.org.uk/living-with-autism/understanding-behaviour.aspx Updated 07/06/10 (accessed 07.06.10).

National Autistic Society, 2009c. The sensory world of the autistic spectrum. Available on: http://www.autism.org.uk/living-with-autism/understanding-behaviour/the-sensory-world-of-the-autism-spectrum.aspx Updated 25/05/2010 (accessed 07.06.10).

National Autistic Society, 2009d. The Autism Bill. Available on: http://www.autism.org.uk/dhstrategy. NAS welcomes new adult autism strategy for England. Updated 12th April 2010 (accessed 07.06.10).

Northfield, J., 2004. Factsheet—What is a learning disability? British Institute of Learning Disabilities, UK. Available on: http://www.bild.org.uk/pdfs/05faqs/ld.pdf (accessed 07.06.10).

Ouldred, E., Bryant, C., 2008. Dementia Care. Part 2: understanding and managing behavioural challenges. Br. J. Nurs. 17 (4), 242–247.

Royal College of Psychiatrists, 2004. Autism and Asperger Syndrome Fact

Sheet for Parents. Mental Health and Growing Up Factsheet 12. Royal College of Psychiatrists. Available on: http: //www.rcpsych.ac.uk/pdf/ Sheet12.pdf Reviewed 03/09 (accessed 07.06.10).

Searson, B., 2008. Meeting the challenges of epilepsy. Learning Disability Practice 11 (9), 29–35.

Thompson, S., 2002. A fragrant message. Learning Disability Practice 5 (5), 15–17.

Wikipedia, 2010. Gillick Competence. Available on: http: //en.wikipedia. org/wiki/Gillick_competence.

Wing, L., 1997. The autistic spectrum. Lancet 350 (9093), 1762.

Care of the elderly

14

Shirley Price   Sandra A Oram

Introduction

This chapter is devoted mainly to dementia and its treatment, but as the elderly may suffer some of the specific conditions also suffered by those with dementia, the essential oils and treatments that apply to the general care of the elderly are also advocated.

For more than a decade a wide range of healthcare professionals in both hospitals and residential or nursing homes have realized the benefits of using essential oils to help elderly people suffering from various types of dementia. There is also awareness of the need to help those in a younger age group with early onset of dementia.

Massage and essential oils

As many elderly people receive little or no caring touch from others, introducing massage can not only improve their quality of life but can also benefit those caring for them, a massage being relaxing for both parties, giving both warmth and comfort. Using essential oils enhances these benefits, as they can assist such problems as anxiety, depression, indigestion, insomnia, constipation etc.

Extra care is necessary when treating more mature clients, as ageing brings about numerous physical, mental and emotional changes. The span of concentration lessens when short-term memory deteriorates, and the massage time may therefore need adjusting.

In 1988 Helen Passant introduced massage to what was then called the 'geriatric ward' at Churchill Hospital, Oxford. She discovered that not only did patients' skin texture improve, becoming stronger and more resistant to bruising and tissue damage, but they became more alert (and calmer when anxious or noisy). Essential oils were later introduced to the treatment, enabling conventional sedative medicines to be reduced (Passant 1990).

The cost of dementia

The cost of dementia to the UK is twice that spent on cancer care, yet the amount spent on research into dementia is 12 times lower than that for cancer (www.dementia2010.org).

The Alzheimer's Research Trust has commissioned the Health Economics Research Centre at the University of Oxford to produce a report on the economic cost of dementia to the UK, and the country's investment in research to find new treatments, preventions and cures. The Oxford team's findings are astonishing, showing dementia to be the greatest medical challenge of our time.

- Over 820 000 people in the UK live with Alzheimer's and other dementias.
- Dementia costs the UK economy £23 billion per year: more than cancer and heart disease combined.
- Dementia research is severely underfunded, receiving 12 times less support than cancer research. www.dementia2010.org

Dementia and its variations

Dementia and related illnesses are a financial strain on the health service and healthcare resources. The Alzheimer's Society states that: 'a quarter of all hospital beds are used by people with dementia but many are not getting the quality of care they deserve'. A *British Medical Journal* editorial of December 2002 states: 'People with dementia are among the most vulnerable in our society. Symptoms often need to be treated and drugs, although moderately effective, can be hazardous. Aromatherapy and bright light treatment seem to be safe and effective and may have an important role in managing behavioural problems in people with dementia.'

In 2010 the BBC announced that around 500 people a day develop Alzheimer's, and a University of Oxford report for an Alzheimer's research trust suggests that there are now around 820 000 people in the UK with dementia (Ketteringham 2010). This is likely to double over the next 30 years, the numbers affected being far greater when one considers the family members of each sufferer.

Dementia is a decline in memory and thinking, present for 6 months or more, which is of a degree sufficient to impair functioning in daily living. Although attention is usually focused on cognitive deficits, more than 50% of people with dementia experience a decline in emotional control, with behavioural and psychological symptoms (BPSD) which are distressing to both the patient (Gilley et al. 1991) and their carers (Rabins et al.

1982). People with dementia may develop mood disorders such as anxiety, depression, aggression and restlessness. These changes can be confusing, irritating or difficult for family members and carers to deal with, leaving them feeling resentful, stressed and helpless. Consequently, treatment of not only the client but all his/her family should be considered.

Dementia can happen to anybody, but is more common after the age of 65 years, with 1 in 14 over the age of 65 being affected. However, people in their 40s and 50s (approximately 16 000) are now being diagnosed with early-stage dementia (www.alzheimers.org.uk). Another factor that may contribute to an increase in dementia in the near future is the increase in alcohol consumption, which can lead to alcohol-related dementia.

The most common cause of dementia is Alzheimer's disease, although there are many categories:

- **Alzheimer's disease** – accounts for between 50% and 70% of all cases – it is a progressive, degenerative illness that attacks the brain.
- **Dementia with Lewy bodies** – a form of dementia with similar characteristics to Alzheimer's and Parkinson's diseases. Professor Ian McKeith (2010) of Newcastle University tells us that it accounts for about 4% of all cases of dementia in older people and is more prevalent in the over-65s. Lewy bodies are tiny spherical protein deposits found inside nerve cells, disrupting the brain's normal functioning (Mental Health Foundation 1999) and are found in approximately a quarter of people with Alzheimer's disease when examined after death. Researchers have yet to understand fully why Lewy bodies occur in the brain and how they cause damage

  Lewy body dementia (LBD) accounts for up to 20% of all late-onset dementia cases (Ballard 2008), with 800 000 patients in the US and 820 000 in the UK (www.dementia2010.org). The sense of smell of people with 'Lewy bodies' is inferior to that of those without them (Alzheimer's Society newsletter 2004). This work involved a detailed series of experiments where the ability to detect the scent of lavender was correlated with changes found in the brain post mortem; in time, it was hoped that by inhalation, a simple patient-friendly' smell test (using lavender) could hopefully make diagnosis of dementia with LBD more accurate (Petit-Zeman (2004).

Research reported in the *Journal of Neuroscience* links the loss of smell with a build-up of amyloid protein, which is a hallmark of Alzheimer's disease. The research suggests that loss of smell could be used as an early indicator of the disease (Wesson et al. 2010).

- **Vascular dementia** – the broad term for dementia associated with problems of circulation to the brain.
- **Huntington's disease** – an inherited, degenerative brain disease that affects the mind and body – dementia occurs in the majority of cases.
- **Frontotemporal lobe degeneration (FTLD)** – a group of dementias involving degeneration in one or both of the frontal or temporal lobes of the brain. This is often associated with motor neuron disease and is slightly more common in men.
- **Alcohol-related dementia** – caused by excess consumption of alcohol, especially with a diet low in vitamin B_1 (thiamine).
- **Parkinson's disease** – a progressive disorder of the central nervous system; some people with Parkinson's disease may develop dementia in the late stages (see text on Parkinson's disease.)

The value of touch with essential oils

Common symptoms of dementia include:
- Apathy and withdrawal
- Progressive and frequent memory loss
- Confusion
- Loss of ability to perform everyday tasks.
- Personality changes and behaviour changes.

It is essential to discriminate between symptoms of dementia and those of a different treatable condition, such as vitamin deficiency, depression, infection, a medication problem or a brain tumour.

Behavioural symptoms in people with dementia (Alzheimer's Society)

- Aggression (verbal or physical)
- Delusions (being disturbed by thoughts, and believing things that are not true)
- Depression
- Hallucinations (seeing or hearing things that are not there)
- Irritability, anxiety or suspicion
- Loss of normal inhibitions – for example, touching their private parts.
- Restlessness or over-activity
- Tendency to shout repeatedly or become noisy.
- Tendency to wander.

Box 14.1

Aromatherapy and Dementia Study
This study was conducted in a multicultural dementia daycare centre over a period of 18 months. It introduced a gentle hand treatment for clients, using three essential oils. The study evolved out of the process of action research, where the family carers and daycare staff participated with the researchers to choose, design, develop and evaluate a hand treatment programme. Data was collected through in-depth interviews pre- and post treatment, focus group discussions, client observation logbooks and a disability scale. The findings indicated a positive strengthening of the relationship between the person with dementia and

their family carer, and an improvement in feelings of health and wellbeing for both. The specific improvements for clients include increased alertness, self-hygiene, contentment, initiation of toileting, sleeping at night and reduced levels of agitation, withdrawal and wandering. Family carers reported less distress, improved sleeping patterns and feelings of calm. They also found the treatment useful in helping them manage the difficult behaviours exhibited by their relative. The benefits of this treatment for nursing practice are that it is safe, effective and easily administered by staff in any setting.

Int J Nurs Pract 1998 Jun; 4(2): 70–83 Kilstoff K, Chenoweth L Faculty of Nursing, University of Technology, Sydney, Australia. For more information: kathy.kilstoff@uts.edu.au

Some successful studies and clinical trials

Controlled clinical trials of aromatherapy in dementia were initiated after promising results were obtained from open trials of historical medical remedies – in folklore, linen bags were filled with lavender flowers and placed under pillows in order to facilitate sleep – one showed that the use of lavender increased sleep patterns in dementia patients who were in residential care (Henry et al. 1994).

Other studies showing that aromatherapy works when used to treat agitated people with dementia:

- Geranium, lavender and mandarin essential oils in an almond oil base applied to the skin of 39 patients over an unspecified period resulted in increased alertness, contentment and sleeping at night – with reduced levels of agitation, withdrawal and wandering (Kilstoff & Chenoweth 1998).
- Essential oils including ylang ylang, patchouli, rosemary and peppermint and others produced a marked decrease in disturbed behaviour in most participants. This led to a reduction in prescribed conventional medicines (Beshara & Giddings 2003).
- Researchers at Oldham Cottage Hospital investigated the potential of essential oil of lavender to aid rest and relaxation, thereby encouraging the healing process. Patients were monitored for 7 days, during which time their sleep patterns, dozing and alertness during the day were recorded. For the following 7 days one drop of *Lavender angustifolia* was put on each patient's pillow at night. No other changes were made to the patients' daily routine or medications that they were receiving. At the end of the 7 days, patients' records were collated and analysed. Interestingly, all patients reacted favourably to the treatment, with increased daytime alertness and improved sleep patterns, and those who had previously experienced confusion were observed to display as much as a 50% reduction in their symptoms (Hudson 1996).

Results of placebo-controlled clinical trials using essential oils for the treatment of residential care residents with advanced dementia:

- Lemon balm and lavender aroma were introduced to six patients and compared to a control

group using sunflower oil for 1 week. The treatment increased functional abilities and communication, and reduced difficult behaviour (Mitchell 1993).
- Lavender aroma and massage with 21 patients were compared to aroma or massage alone for 1 week. Aromatherapy with massage significantly reduced the frequency of excessive motor behaviour (Smallwood et al. 2001).
- Lavender oil was given to 15 patients via AromaStream and placebo (water) on alternate days for 10 days. Inhalation of the lavender significantly reduced agitated behaviour (as assessed using the Pittsburgh Agitation Scale) versus placebo (Holmes et al. 2002).

Box 14.2

Melisssa officinalis and agitation in dementia

Ballard et al. (2002) carried out a double-blind placebo-controlled trial to establish whether *Melissa officinalis* would have a positive effect on agitation in people with severe dementia. Seventy-two people with clinically significant agitation were randomly assigned either to an aromatherapy group, receiving massage on their hands and arms twice a day with a base lotion containing melissa essential oil, or a placebo group, receiving the same massage with a base lotion containing sunflower oil.

The blends were applied to the faces and arms of the patients in both groups, twice a day. No significant side effects were observed and 71 patients completed the trial.

Results

The results were compared between the groups over a period of 4 weeks. Those who received the lemon balm [melissa] treatment became less agitated than those who had the sunflower oil.

The improvements were clear in the first week and continued so for a full 3 weeks.

Sixty per cent (21 out of 35) of the melissa group experienced a significant improvement in their agitation scores following treatment, compared to 14% (5 out of 36) of the placebo group. The authors concluded that aromatherapy with the essential oil of *Melissa officinalis* is safe and effective for clinically significant agitation in people with severe dementia, and that there is a need for further controlled trials (Ballard et al. 2002).

- Lemon balm (melissa) lotion was applied to the face and arms of 36 patients, and another 36 had sunflower oil applied. Melissa was associated with highly significant reductions measured on the Cohen–Mansfield Agitation Inventory (CMAI) and social withdrawal, together with an increase in constructive activities (dementia care mapping) (Ballard et al. 2002).
- Lavender, marjoram, patchouli and vetiver were applied as a cream to the body and limbs of 36 patients and compared with inert oil. The essential oil combination significantly increased the Mini Mental State Examination (MMSE) but also increased resistance to care (considered to be due to increase in alertness), compared to inert oil (Bowles-Dilys 2002).

What is remarkable is that all treatments resulted in significant benefit, including (in most instances) reductions in agitation, sleeplessness, wandering and unsociable behaviour (Snow et al. 2004) www.alzheimers.org.uk 2007.

Considerations when treating the elderly

When treating elderly clients it is a good idea for the therapist to have the same pleasant-smelling oil blend on his/her hands at each visit, as this can help to create a bond with the client.

Comfort

Each aromatherapy treatment needs to be adapted according to the health of the client; a full body massage may be too much for some elderly people, and if lying down is difficult or uncomfortable, targeting specific areas such as the hands or feet is also beneficial. If massage is inappropriate or not wanted, essential oils can be applied in a lotion daily, vaporized, used in the bath or with a compress.

As the skin of an elderly client may be wrinkled, slightly more carrier oil may be needed for a massage to minimize stretching. Care must be taken not to leave any oil residue on clients' hands or feet, as this could cause them to drop things or fall if they slip or lose their grip.

Treating common ailments

Appetite stimulation

Older people may sometimes need encouragement to eat if they are suffering from a loss or lack of appetite. Unlike conventional drugs, essential oils do not have side effects; neither are they as invasive as inserting a feeding tube.

A blend of *Citrus bergamia* [bergamot] and *Citrus aurantifolia* [lime] produces a mouth-watering aroma when used in a vaporizer before meals.

Other oils useful in this respect include *Carum carvi* [caraway], *Foeniculum vulgare* [fennel], *Mentha spicata* [spearmint], *Myristica fragrans* [nutmeg] and *Zingiber officinale* [ginger].

A study using indirect inhalation and/or topical application proved to be effective in promoting patients' appetites, often within 24 hours. Meals monitored by staff showed an increase of food intake from zero the first day to 25% by the third day, and up to 75% and more by the 10th day. These are measurable, effective outcomes without harmful side effects (O'Haynes 2010).

Anxiety and depression

Studies have shown that generalized anxiety disorder (GAD) may be the most common mental disorder among the elderly and is more common than depression in that group (7% and 3%, respectively) (Warner 2006). Anxiety can take many forms and have many causes, perhaps due to loss of mobility and independence, fear over finances, gradual deterioration in health or the decline of a loved one – when it is not surprising that anxiety disorders may develop. Aromatherapy with direct and indirect inhalation is able to reduce anxiety, agitation and other symptoms of the elderly, improving patients' quality of life and making them more relaxed and less stressed. Patients wander less, are more easily redirected by staff and less likely to fall (Perry 2007). Traditional drugs for Alzheimer's often have side effects such as dizziness, which can also be helped by the use of essential oils (O'Haynes (2010); therapeutic essential oils have no side effects and enhance psychological and physical wellbeing.

Some people with behavioural and mood changes due to dementia (more common in the middle and later stages) can become quite distressed if they are aware that they are acting inappropriately, but for those who are unaware this may not be a problem. Considerable distress may be seen in the family, friends and carers of those with dementia. Therefore it is important when treating dementia patients to be aware of their families and carers, giving them treatment too if necessary to relax their stress.

Depression

This is common when patients are stressed or anxious, and 1 drop of *Thymus vulgaris* ct. *thymol* [phenolic thyme] rubbed on the back of the hands is most effective. A blend of two or three of the following oils – which treat both anxiety *and* depression – can be given by inhalation, in the bath or by hand, foot or scalp massage: *Abies balsamea* [Canada fir], *Aloysia triphylla* [verbena], *Chamaemelum nobile* [Roman chamomile], *Leptospermum scoparium* [manuka], *Litsea cubeba* [may chang] – also helpful to insomnia and memory loss, *Mentha spicata* [spearmint], *Nepeta cataria* [catmint], *Ocimum basilicum* [European basil] and *Origanum majorana* [sweet marjoram].

Circulation

As age progresses people move around less and the speed of circulation through the body is reduced, which can lead to health problems. An aromatherapy massage (towards the heart) stimulates the circulation, helping to maintain and improve health. Foot baths and foot massage are also helpful. To enhance the treatment the carer can be given a lotion to apply daily. Lower leg massage – not forgetting that pressure must be on the upward movement only – is also beneficial. Circulation-stimulating essential oils include: *Citrus aurantium* var. *amara* [bitter orange], *Citrus limon* [lemon], *Cupressus sempervirens* [cypress], *Rosmarinus officinalis* [rosemary], *Foeniculum vulgare* [fennel], *Salvia officinalis* [sage].

Foot baths can be given as a preliminary to aromatherapy massage, when the essential oils should be dissolved in a teaspoonful of honey, cream or white lotion before adding to the water, swishing well. The feet should be soaked for 10 minutes.

Constipation

Many elderly people do not drink enough water, which can contribute to constipation. A blend of citrus essential oils in a carrier oil applied with gentle abdominal massage can be helpful, and they should also be encouraged to drink plenty of fluids to soften stools further. The digestive system reflex points on the feet can be massaged (see Swiss reflex treatment in Ch. 8), which may be a preferred treatment for some.

It has been said that clearing the bowels can rectify mild cases of confusion almost immediately.

Essential oils which both stimulate the digestive system and ease constipation are *Rosmarinus officinalis*, *Zingiber officinale* [ginger], *Mentha spicata* [spearmint]

Digestion-stimulating oils: *Coriandrum sativum* [coriander], *Myristica fragrans* [nutmeg], *Piper nigrum* [black pepper], *Salvia officinalis* [sage].

Oils that relieve constipation: *Citrus aurantium* var. *amara* [bitter orange], *Citrus reticulata* [mandarin], *Citrus sinensis* [sweet orange], *Foeniculum vulgare* [fennel].

A massage blend containing these oils can be applied to the abdomen. Massage should be in gentle circles in a clockwise direction around the abdomen following the line of the digestive tract. Alternatively, the relevant digestive reflex points on the feet or hands can be massaged. These treatments can easily be shown to carers so that they may continue the massage in the therapist's absence to ensure ongoing relief.

Diarrhoea

This condition can be just as upsetting to a patient as constipation, and the following essential oils will be found helpful:

Origanum majorana [sweet marjoram] and *Citrus limon* [lemon] are effective where the diarrhoea is of nervous origin, as they also have tranquillizing effects.

Melaleuca viridiflora [niaouli] – also anti-inflammatory

Mentha x piperita [peppermint] – also anti-inflammatory and will help against nausea

Pelargonium graveolens [geranium] – also anti-inflammatory and calming.

The anti-inflammatory oils above are useful where there is colitis or gastroenteritis, and *Syzygium aromaticum* (flos) [clove bud], *Pimpinella anisum* [aniseed], *Melaleuca cajuputi* [cajuput] and *Myristica fragrans* [nutmeg] relieve the spasms (Valnet 1992 pp. 114, 95, 101, 161).

A blend which has been found to work well for both enteritis and irritable bowel syndrome (frequently used with success by S Price) and mostly administered internally diluted in a dispersant e.g. honey, then water, is equal quantities of *Foeniculum vulgare* var. *dulce* [fennel], *Mentha* x *piperita* and *Piper nigrum* [black pepper].

Diverticulitis (Diverticulosis)

This is where small, harmless bulges occur in weak points in the large intestine and exists in most elderly people (Wingate & Wingate 1996). It is only when one or more of these diverticula becomes inflamed that chronic diverticulitis can set in – and constipation, abdominal pain and bleeding may manifest.

The diet should be changed to one rich in fibre, and massage with anti-inflammatory essential oils such as rosemary and bitter orange (in Constipation above) would be beneficial. Other anti-inflammatory oils that act on the digestive system are: *Commiphora myrrha* [myrrh], *Chamomilla recutita* [German chamomile], *Juniperus communis* fruct. [juniper berry], *Melissa officinalis* [melissa].

Headaches and migraines

The causes of headaches and migraines are many. To relieve symptoms, a few drops of essential oil can be vaporized or dropped onto a tissue or the palms of the hands (one drop in this case is sufficient) and then inhaled.

Lavandula angustifolia [lavender] (analgesic and anti-spasmodic) massaged into the temples can work wonders, or a cold compress of *Mentha* x *piperita* [peppermint] (analgesic and antispasmodic) applied to the forehead or the back of the neck can bring relief.

Migraines that appear to be caused by restricted blood supply may respond positively to warm compresses applied to the back of the neck, using *Origanum majorana* [sweet marjoram], which is a vasodilator.

Suitable oils for headache and migraine treatments include: *Lavandula angustifolia* [lavender], *Chamaemelum nobile* [Roman chamomile], *Ocimum basilicum* [basil], *Mentha* x *piperita* [peppermint], *Origanum majorana* [sweet marjoram], *Rosmarinus officinalis* [rosemary], *Aniba rosaeodora* [rosewood].

High blood pressure

A small pilot study was conducted by Basnyet (1999), aromatherapist at the Natural Health Centre in Preston, Lancashire, UK. Twenty patients were divided into two groups of 10, the first group to receive five 45-minute aromatherapy treatments using 15 mL of unrefined grapeseed carrier oil containing one drop of each of *Cananga odorata* [ylang ylang], *Salvia sclarea* [clary sage] and *Origanum majorana* [sweet marjoram] over a period of 6 weeks. The second group received the same massage but without the essential oils.

The massage techniques used were effleurage (stroking), petrissage (kneading), gentle friction, vibration and feathering, using 15 mL of grapeseed carrier oil, which in the aromatherapy group contained one drop of each essential oil.

At the end of the treatment period the improvement in pulse rate of patients in the treatment group was consistently higher than that observed in the control group: seven out of 10 in the treatment group and six out of 10 in the control experienced a reduction in their raised blood pressure.

The report concludes that 'overall blood pressure readings in both groups improved successfully, which would indicate that this type of tactile treatment can have a beneficial effect on the raised arterial blood pressure' (Internet Health Library 2006).

Insomnia

The older and less active people become the less sleep they may require, especially as many have 'forty winks' during the day, possibly detracting from a complete night's sleep. The amount of essential oils used for insomnia is important, as one or two drops of *Lavandula angustifolia* [lavender] can be relaxing and soporific, but a high dose can have the opposite effects. Two to four drops can be inhaled from a tissue or put into a vaporizer or bath. A simple neck and shoulder massage with – or application of – a blend of oils is very effective. Other oils beneficial for insomnia include: *Cananga odorata* [ylang ylang], *Chamaemelum nobile* [Roman chamomile], *Origanum majorana* [sweet marjoram], *Citrus aurantium* var. *amara* flos [neroli bigarade], *Citrus bergamia* [bergamot], *Citrus limon* [lemon], *Citrus reticulata* [mandarin], *Citrus sinensis* [sweet orange], *Lavandula angustifolia* [lavender].

Short- and long-term memory loss and reminiscence

Essential oils can stimulate the mind and improve memory recall (Moss et al. 2003), which is useful not only for students when revising but also for the elderly, especially those suffering from Alzheimer's disease. Introducing essential oils can trigger nostalgic memories, bringing them to the fore where they can be enjoyed by all – clients, carers and family.

Rosmarinus officinalis [rosemary] and *Mentha* x *piperita* [peppermint] are reputed to stimulate the memory, others often used being *Litsea cubeba* [cubeb], *Mentha* x *piperita* [peppermint], *Rosmarinus officinalis* [rosemary] and *Syzygium aromaticum* [clove bud].

In illnesses such as Alzheimer's disease, essential oils can help to stimulate the mind and improve the memory. *Rosmarinus officinalis* [rosemary] is reputed to stimulate the memory, as is *Mentha* x *piperita* [peppermint]. *Salvia officinalis* [sage] is also said to boost the memory – it has been found to possess acetylcholinesterase (Ach) enzyme inhibition activities, which help to raise Ach levels in the brain. Ach improves concentration and may play a role in the treatment methods for memory loss associated with diseases such as Alzheimer's. www.nutrition-and-you.com 2010. It has been shown that it acts as an enzyme inhibitor (cholinesterase) – as shown by three licensed drugs for Alzheimer's disease. www.betterhealth.vic.gov.au

Pain relief (arthritis/rheumatism)

Patients with high levels of pain (after hip, knee or back surgery, or who suffer arthritis, rheumatism or osteoporosis) find it difficult to participate in their daily rehabilitation regime. The application of essential oils on or around the pain area(s) at designated times of the day and night results in a definite decline in the perception of pain and an increase in comfort levels. Compresses can also be applied, followed by warm towels or heat pads, or a bag of frozen peas wrapped in a tea towel if the joints are inflamed. After treatment, the client or carer should be given a lotion containing the relevant oils to apply twice a day to maintain the benefits – the overall effect is not only beneficial, but they respond better to the rehabilitative process and have a speedier recovery (O'Haynes 2010).

Case 14.1

Pain and osteoporosis

Kate Nellist – Aromatologist

Assessment

Mrs O (aged 80) was diagnosed with osteoporosis in her late 60s. She had been very active and disliked being incapacitated and dependent on her family; however, as the years progressed she had to accept this more and more. By her early 80s Mrs O had had several fractures of the ribs and spine and was using a TENS machine for pain management, as well as paracetamol and Voltarol (diclofenac), although she tried to take as little medication as possible; other medicines included fosimax and lactulose. Owing to her lack of mobility her circulation was poor and she suffered from constipation. As her bone condition worsened her pain increased, and in the late stages, when it was severe, she was using morphine patches.

Intervention

Mrs O's wish was always to feel less pain, and this was achieved by massaging her hands, arms and legs three times per week. The essential oils used were:

- *Rosmarinus officinalis* [rosemary] – analgesic, anti-inflammatory, circulation stimulant, laxative
- *Citrus aurantium* var. *amara* [bitter orange] – anti-inflammatory, circulation stimulant, laxative
- *Lavandula angustifolia* – analgesic, anti-inflammatory, calming
- *Origanum majorana* – analgesic, calming, digestive stimulant.

The blend was chosen to support the circulation and relieve the pain. A home application lotion was made with the same essential oils in a base enhanced with 10% wheatgerm and 10% avocado oils to feed her dry skin, and Mrs O applied this herself every day morning and night.

Outcome

Although there was never to be a full recovery, Mrs O looked forward to her treatments – her face would light up, and afterwards she was able to move more easily; the daily application of the lotion and the regular massages meant she could go longer between pain relief medications, which pleased her greatly. The pleasure of being able to relieve Mrs O's severe pain through her final weeks of life was very rewarding for the therapist.

Case 14.2

Leg ulcer

Kate Nellist – Aromatherapist/aromatologist

Assessment

Mrs R (71 years) had had cellulitis and a leg ulcer 4 years previously and visited her GP when the symptoms recurred. She was prescribed antibiotics for 1 week, and on the second visit a cream for a further week, but the symptoms did not abate.

After 2 more weeks Mrs R was admitted to hospital – a small ulcer had appeared on lower left leg and she was put onto IV antibiotics for 4 days. The leg was so painful by this stage that she was unable to walk (the ulcer was treated and dressed each day).

Mrs R was moved to another hospital for a week then discharged with a course of oral antibiotics – doxycycline – for 11 days.

Because the situation was worsening rather than improving with medical intervention, Mrs R made an aromatology appointment: she was angry, saying the doctor just did not listen to her. After listening and taking notes, the therapist gave Mrs R a glass of rose hydrolat (10 mL in 100 mL water) while her legs were examined and a treatment plan was prepared. Her lower left leg was hot, reddish-purple and itchy, with dry flaky skin; one small area was slightly open; it was shiny and felt taut, and the ankle was swollen and stiff with oedema and poor circulation. The right leg felt soft and warm, with slight oedema round the ankle, and the circulation was sluggish.

Intervention

The left leg was sprayed liberally with undiluted hydrolat of *Chamaemelum nobile* to cleanse the area. Within 5 minutes the leg felt softer and cooler, and Mrs R commented that the itchiness had gone. The open area was the size of a 10p coin, with five other pinhead areas that could break

down. Mrs R, having finished her drink, was calmer and becoming relaxed, her face less tense and cooler.

A compress was made for the main ulcer, using oils for pain, inflammation, infection, circulation and cell regeneration (the main chemical components were alcohols, esters and sesquiterpenes). The essential oils chosen were:
- *Aniba rosaedora* [rosewood] – 95% linalool
- *Chamaemelum nobile* [Roman chamomile] – 80% esters,
- *Matricaria recutita* [German chamomile] – 35% sesquiterpenes, 20% alcohols, 35% oxides
- *Piper nigrum* [black pepper] – 30% sesquiterpenes, 60% monoterpenes.

After the compress a gentle massage was given using macerated passion flower, hypericum and calendula oils – 10 mL of each, with 2 drops each of the essential oils. The lower left leg was massaged, avoiding the ulcer and with particular care on the five pinhead areas (the right lower leg was also massaged to balance the body). Finally, a melonin dressing was put on the open ulcer, using 2 drops of *Mentha arvensis* [cornmint] to soothe and protect it; it was to be left open to the air when possible and covered with the dressing when moving or going out. Mrs R was given a bottle of rose hydrolat to make a daily drink with water.

Over the next 4 weeks Mrs R returned for weekly treatments following the same regime.

Outcome

After 4 weeks of aromatology and home treatment the ulcer closed and the pinhead areas had cleared. Mrs R continues to look after her legs daily with Nurture Circulation lotion from Penny Price Aromatherapy.

For problems such as these, therapists aim to help relieve inflammation and pain, and gentle massage and daily application of a lotion is beneficial. Analgesic and anti-inflammatory essential oils have been found to be helpful: *Lavandula angustifolia* [lavender], *Origanum majorana* [sweet marjoram], *Rosmarinus officinalis* [rosemary], *Ocimum basilicum* [basil], *Citrus limon* [lemon], *Piper nigrum* [black pepper], *Zingiber officinale* [ginger].

Pressure sores and wounds

Bed sores can occur when long periods are spent in bed (often the case in an old peoples' home), the sacrum and buttocks being the most affected. If they

are not treated early enough ulcers can form, which take longer to heal.

Always consult the client's GP before treating open wounds, and for methods of treatment and beneficial essential oils see Chapter 10, which deals specifically with wounds and pressure sores.

Respiratory problems

The conifer family is chiefly acknowledged in textbooks as having expectorant properties (Boyd & Pearson 1946), although essential oils from other families also possess them.

Elderly people suffering from catarrhal problems, chronic bronchitis or asthma can benefit from a daily application of essential oils in a carrier lotion onto the chest and neck, and the thin skin behind the ears facilitates percutaneous penetration.

Eucalyptus smithii [gully gum] is an excellent preventive measure for winter coughs and colds. Not only does it increase the resistance of the respiratory system to infection, it is also anticatarrhal, antiviral and an effective expectorant. It has a pleasant aroma, is inexpensive and can be vaporized daily in the lounge area of the ward, and/or in the ward (or bedrooms, as many of the newer hospitals name the rooms of the elderly or patients with learning difficulties).

Boswellia carteri [frankincense], *Melaleuca viridiflora* [niaouli] and *Myrtus communis* fol. [myrtle] are all anti-infectious, anticatarrhal and expectorant – niaouli is an excellent choice for chronic cases.

Other essential oils with useful properties for chest problems are:

- *Abies alba* fol. [silver fir] – anticatarrhal, expectorant
- *Eucalyptus staigeriana* [lemon scented iron bark] – anti-inflammatory
- *Hyssopus officinalis* [hyssop] – anticatarrhal, anti-infectious, anti-inflammatory antitussive, expectorant, mucolytic. NB Not suitable for epileptic patients
- *Lavandula angustifolia* [lavender] – antiseptic, antispasmodic

- *Mentha* x *piperita* [peppermint] – anti-infectious, anti-inflammatory, antispasmodic, expectorant and mucolytic (useful where there are sinus problems)
- *Ravansara aromatica* [ravensara] – anti-infectious, expectorant
- *Thymus vulgaris* ct. *linalool* [sweet thyme] – anti-infectious, antispasmodic.

Eight drops of essential oils selected from the above (see also Appendix B1 on the CD-ROM) should be added to 50 mL carrier lotion for application.

Skin

As people get older the skin loses its tone and elasticity owing to a decrease in collagen and elastin, the skin of elderly people becoming thinner and often deeply wrinkled. Because of this more oil needs to be applied for massage, to prevent dragging the skin, preferably selecting carrier oils that will benefit the skin, such as apricot or peach, avocado, calendula, evening primrose and wheatgerm. Essential oils which help to improve dryness and elasticity are *Aniba rosaeodora* [rosewood], *Chamaemelum nobile* [Roman chamomile], *Helichrysum angustifolium* [everlasting], *Rosa centifolia* [rose], *Salvia sclarea* [clary sage] (helps cell regeneration), *Santalum album* [sandalwood].

Case 14.3

Itchy skin

Christopher Hassall – Aromatherapist

Client assessment

In 2008 Mary (90) was referred to the Day Hospice with a primary cancer of the thyroid, plus several other medical issues, including a hiatus hernia. When she first came she was apprehensive, thinking she would not 'fit in', but after a while she relaxed and joined in with a number of activities. Mary lives on her own, with a weekly visit from her daughter-in-law.

After 3 months of attending the Day Hospice Mary started a course of chemotherapy, which caused a widespread itchy rash on her back. Because of her age her skin was very dry and wafer thin; she had been rubbing the area with a small stick to obtain relief from the itching, which had caused the skin to break and become sore, bleeding in places.

She was prescribed Conotrane cream by her GP, but after using it for more than 2 weeks there was no

improvement, so a nurse asked whether anything could be done with aromatherapy.

Intervention

A lotion was applied to the area morning and evening, containing:

- *Mentha* x *piperita* [peppermint] – soothing to irritated skin (in high dilution)
- *Santalum austrocaledonicum* [sandalwood] – dry skin
- *Commiphora myrrha* [myrrh], *Lavandula angustifolia* and *Matricaria recutita* [German chamomile] – anti-inflammatory, cicatrizant

Outcome

Within 2–3 days the itching had subsided. Mary continues to use the blend and has since had more chemotherapy sessions without the side effects of itchy skin.

Parkinson's disease

Aromatherapy can be of benefit in Parkinson's disease to promote general relaxation and relieve muscular rigidity. In a preliminary trials S Price (1993) used the following oils with a good measure of success (100% in two of the symptoms) and the blend was found to give relief to several symptomatic side effects. The aim was to achieve relaxation in the patients and help relieve anxiety, with the added effects of reducing pain, improving digestive functioning and aiding sleep.

Equal quantities of the three essential oils below were blended together and added at a concentration of 1.5% to either carrier oil for a weekly massage or base lotion for daily application:

- *Salvia sclarea* (clary) – relaxant, nerve tonic, phlebotonic
- *Origanum majorana* (sweet marjoram) – analgesic, antispasmodic, digestive tonic, hypotensor, nerve tonic, relaxant, sleep inducing
- *Lavandula angustifolia* – analgesic, antispasmodic, digestive stimulant, hypotensor, sedative, sleep inducing.

Muscular rigidity and changes in gait are a major difficulty for Parkinson's disease sufferers and aromatic baths have been found to be helpful (the use of a specialist hoist for bathing may be needed for safety). Regular massage to promote general relaxation will also help stimulate functional ability, and regular facial massage can help to relieve the lack of facial expression caused by neuromuscular change.

Summary

As people today are living well beyond three score years and ten, a greater number will probably develop some form of dementia, and the value of essential oils can be considerable – their aroma and specific chemical properties may be applied to many conditions and aspects of life and care.

Aromatherapy is an effective complementary therapy in the care of the elderly and is increasingly accepted at varying levels in care homes. The aromatic qualities of essential oils can be used to deliver their therapeutic qualities through vaporizers to improve the mood and atmosphere of the home, and are invaluable when used directly on clients for their individual needs. Aromatherapy and massage can provide a useful addition to psychological therapeutic interventions with clients suffering from dementia.

References

Alzheimer's Society Newsletter, 2004. February.

Ballard, C.G., O'Brien, J.T., Reichelt, K., Perry, E.K., 2002. Aromatherapy as a safe and effective treatment for the management of agitation in severe dementia: the results of a double-blind, placebo-controlled trial with melissa. J. Clin. Psychiatry 63 (7), 553–558.

Ballard, C., 2008. Translational Neuroscience. www.alzheimers.org.uk.

Basnyet, J., 1999. Aromatherapy Issue 39, April www.positivehealth.com.

Beshara, M.C., Giddings, D., 2003. Use of plant essential oils in treating agitation in a dementia unit: 10 case studies. Int. J. Aromather. 12, 207–212.

Bowles-Dilys, E.J., Griffiths, M., Quirk, L., et al., 2002. Effects of essential oils and touch on resistance to nursing care procedures and other dementia-related behaviours in a residential care facility. Int. J. Aromather. 12, 1–8.

Boyd, E.M., Pearson, G.L., 1946. The expectorant action of volatile oils. Am. J. Med. Sci. 211, 602–610.

Gilley, D.W., Whalen, M.E., Wilson, R.S., et al., 1991. Hallucinations and associated factors in Alzheimer's disease. J. Neuropsychiatr. 3, 497–500.

Henry, J., Rusius, C.W., Davies, M., 1994. Lavender for night sedation of people with dementia. Int. J. Aromather. 6 (2), 28–30.

Holmes, C., Hopkins, V., Hensford, C., 2002. Lavender oil as a treatment for agitated behaviour in severe dementia: a placebo controlled study. Int. J. Geriatr. Psychiatry 17, 305–308.

Hudson, R.T., 1996. The value of lavender for rest and activity in the elderly patient. Complement. Ther. Med. 4, 52–57.

Internet Health Library, 2006. Alternatives in Health 3, 4. www .internethealthlibrary.com.

Ketteringham, A., 2010. Alzheimer's Society comment (3rd Feb)www. alzheimers.org.uk.

Kilstoff, K., Chenoweth, L., 1998. New approaches to health and well-being for dementia day-care clients, family carers and day-care staff. Int. J. Nurs. Pract. 4, 70–83.

McKeith, I., 2010. www.alzheimers.org.uk.

Mental Health Foundation, 2010. Factsheet 403.

Mitchell, S., 1993. Aromatherapy's effectiveness in disorders associated with dementia. Int. J. Aromather. 4, 20–23.

Moss, M., Cook, J., Wesnes, K., Ducket, P., 2003. Aromas of rosemary and lavender essential oils differentially affect cognition and mood in healthy adults. Int. J. Neurosci. 113 (1), 15–38.

O'Haynes, O., 2010. www.ifaroma.org.

Passant, H., 1990. A holistic approach in the ward. Nurs. Times 86 (4), 26–28.

Perry, E., 2007. Aromatherapy for the treatment of Alzheimer's Disease. Journal of Quality Research in Dementia Issue 3.

Petit-Zeman, 2004. Sniffing out dementia. Alzheimer's Society Newsletter (February 8th) www. alzheimers.org.uk.

Price, S., 1993. Parkinson's disease project: is aromatherapy an effective treatment for Parkinson's disease? The Aromatherapist 1 (1), 14–21.

Rabins, P.V., Mace, N.L., Lucas, M.J., 1982. The impact of dementia on the family. J. Am. Med. Assoc. 248, 333–335.

Smallwood, J., Brown, R., Coulter, F., 2001. Aromatherapy and behaviour disturbances in dementia: a randomized controlled trial. Int. J. Geriatr. Psychiatry 16, 1010–1013.

Snow, L.A., Hovanec, L., Brandt, J., 2004. A controlled trial of aromatherapy for agitation in nursing home patients with dementia. J. Altern. Complement. Med. 10, 431–437.

Valnet, J., 1992. The practice of aromatherapy. Daniel, Saffron Walden.

Warner, J., 2006. More older adults affected by anxiety disorders than depression.

Wesson, D.W., Levy, E., Nixon, R.A., Wilson, D.A., 2010. Olfactory Dysfunction Correlates with Amyloid-β Burden in an Alzheimer's disease Mouse Model). J. Neurosci. 30 (2), 505–514.

Wingate, P., Wingate, R., 1996. Medical Encyclopedia. Penguin Books Ltd, London, p. 185.

www.alzheimers.org.uk.

www.betterhealth.vic.gov.au.

www.dementia2010.org.

www.nutrition-and-you.com2010.

Palliative and supportive care

Sue Whyte   Elaine Cooper

15

CHAPTER CONTENTS

Introduction

The approaches to palliative and supportive care are holistic; they differ in philosophy from curative strategies in that they focus primarily on the consequences of a disease rather than on its cause or specific cure – they are pragmatic and multidisciplinary, with very little distinction between palliation and support (National Council for Hospice and Specialist Palliative Care Services [NCHSPCS] 2000). This chapter gives an insight into palliative and supportive care, together with the use of essential oils. With the help of aromatherapy, people have enjoyed a quality of life better than they might otherwise have experienced.

Defining palliative and supportive care

Although originally written for those with cancer, the definitions of palliative and supportive care '...can be used for people with any life-threatening illness.' (National Council for Palliative Care [NCPC] 2010)

Supportive care helps patients and their families to cope with cancer and its treatment – through the process of diagnosis and treatment, to continuing illness, possible cure or death and into bereavement (NICE 2004). Where cure is not an option, care is focused on helping them through the difficult times ahead and maintaining optimum independence with the best quality of life possible. Supportive care is an integral part of palliative care.

Palliative care involves the total care of patients with advanced progressive illness which no longer responds to curative treatment. It is needed when the best quality of life for them and their families becomes the most important issue, and where the management of pain and other symptoms, and the provision of psychological, social and spiritual support, are paramount. Palliative care neither hastens nor postpones death: it merely recognizes a patient's right to spend as much time as possible at home, and pays equal attention to physical, psychological, social and spiritual aspects of care wherever the patient is (World Health Organization [WHO] 1990).

Palliative and supportive care does not see the patient in isolation but as part of a family unit – whatever that family unit might be. Many patients die in residential care where members of staff and other residents are part of the 'family': indeed, they may be the only 'family', and therefore experience the loss themselves. Those providing day-to-day care and support to patients and carers are facing the reality of death – it is often forgotten that they too need support.

Aromatherapists could teach a simple massage technique to these people – even the patient – to give them the opportunity to give and receive caring touch. It can be a transforming experience, as so often the loved ones feel helpless in not knowing how to show they care, or are frightened of 'doing the wrong thing'. Similarly, the patient often feels s/he is giving nothing in return for the love and care shown, and being able to participate in a simple massage can make a world of difference.

End of life care – the definition suggested by the NCPC states that: '....*all* those with advanced, progressive, incurable illness....' should be given such care. When this final stage begins is difficult to determine as it depends on many factors, not least on individual personal and professional points of view and the nature of the condition.

Decline at the end of life (see also, below, under Common characteristics) falls broadly into three main categories, those who will:

- remain in reasonably good health until shortly before death, with a steep decline in the last few weeks or months
- decline more gradually, with episodes of acute ill health
- be very frail for months or years before death with a steady, progressive decline

(Department of Health [DOH] 2008 End of Life Care Strategy).

Palliative and supportive care requires the expertise of a multidisciplinary team whose members include doctors, nurses, physiotherapists, occupational therapists, social workers, clergy, counsellors, complementary therapists etc., but to be effective it must be tailored to the needs of patients and their families. Often both palliative and supportive care are provided by the patient's family and other carers, and not exclusively by professionals (NICE 2004). The aromatherapist, even if treating a patient independently, is still part of the team and should recognize the importance of keeping the team informed of his/her part in the patient's care.

The disorders involved

Until now, palliative and supportive care has been largely confined to those with cancer – at least 50% of all patients in the UK with this condition will have had such care at some time in the course of their illness (Addington-Hall 1998). However, in developed countries more people die of chronic circulatory and respiratory conditions such as chronic heart disease (CHD), stroke and chronic obstructive pulmonary disease (COPD). Few palliative care services have focused on their needs or those of others with non-cancerous life-limiting conditions when they near the end of their life (NICE 2003; Ahmedzai 2006; Gore et al. 2000).

The ageing population is increasing rapidly – it is estimated that by 2033 in the UK, 23% of the population will be over the age of 65 (Office of National Statistics 2009). Many, if not most, will have two or more coexisting chronic conditions that will significantly impair their quality of life. Palliative and supportive care has now broadened to include all those with life-limiting conditions, notably:

- cancer
- infection with human immunodeficiency virus (HIV) and acquired immunodeficiency syndrome (AIDS)
- degenerative neurological disorders such as motor neuron disease (MND), multiple sclerosis (MS) and Parkinson's disease (PD)
- chronic circulatory conditions, including CHD and stroke
- chronic respiratory conditions, e.g. COPD
- chronic organ failure such as kidney and liver
- disorders that occur only in childhood, e.g. cystic fibrosis
- various genetic and congenital disorders, e.g. Huntington's disease

Common characteristics

These disorders have some or all of the following characteristics in common:

- an increased likelihood of fear, psychological, social and spiritual distresses
- unpredictable symptoms, which are always changing and can be very distressing. There will be good days and bad days, which can add to the frustrations and stress of the patient, family and carers

- a lack of understanding of these disorders by some healthcare workers and by society in general, can unwittingly contribute to the person's distress
- life-threatening, with shortened life expectancy – often quite significant, and the last phase of the illness probably being relatively short
- a 'life' pattern which can fluctuate quite markedly both in the individual and from person to person, e.g. there may be periods of remission, exacerbation or stability, or there may be a slow progressive decline; nevertheless, people may also appear fit and well with little or no change to their way of life
- the rate and manner of decline can fluctuate and varies considerably from person to person. The point comes when death is likely to occur in a matter of hours or days rather than weeks.

Symptoms

Below are some examples of distressing symptoms caused directly or indirectly by the disease or its treatment and commonly encountered in palliative care. Most, except possibly those marked with * can be helped or alleviated in some way by the essential oils listed alongside the individual symptoms in Appendix A II on the CD-ROM. More detailed information on the emotional aspects can be found in *Aromatherapy and Your Emotions* (Price 2000).

Physical examples

- Pain
- Fatigue – no energy – always feeling tired/weak
- Weight loss*/gain*
- Poor appetite – loss of interest in food – nothing tastes or smells the same
- Feeling sick most/all of the time – smells, especially food/or sight/thought of food
- Vomiting* with or without nausea/with or without effort
- Sleep problems – can't get to sleep/keep waking up
- Feeling out of breath all the time – and at rest/ can't breathe – panic attacks
- Mouth problems – dry – sore /ulcerated/infected – nasty taste
- Hot flushes/sweats
- Skin problems – dry/papery/marks or tears easily/ lesions/bruising/rashes/sore/red

- Wound/stoma smells/'I smell'
- Muscle spasms/rigidity/weakness/loss of control* – difficulty in swallowing*/dribbling of saliva*/ attacks of choking*
- Impaired speech*
- Loss of bladder control/constipation/diarrhoea
- reduced mobility – reduced dexterity
- Impaired sensation* – reduced/increased/altered – numbness/pins and needles
- Swollen limb(s)/swollen body
- Joint contractures*
- General impaired body function.

Psychosocial examples

- Shock and disbelief at the diagnosis, unable to make sense of what is happening – often described as 'a whirlpool of emotions'
- Anger and frustration with delays in diagnosis, etc.
- Anxiety and fear of pain, the unknown, death itself, how, when and where they will die, fear of being alone when that time comes
- Tense, depressed, anxious, frightened and panicky – not able to say why
- Feeling helpless and no longer in control
- Worry about the future, how will their loved ones cope, how will it affect them
- Loss, grief, appearance, independence, different future
- Feeling alone and isolated
- Confusion, including disorientation (usually associated with brain tumours or dementia, can be due to medication)
- Marked fluctuations in mood
- Withdrawing from people, not talking about their illness, keeping loved ones at a distance
- Low morale and self-esteem – 'can't be bothered', 'what's the point' etc.

Anxiety and panic

There is some evidence to show that aromatherapy massage can help relieve anxiety and aid relaxation (Hadfield 2001, Imanishi et al. 2007, Wilkinson et al. 2007). When patients are experiencing severe anxiety and panic there are many calming and sedative essential oils to choose from, such as *Chamaemelum nobile* [Roman chamomile], *Canarium luzonicum* (elemi), *Cananga odorata* [ylang ylang], *Citrus aurantium* var *amara* per. [orange bigarade] and

Case 15.1

Pain relief

Elaine Cooper – Aromatologist

Assessment

Jane is married with school-aged children and worked as a cleaner. At 47 years of age a small lump was growing on her right hip. She was diagnosed with neurofibrosarcoma and received radiotherapy followed by chemotherapy.

Jane has now developed bone metastases in the hips, ribs and sternum, and is aware that her disease is incurable. She attends NHS day hospice one day per week for supportive and palliative care; she has increasing pain and tenderness over her sternum and shoulder. Sleep was poor because of the pain despite medication of fentanyl patch 25 mg, diclofenac 50 mg and morphine liquid 10 mg for breakthrough pain.

The worst pain was in her shoulder and she could not relax or sleep because of it; her mood was very low. Jane had several swellings and many small lumps in her tissues.

Intervention

Massage was out of the question, so it was decided to use an essential oil compress on the shoulder, blending essential oils of:

- *Origanum majorana* [sweet marjoram] – calming to the nervous system, analgesic for aching muscles
- *Juniperus communis* (fruct) [juniper berry] – helpful for painful joints and insomnia
- *Chamaemelum nobile* [Roman chamomile] – sedative, anti-inflammatory.

After 10 minutes she looked comfortable and relaxed, with no response when spoken to softly.

Outcome

Jane slept for a half hour, and on waking she felt relaxed and had less pain, telling the day hospice manager and her husband (with a smile) how much better she felt. Jane has a compress applied weekly at the day hospice and has a blended lotion containing the above oils plus *Lavandula angustifolia* to apply daily at home on areas of pain and to aid sleep. This intervention was simple and gave effective symptom relief.

Citrus reticulata [mandarin] (also see Appendix B.9 on the CD-ROM). The patient can be asked to choose the aroma they find the most pleasing from a small selection of single oils, and/or a blend of two or three.

Patients can be given a 10 mL bottle of the chosen oil/s blended in a carrier to use themselves on pulse points during periods of anxiety. If they feel a panic attack pending they can inhale the oils from an inhaler stick or a tissue – many patients have experienced a reduction in anxiety simply by inhaling their chosen oil. Elaine Cooper has worked closely with a clinical psychologist in oncology and palliative care where she works in an NHS palliative care team, with referrals requesting to aid relaxation and reduce anxiety with aromatherapy, and there have been some outstanding results with some patients.

Essential oils chosen most frequently are *Rosa damascena* [rose otto], *Citrus aurantium* var. *amara* flos [neroli], *Boswellia carteri* [frankincense], *Lavandula angustifolia* and *Chamaemelum nobile* [Roman chamomile].

Spirituality

Being confronted with their own mortality often makes a person turn inwards and question their innermost thoughts, beliefs and values in an attempt to make sense of what is happening. The less a person is able to do physically, the more time they have for thinking, which can lead to much anguish and torment. Aromatherapy treatment may afford help in spiritual care, bringing comfort and peace in the form of deep relaxation. Patients may then be able to focus on their own spirituality. Essential oils that would help here are those which are both uplifting and soothing, analgesic and/or tonic to the heart, relieving any fears, e.g. *Boswellia carteri* [frankincense], *Chamaemelum nobile* [Roman chamomile], *Citrus bergamia* [bergamot], *Lavandula angustifolia* [lavender], *Ocimum basilicum* [sweet European basil] and *Origanum majorana* [sweet marjoram] (Price 2000; Tisserand 1992).

For the patient and their family, social problems and issues arise from the changes and adjustments that have to be faced in their relationships and daily life, whether they are temporary or permanent.

Pain – an example of the complex nature of a symptom

According to Twycross and Lack (1984) the perception of pain is modulated by the patient's mood and morale, the meaning of pain to the patient and the

Case 15.2

Fungating lesion

Sarah Wright – Aromatherapist

Assessment

This patient, who took pride in her appearance, had cancer of the vulva, with local spread causing a fungating lesion in her left groin. She was very distressed by this, due to its appearance and the malodour, of which she was very conscious and tried to disguise it with perfume.

Intervention

The aromatherapist discussed the use of essential oils to disguise odour and the patient was happy for any help she could get. Oils were chosen together, selecting the aromas she liked. The aromatherapist advised the use of more than one oil to increase the efficacy through synergy. The essential oils chosen were:

- *Lavandula* x *intermedia* [lavandin] – antiseptic, deodorant, calming, cicatrizant
- *Citrus aurantium* var. *sinensis* [sweet orange] – antiseptic, calming
- *Myristica fragrans* [nutmeg] – deodorant, analgesic, antibacterial

- *Cupressus sempervirens* [cypress] – deodorant, antiseptic, antibacterial

The patient was provided with a 5 mL bottle of each and instructed to use two drops on a tissue to inhale as needed, or tuck it into her clothes near to the wound. Written instructions were also provided.

To help aid relaxation, shoulder massage was carried out in a 1% dilution in sweet almond oil with:

- *Citrus paradisi* [grapefruit] – refreshing,
- *Boswellia carteri* [frankincense] – analgesic, anti-inflammatory, cicatrizant.

Outcome

The following week the patient reported that she had coped much better with the odour from her wound, had enjoyed using the oils and felt more confident when in company.

The patient enjoyed and looked forward to her massage, feeling relaxed and calm after a treatment; she felt pampered and more 'normal', despite suffering such a disfiguring disease.

---

fact that pain may remain intractable if mental and social factors are ignored (see Box 15.1).

Pain is a warning of actual or potential tissue damage or pathology and creates some muscle tension (guarding) to protect the area. It elicits an arousal and an emotional response, and is modified by mental state and emotions (Marieb 1998). Most people with pain usually become anxious about the possible implications; this leads to more muscle tension, and muscle tension increases the pain that increases the emotional response, and so on, each perpetuating the other into a vicious circle that can become a spiralling process (McCaffery & Beebe 1989).

Localized pain and essential oils

Massage with analgesic essential oils brings its own benefits, but if massage is not advisable the application of essential oils in a lotion – or with a compress or spray – can also bring a reduction in pain.

Factors to be considered that might be contributing to the pain include inflammation, tension, swelling or nerve involvement etc. A significant reduction in pain may possibly be achieved by using the following.

Oils containing esters and sesquiterpenes, which are generally regarded to be anti-inflammatory, antispasmodic and calming, making them very useful for pain, include *Chamaemelum nobile* [Roman chamomile], *Lavandula angustifolia* [lavender] and *Citrus aurantium* var. *amara* (fol) [neroli].

Box 15.1

Some factors affecting pain threshold

Threshold lowered by:	Threshold raised by:
Discomfort	Relief of symptoms
Insomnia	Sleep
Fatigue	Rest
Anxiety	Sympathy
Fear	Understanding
Anger	Companionship
Sadness	Diversional activity
Depression	Reduction of anxiety
Boredom	Elevation of mood
Introversion	Analgesics
Mental isolation	Anxiolytics
Social abandonment	Antidepressants

Pogostemon patchouli [patchouli] and *Commiphora myrrha* [myrrh] are also anti-inflammatory, and *Lavandula angustifolia* [lavender] and *Zingiber officinale* [ginger] are useful for their analgesic properties.

Where there is pain combined with anxiety or depression Cooper has found a blend of *Boswellia carteri* and *Commiphora myrrha* to be most helpful.

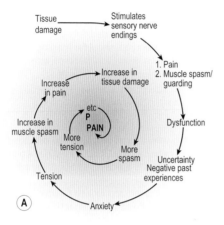

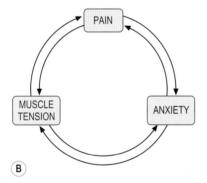

Figure 15.1 • Pain spiral. From McCaffery and Beeb 1989.

From observing, listening and talking to patients over many years, Whyte believes that the principle of the pain spiral (see Figure 15.1) may apply to other physical symptoms the patient may experience. Similarly, their general outlook on life will contribute to their mood and confidence; the coping strategies they use – and their personality – do not usually change because they are ill, although they may subsequently do so. The effects of the close, subtle interplay between the physical, psychological, social and spiritual aspects should never be underestimated. Any negative factors in the person's life will lower their tolerance level to symptoms, whereas positive

ones will raise it. Most people, when in low spirits, find that everything seems to be worse; likewise, when feeling full of the joys of spring, they can cope with anything. Illness is no different. However, even the most cheerful and positive of people can be knocked off balance and succumb to physical symptoms that nothing seems to ease. For example, feeling sick all the time – made worse by the sight, smell and sometimes even just the thought of certain things – can be a major problem for some patients, making them more anxious and distressed.

In Ch. 7, Price discusses the effects that essential oils have on the emotions, which may or may not be a placebo response: according to Tisserand, if a smell is appealing, it soothes the mind (Tisserand 1992 p. 99). Placebo or not, if the experience of aromatherapy is pleasant and relaxing, even for a short time, it will surely have some beneficial effect on the patient's mood and morale long enough to interrupt the vicious circle, thus helping them relax (Hadfield 2001), enhancing factors that raise a person's tolerance level to their situation. This has a dual effect:

- it enables the patient to cope more effectively with their illness and day to day problems
- by reducing stress alone, pressure on the immune system is lessened (Alexander 2001, Fujiwara et al. 2002, Kuriyama et al. 2005).

Evidence from various studies discussed and cited by Tavares (2003) is encouraging, as it supports much of the anecdotal evidence given in many books and articles regarding the positive effect aromatherapy and massage can have on symptoms and quality of life (Bowers 2006, Corner et al. 1995; Downer et al. 1994; Gatti & Cajola 1923; Grealish et al. 2000; Lee & Lee 1992; Pan et al. 2000; Wilkinson et al. 1999; Wilkinson S. et al. 2007).

Aromatherapy intervention

Cancer, HIV/AIDS, MND etc. are not in themselves a contraindication to massage or aromatherapy treatment. Irrespective of the disorder, holistic principles still apply – it is the person who is being treated, not the disease. This does not mean that specific problems cannot sometimes be helped by the judicious use of essential oils with or without massage. If in doubt, do not treat the person without discussing the situation with an experienced aromatherapist working in palliative care, nursing or medical staff. In many cases the doctor or nurse will have limited understanding of the use of massage and essential oils, unless the practice of aromatherapy has been established in the service. There is, however, a growing number of specialist aromatherapists who have worked in palliative care for many years who may be contacted through the local hospice or professional aromatherapy organizations such as IFPA or the National Association of Complementary Therapists in Hospice and Palliative Care (NACTHPC).

Nevertheless, when a patient is expecting aromatherapy, it is important that they receive some form of treatment, providing it is safe and likely to give benefit. If it is unsuitable, an explanation should be given as to why, along with possible alternatives or an appropriate referral.

Aromatherapists need to be sensitive to complex situations and be able to adapt their approach and treatments accordingly. Working with patients in palliative care requires some knowledge and understanding of the disease processes, the medical interventions involved, and how these affect patients and their families. This will then enable the therapist to assess a patient fully and determine the most appropriate aromatherapy treatment.

- Referrals to the aromatherapy service may be for either the patient or the carer, and may come from the patient or carer themselves, a family member or a health professional. Where patients are seen will depend on the particular setting in which the therapist is working, and how the service is organized.

Use of essential oils

Essential oils may be considered safe, as they are used in low concentrations. However, where a boost is needed, the careful clinical application of a higher concentration has proved safe and effective.

Although there is no conclusive evidence that some oils have oestrogen-like properties, it is preferable to err on the side of caution in their use with patients who have oestrogen-dependent tumours (Tisserand & Balacs 1995, Sheppard-Hanger et al. 1994). If there is doubt about the significance of any symptoms and signs found during consultation or the safety of using essential oils and/or massage, the aromatherapist must discuss this with the other professionals on the team.

A 'nite-lite' vaporizer with a naked flame is not permitted in hospitals, but may be encountered in the home. It should always be placed in a safe position and never left unattended.

Cautions and contraindications

As the purpose of aromatherapy is to bring a net gain to patients, weighing up any contraindications to the use of essential oils or massage against the potential benefits is very important, especially at a distressing time for a patient.

- Some diseases and/or their treatments can alter a person's sense of smell and taste, the fragrance of some essential oils perhaps being intensely disliked; although some patients are able to tolerate oils which may bring relief, others find even pleasant smells abhorrent.
- Nausea may be a contraindication, especially if severe or likely to be recurrent, because:
  ○ just the thought of smelling anything can be nauseating
  ○ an essential oil (smell) given to relieve nausea – especially if repeated – may at a later date evoke unpleasant memories and/or precipitate nausea and vomiting, i.e. the Pavlov response. The likelihood of this happening is reduced if a blend of two to four oils is used, e.g. *Pimpinella anisum, Foeniculum vulgare var. dulce* [sweet fennel], *Mentha x piperita* [peppermint] and *Anthemis nobilis* [Roman chamomile] (Gilligan 2005).
- Account should be taken of the possible adverse effect the aroma might have on other patients in the room.
- Seizures and epileptic fits can be precipitated by smells – check with staff or family if this is a possibility.
- Skin allergies or sensitivities: patients undergoing palliative chemotherapy often have increased skin sensitivity – if in doubt do a patch test first.
- Be aware of patients with asthma or other respiratory conditions, as volatile substances can precipitate coughing or aggravate breathing difficulty. However, chosen with care, essential oils can bring fast relief. They can help panic attacks associated with severe breathing difficulties (both Whyte and Cooper have found that *Myrtus communis* [green myrtle] inhaled from a tissue has a calming effect on breathing, especially when severe anxiety is present.
- Cooper has found the following essential oil blend to be useful for respiratory symptoms that occur

frequently in lung cancer – shortness of breath, discomfort, upper body tension, potential infection and coughing:

- *Pinus sylvestris* [pine], *Cedrus atlantica* [cedarwood], *Boswellia carteri* [frankincense] and *Melaleuca viridiflora* [niaouli] (see also Appendix A2 on the CD-ROM).
- The essential oil blend alone can be used in inhalation; it can also be put into carrier oil for gentle upper body massage or into a lotion as a chest rub. Using these methods, patients have frequently reported less upper body tension and discomfort, easier breathing and a feeling of control. Having something to use themselves which is not a medical intervention and for which they have a choice appears to empower the person.
- Another blend, *Picea mariana* [black spruce] and *Abies balsamea* [Canadian balsam], can be useful for inhalation by breathless, fatigued patients.

Massage

There is confusion in many people's minds concerning the use of massage with those who have cancer. Books and courses often say that it is contraindicated, yet massage and aromatherapy are two of the most popular and frequently used therapies in palliative and supportive care (Lewith et al. 2002, Macmillan 2002). This paradoxical situation has arisen because many believe that massage can spread cancer cells through the body by stimulating the lymphatic and vascular circulation. Breathing and the normal physical activity of daily life also stimulate the flow of blood and lymph, and if patients feel well enough they are encouraged to take exercise within their own tolerance level (Sikora K personal communication). Massage would appear to be safe as long as it is gentle and pressure over tumour sites and lymph glands is avoided (Holey &Cook 2003, McNamara 2004).

Unless people with a chronic illness are fairly robust physically and feeling reasonably well, it is unlikely they would tolerate a whole body massage, and in those who can, it would probably be modified – omitting particular areas such as the abdomen or chest. For others, it is more likely to be a part body massage such as the feet or back and shoulders etc., or, in the case of the very frail, holding hands and perhaps stroking.

Contraindications to massage (see also Ch. 8)

In the situations listed below, unaffected areas can be massaged, e.g. the hands or feet, a careful, light 'holding touch' can be comforting if tolerated. Remember too, that compresses, sprays or inhalation can all be used when massage is not appropriate:

- unexplained lumps, bumps, swelling or areas of heat – these may be disease related and need to be discussed with the patient's doctor
- areas where there is unexplained pain, especially over bones, as this may indicate spread of disease to the bone, especially in cancer
- high fever, infection or sepsis, as there is a risk of spreading infection, making the patient feel worse
- areas of the body receiving radiotherapy (and for up to 5 or 6 weeks afterwards), as the skin is extra sensitive after treatment. However, massage with essential oils such as *Melaleuca viridiflora* [niaouli] is recommended a short time (not immediately) before treatment, to strengthen the area (Franchomme & Pénoel 2001 p. 398), but only after discussing it with the patient's oncologist and radiotherapist to obtain their permission. (See also Appendix A1 on the CD-ROM, *Melaleuca viridiflora*, observations.)
- a limb or foot where deep vein thrombosis (DVT) is suspected or recently diagnosed – there may be general swelling of the part, with redness and cramp-like pain. People with advanced progressive disease are more susceptible to DVT, especially when they are frail, ill, and have reduced mobility, and it might be there without symptoms (Johnson et al. 1999)
- skin lesions, rashes, recent scar tissue; a red, painful and inflamed patch could indicate cellulitis
- stoma sites, catheters, medication patches; TENS machine pads, syringe driver cannulae and tubing or any other attached medical device
- certain conditions of the heart, lungs, kidneys and liver, as well as cancers, can cause oedema (swelling) of the limbs or other parts of the body – massage could further compromise the heart and lungs
- muscle spasm, rigidity and pain in neurological conditions such as MND, MS and PD: Tavares (2003 p. 34) suggests that massage may be contraindicated, as it can provoke or increase the spasm. However, if tolerated, light gentle treatment has been found to be beneficial.

Use massage with caution in the following circumstances:

- the presence of petechiae on the skin (pin-prick bruising, which indicates a low platelet count); use gentle stroking, or light holding touch only, unless working in a specialist area and able to discuss this with the medical team (Tavares 2003)
- limbs or areas with lymphoedema, when direction and pressure (lack of) are important. Without previous experience, it may be advisable to work in conjunction with a lymphoedema nurse specialist or physiotherapist (Tavares 2003)
- possible side effects of radiotherapy, which can include sore skin, fatigue and local effects depending on the site of irradiation, e.g. neck area (may result in sore, dry mouth and difficulty in swallowing); stomach area (digestive disturbances)
- avoid radiotherapy entry and exit sites for 3–6 weeks, as the effect on the skin is dose related
- frail patients, or those suffering side effects of treatment (see above); massage should be modified in relation to the duration of treatment, the pressure used and the area of the body to be worked on.

Changes affecting treatment

The aromatherapist needs to be aware of situations – some fortunately very rare – that might arise while treating a patient. They need to know what action to take, and who to inform should there be any change in the patient's condition. The aromatherapist may be the only person who has an opportunity of seeing changes in parts of the patient's body normally covered with clothing, such as skin lesions or swellings. Consultation with the professional team will decide what changes need to be referred, whom to notify when necessary, and what advice to give patients who report a change in their condition, which could include:

- recurrence of pain
- nausea and/or vomiting
- breathlessness or other breathing problems, severe panic attacks or choking
- epileptic fit or other form of seizure (usually associated with brain tumours).

Rare occurrences are:

- haemorrhage: this can be via the mouth, due to coughing or vomiting; from the stomach, nose, vagina, rectum; or from the site of a stoma or wound
- pathological fracture – usually associated with bony cancer metastases
- spinal cord compression occurs in 5–10% of people with cancer (Doyle et al. 1999) and is a neurological emergency. Symptoms may be present for weeks or may occur suddenly, and include pins and needles, sensory loss and weakness (usually in the lower extremities), starting in the feet and moving upwards. If this remains untreated paralysis will ensue, so urgent medical advice should be sought.

Aromatherapists should be able to support the patient through any distressing emotions that may arise, and also be aware of other available options for support and the means of referral. (Those who work in palliative and supportive care, including aromatherapists, may need support themselves, and some form of supervision may be available in their area.)

Therapists should at all times recognize and acknowledge not only their own limitations but also those of aromatherapy, and should know when to refer a patient.

Preventing cross-infection

As a result of their condition and/or treatments, patients' immune systems are often highly compromised, making them more vulnerable to infection. This is more likely to occur when they are debilitated. It is incumbent on therapists to make themselves familiar with universal infection control procedures if they are working in an environment such as a hospital or hospice, where they may come into contact with patients' body fluids. Similarly, if treating people with infections such as methicillin-resistant *Staphylococcus aureus* (MRSA), advice should be sought on local infection control procedures.

An aromatherapist in good health with good energy levels, following a high standard of hygiene and infection control practices, will have a minimal risk of cross-infection. To prevent this, aromatherapists should follow basic hygiene practices at all times, the most important being thorough hand washing before and after treating a patient (even if gloves have been used), plus the judicious use of essential oils, many of which have been proved to suppress *S. aureus* and other microorganisms (Moon, Wilkinson, & Cavanagh 2006, Williams et al. 1998, Caelli et al. 2000).

Essential oil blends

The following information is based on Cooper's experience over more than 16 years of using essential oils in an NHS integrated supportive and palliative care service:

Mouth ulcers due to chemotherapy or disease in the mouth

5 mL *Calendula officinalis* macerated [marigold] – promotes healing and reduces inflammation (Fleischner 1985, ESCOP, 2003, Price & Price 2008)

2 drops *Commiphora myrrha* [myrrh] – contains a high proportion of anti-inflammatory and slightly analgesic sesquiterpenes and antiseptic alcohols

Apply 1 drop directly to the mouth ulcer using a cotton bud three times a day.

Candida in the mouth

1 drop *Aniba rosaeodora* [rosewood] (or *Melaleuca alternifolia* [tea tree]) in honey and water – to be used as a mouth rinse 3–5 times a day.

Tea tree is perfect for treating mucous membrane infections of the mouth and gums, and for *Candida*-related infections (Schnaubelt 1998). Rosewood contains up to 90% alcohols, which are antifungal, antiseptic and free from irritation.

Vaginal *Candida*

3 drops *Aniba rosaeodora* – antifungal, anti-infectious, antiviral

2 drops *Lavandula angustifolia* [lavender] – antiviral, antiseptic

Use in the bath frequently and in white lotion for direct application.

Malodour due to discharging or fungating wounds

The following oils appear to be useful in practice although they have not been tested for their odour fighting effects.

Vaporize *Thymus vulgaris* ct. thymol, ct. linalool [sweet thyme] with *Eucalyptus citriodora* [lemon scented gum], or *Citrus bergamia* [bergamot] with *Lavandula angustifolia*

As an alternative or addition to vaporization, place a few drops of the oils on a pad and place over the top of any wound dressings.

Case 15.3

Dry cracked skin on feet and legs

Rachel Clark – Aromatherapist

Assessment

Mrs B (62) was diagnosed with chronic obstructive pulmonary disease. She used to be active and finds it difficult to cope with the present loss of independence. She is on portable oxygen, enabling her to get out of the house, but is frustrated by being unable to do things she would like to do and wants to get back to work. Mrs B becomes very breathless on exertion and feels panicky in enclosed spaces; most of her joints ache, she aches particularly in her chest, and gets cramp regularly (a side effect of seretide inhalers).

Mrs B has suffered with painful, cracked and dry skin on her feet and elbows for the last 2½ years, during which time she has tried numerous proprietary lotions and creams, with little or no relief.

Intervention

An aromatherapy blend was prescribed for her to apply morning and night:

70 mL white carrier lotion, 20 mL shea butter and 10 mL *Calendula officinalis* (to aid healing) were blended to create an emollient base to retain moisture. Essential oils added were:
- 5 drops *Lavandula angustifolia* – antibacterial, anti-inflammatory
- 5 drops *Boswellia carteri* [frankincense] – calming, anti-inflammatory, cicatrizant
  2 drops *Melaleuca alternifolia* [tea tree] – antifungal, anti-inflammatory, phlebotonic
- 2 drops of *Santalum album* [sandalwood] – skin healing (anecdotal evidence).

Outcome

Mrs B used the cream twice daily for 3 months, the improvement being noticeable after 2 weeks, and the texture of her skin gradually improved. She now uses the blend less often: the skin on her legs, feet and elbows is visibly better. She is pleased with the result and was able to enjoy Christmas free from the usual discomfort and pain.

Pruritus (skin itching)

A specific blend of essential oils may be combined with a lotion base for symptoms that may not be responding to medical treatment, for example itchy skin complaints, or to help with pain relief (Clark, 2010).

In 15 years Cooper has not found anything better than the Shirley Price's recipe of *Santalum album*, *Lavandula angustifolia* and *Mentha* x *piperita* in white lotion; she uses it extensively for pruritus associated with liver disease and jaundice. It often gives more relief than any prescribed medication, and patients frequently say it is the best relief they have had. The excellent effect is well known in the Walsall area, with Macmillan nurses, hospice nurses and palliative care consultants all requesting it for their patients.

For patients with a sensitivity to menthol, *Anthemis nobilis* [Roman chamomile] has been used to good effect in place of *Mentha piperita*.

The following blends have been used by the specialist complementary therapy team in NHS Walsall working with Cooper after receiving positive evaluation and feedback from users.

Bone/joint pain or discomfort

A blend of 50 mL carrier lotion with the following essential oils has consistently proved effective in relieving this type of pain.

> *Commiphora myrrha* [myrrha] – anti-inflammatory
>
> *Boswellia carteri* [frankincense] – analgesic, anti-inflammatory
>
> *Melaleuca viridiflora* [niaouli] – analgesic, anti-inflammatory

In an audit carried out in NHS Walsall during 2009 it gave partial or good relief to 100% of patients who used it, being the only one in the audit to give relief to all users (see Box 15.2).

Box 15.2

NHS Community Health – Complementary Therapy Audit

Aromatherapy Prescription Blends audit – April 2009 – December 2009

Aromatherapy blends are given to patients as a support to symptom control in cancer care, palliative and end of life care.

Standard blends developed by the team have previously shown effectiveness to help relieve the following common problems: anxiety, insomnia, bone/joint pain, dry skin, pruritus (itching) and hot flushes.

Other blends are provided for other symptoms or for the above problems as an alternative if needed.

Each blend is based on the chemical components present in essential oils and these are blended to give the best synergy and chemical combination for optimum therapeutic effect.

Reasons for the audit

a) To discover to what degree patients felt the blend had relieved their problem or symptom, i.e. good relief, partial relief, no relief or made symptoms worse

b) To discover if the patients experienced any negative side effects from the prescription blend

c) To obtain patients' comments of the effectiveness of aromatherapy blends supplied by the complementary therapy team

A simple audit questionnaire was developed and given to each patient who received a blend (see Box 15.3).

Sample of comments made by patients on audit questionnaires

- Excellent service and I would like to thank the NHS for making it available.
- The blends helped with relaxation – I did not feel so tense after using blends.
- Inhaling the oil gives me an uplifting experience and relieves the nausea.
- Eases pain – no analgesic pain killers taken now due to this cream.
- It does help with sleeping.
- Feels much more comfortable, skin less dry, less itching and feet no longer feel like the skin is cracking – appear better visually.
- Just to say thank you for this cream – it really works. Thank you for the therapy and such fantastic service and staff.
- Very effective to help with nausea after chemotherapy.
- Very pleasant smell and very easy to use, easily absorbed – helps peripheral neuropathy.

Findings and recommendations

The outcome of the audit is extremely positive, indicating that patients welcome these complementary approaches as a beneficial supportive treatment option in their care. Figures from the audit indicate that 91% of patients had relief

Continued

from symptoms by using these blends, 58% had good relief and 33% had some relief. Only two patients out of 139 answered yes to negative effects as a result of using blends.

It appears that individual blending for patients on a one to one basis is slightly more effective than standard blending. The team recommends, however, that all but one standard blend should continue to be used as the success rate is good.

The blend provided for bone and joint pain gave relief to 100% of patients, which may indicate a case for further research, as some patients felt that it was better than non steroidal anti-inflammatory drugs.

It is recommended that:

- the standard blend for hot flushes be removed as this appears to be the least effective
- individual aromatherapy blends should continue to be provided on a needs basis
- the therapist should use their professional judgement in deciding on a standard or individual blend.

Box 15.3

Results for standard blends

	Good relief	Partial relief	No relief
Sleep blend	11	12	2
Dry skin	2	0	0
Bone/joint pain	6	14	0
Pruritus/itching	5	0	1
Sweats/flushes	0	3	1
Anxiety	2	1	1
Total 61	26	30	5
Other blends			
Total 93	63	21	9
Total blends			
Total 153	89	50	14

Results for standard blends are as follows

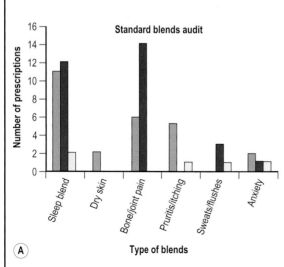

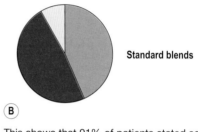

B

This shows that 91% of patients stated some relief, 43% being good and 48% being partial; 8% showed no relief.

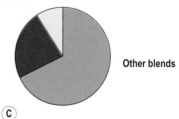

C

Other non-standard blends as above showed 91% of patients reporting some relief from symptoms: 68% received good relief, 23% partial relief and 9% indicated no relief.

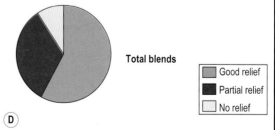

D

Overall blends indicated by patients: 58% gave good relief, 33% gave partial relief and 9% gave no relief. This shows that 91% of patients had some relief of symptoms from treatment with aromatherapy blends.

Case 15.4

Myeloma

Gill Price – Aromatherapist

Assessment

Sarah (52) was diagnosed with myeloma. She was low in mood, tearful, suffering from anxiety, and had considerable pain in her shoulders. In 2002 she received radiotherapy and spinal surgery with rods and plates, and also had a spinal fusion of T4–T7.

Intervention

A course of reflexology did not help the pain. Aromatherapy was tried to help reduce the discomfort between the shoulders and the pain to the right shoulder and side of neck.

A blend of essential oils in sunflower oil was used.

- *Zingiber officinalis* [ginger] – analgesic, general tonic
- *Citrus limon* [lemon] – anti-inflammatory, calming
- *Origanum majorana* [marjoram] – analgesic, calming.

Gentle effleurage was given to the upper back and trapezius muscle, which was very hard and tense. After a few minutes Sarah commented that she could feel the heat penetrating the muscle and she began to relax.

For 5 weeks Sarah had a weekly 20-minute massage treatment and was given a lotion incorporating the same oils for use every morning and evening.

Outcome

Sarah reported a significant reduction in pain in her right shoulder and upper back; she also appreciated the feeling of wellbeing gained from the treatment.

Case 15.5

Skin soreness

Tracey Dickie – Aromatherapist

Client assessment

T was a 75-year-old man diagnosed with cancer of the larynx; he had had surgery for tumour removal 6 months ago and had completed a course of radiotherapy to the neck and right side of his face. He was now 7 days post radiotherapy.

T's main complaint was a soreness and burning sensation to his face and neck, which meant he was unable to shave. This upset him greatly, as he took pride in his appearance: wearing a shirt and tie was difficult as this rubbed on the skin on his neck. Use of an aqueous cream had not helped.

Intervention

An aromatherapy blend was mixed to alleviate T's discomfort and was applied twice daily to his cheeks, chin and neck for 1 week.

- 60 g aloe vera gel – soothing to the skin
- 30 drops *Chamaemelum nobile* [Roman chamomile] – anti-inflammatory, soothes irritation.

Outcome

A week later T was clean shaven and wearing his tie. The gel had provided relief from the burning and soreness (he said 'the scent wasn't too bad either'!). T continued to use the gel for 1 month, reducing the application to once daily, after which he discontinued it. No further soreness of burning sensation was experienced.

Dry, cracked, fingertips (often seen as a side effect of cancer drug treatments)

Excellent results were achieved from a blend of:

100 mL carrier lotion, 25 mL shea butter and 15 mL calendula oil with 5 drops each of the following analgesic, anti-inflammatory and cicatrizant oils:

Boswellia carteri [frankincense] and *Lavandula angustifolia*

2 drops of *Melaleuca alternifolia* [Tea tree] – also anti-infectious

2 drops *Santalum album* [sandalwood] – anti-infectious, decongestant and moisturizing to the skin.

Evaluation stated relief of symptoms in 48 hours.

Further use of this blend has proved helpful for very dry skin and also on patients prone to cellulites; definite improvements were noted.

Inflamed sore, cracked, fingers and toes (Possible side effect of chemotherapy tablets)

90 mL carrier lotion, 10 mL evening primrose oil with 5 drops each of:

Rosa damascena [rose otto] – anti-infectious, anti-inflammatory, cicatrizant

Santalum album – properties as above

Pelargonium graveolens [geranium] – analgesic, anti-infectious, anti-inflammatory, antiseptic, cicatrizant

Good results have been achieved after 7 days use of this blend – hands softened and healed and feet able to be walked on again.

Summary

With its popularity continuing to grow, aromatherapy is one of the three most frequently used complementary therapies provided by hospices and palliative care units in the UK – the other two being massage and reflexology (Wilkes 1992; Macmillan Cancer Relief 2002).

The effects of caring touch should never be underestimated, the shared experience between the giver and the recipient being to their mutual benefit. Aromatherapy massage and therapeutic touch are pleasant, non-clinical experiences, and the use of essential oils provides another clinical tool in healthcare practice, giving both professionals and patients a further choice along the healing or therapeutic pathway.

References

Addington-Hall, J., 1998. Reaching out: specialist palliative care services for older adults with non-malignant diseases. NCHPCS, London.

Ahmedzai, S.H., 2006. COPD and Palliative and Supportive care. NHS Evidence–respiratory. Respiratory Specialist Library.

Alexander, M., 2001. Aromatherapy and immunity: how the use of essential oils aids immune potentiality. Int. J. Aromather. 11 (4), 220–224.

Bowers, L.J., 2006. To what extent does aromatherapy use in palliative care improve quality of life and reduce levels of psychological distress? A literature review. Int. J. Aromather. 16 (1), 27–35.

Caelli, M., Porteous, J., Carson, C.F., Heller, R., Riley, T.V., 2000. Tea tree oil as an alternative topical decolonisation agent for methicillin-resistant *Staphylococcus aureus*. J. Hosp. Infect. 46 (2000), 236–237.

Clark, R., 2010. Care of the dying and deceased patient. A practical guide for nurses. P. Jevon, (Ed.), Wiley Blackwell, UK.

Corner, J., Cawley, N., Hildebrand, S., 1995. An evaluation of the use of massage and essential oils on the well-being of cancer patients. Int. J. Palliat. Nurs. 1 (2), 67–73.

DoH, 2008. End of Life Care Strategy – promoting high quality care for all adults at the end of life. Department of Health, London.

Downer, S.M., Cody, M.M., McCluskey, P., Wilson, P.D., Arnott, S.J., Lister, T.A., et al., 1994. Pursuit and practice of complementary therapies by cancer patients receiving conventional treatment. Br. Med. J. 309 (6947), 86–89.

Doyle, D., Hanks, W.C., MacDonald, N. (Eds.), 1999. Oxford Textbook of Palliative Medicine. second ed. Oxford University Press, Oxford, p. 729.

Escop, 2003. vol. 3. Proposals for European monographs on *Calendulae flos / Flos cum herba*.

Fleischner, A.M., 1985. Plant extracts: to accelerate healing and reduce inflammation. Cosmetics ad Toiletries 100, 45.

Franchomme, P., Pénoël, D., 2001. l'Aromathérapie exactement. Jallois, Limoges.

Fujiwara, R., Komori, T., Yokoyama, M.M., 2002. Psychoneuroimmunological benefits of aromatherapy. Int. J. Aromather. 12 (2), 77–82.

Gatti, G., Cajola, R., 1923. L'azione della essenze sul sysema nervosa. Rivista Italiana delle Essenze e Profumi 5 (12), 133–135.

Gilligan, N.P., 2005. The palliation of nausea in hospice and palliative care patients with essential oils of *Pimpinella anisum* [aniseed], *Foeniculum vulgare var. dulce* [sweet fennel], *Anthemis nobilis* [Roman chamomile] and *Mentha x piperita* [peppermint]. Int. J. Aromather. 15, 163–167.

Gore, J.W., Brophy, C.J., Greenstone, M.A., 2000. How well do we care for patients with end stage chronic obstructive pulmonary disease (COPD)? A comparison of palliative care and quality of life in COPD and lung cancer. Thorax 55, 1000–1006.

Grealish, L., Lomansney, A., Whiteman, B., 2000. Foot massage. Cancer Nurs. 23 (3), 237–243.

Hadfield, N., 2001. The role of aromatherapy massage in reducing anxiety in patients with malignant brain tumours. Int. J. Palliat. Nurs. 7 (6), 279–285.

Holey, E., Cook, E., 2003. Evidence-Based Therapeutic Massage a practical guide for therapists. Churchill Livingstone.

Imanishi, J., et al., 2007. Anxiolytic Effect of Aromatherapy Massage in Patients with Breast Cancer. Evidence-based Complementary and

Alternative Medicine eCAM 2009 6 (1), 123–128.

Johnson, M.J., Walker, I.D., Sproule, M.W., et al., 1999. Abnormal coagulation and deep vein thrombosis in patients with advanced cancer. Clin. Lab. Haem. 21, 51–54.

Kuriyama, H., Watanabe, S., Nakaya, T., Shigemori, I., Kita, M., Yoshida, N., et al., 2005. Immunological and psychological benefits of aromatherapy massage. Advance Access Publication eCAM 2 (2), 179–184. Oxford University Press.

Lee, W.H., Lee, L., 1992. The book of practical aromatherapy. Keats, New Canaan, CT, p. 125.

Lewith, et al., 2002. Complementary Cancer Care in Southampton: a survey of staff and patients. Complement. Ther. Med. 10, 100–106.

Macmillan Cancer Relief, 2002. Directory of Complementary Therapy Services in UK Cancer Care. Macmillan Cancer Relief, London.

Marieb, E., 1998. Human Anatomy and Physiology, fourth ed. Addison Wesley World Student Series.

McCaffery, M., Beebe, A., 1989. Pain, Clinical Manual for Nursing Practice. The CV Mosby Company.

McNamara, P., 2004. Massage for people with cancer, third ed. The Cancer Resource Centre, Wandsworth, London.

Moon, T., Wilkinson, J.M., Cavanagh, H. M.A., 2006. Antibacterial activity of essential oils, hydrosols and plant extracts from Australian grown Lavandula spp. Int. J. Aromather. 16, 9–11.

National Council for Palliative Care, 2010. Palliative and Supportive Care Explained. National Council for Palliative Care, London.

National Statistics Online, 2009. Ageing – fastest increase in the oldest yet. Office of National Statistics.

NHS Evidence – supportive and palliative care, 2007. Introduction to end-stage renal disease in palliative and supportive care. National Institute of Clinical Excellence, London.

NICE, 2003. Guidelines for heart failure. National Institute for Clinical Excellence, London.

NICE, 2004. Guidance on Cancer Services: Improving Supportive and Palliative Care for Adults with Cancer. National Institute for Clinical Excellence, London.

Pan, C.X., Morrison, R., Ness, J., Fugh-Berman, A., Leipzig, R.M., 2000. Complementary and alternative medicine in the management of pain, dyspnoea, and nausea and vomiting near the end of life. A systematic review. J. Pain Symptom Manage. 20 (5), 374–387.

Price, L., Price, S., 2008. Carrier oils for aromatherapy and massage. Riverhead, Stratford-upon-Avon.

Price, S., 2000. Aromatherapy and your emotions. Thorsons, London.

Schnaubelt, K., 1998. Advanced Aromatherapy. Healing Arts press, Vermont.

Sheppard-Hanger, S., 1994. The Aromatherapy Practitioner Manual. Atlantic Institute of Aromatherapy, Tampa, Florida, USA.

Tavares, M., 2003. National Guidelines for the Use of Complementary Therapies in Supportive and Palliative Care. The Prince of Wales Foundation for Integrated Health and The National Council for Hospice and Supportive Care Services May.

Tisserand, R., 1992. The Art of Aromatherapy. The C.W. Daniel Ltd, Saffron Walden, UK.

Tisserand, R., Balacs, T., 1995. Essential Oil Safety Guide, A guide for Health Care Professionals. Churchill Livingstone.

Twycross, R.G., Lack, S., 1984. Therapeutics in Terminal Cancer. Churchill Livingstone.

WHO, 1990. Cancer pain relief and palliative care. A report of the WHO Expert Committee. WHO Technical report series 804, WHO.

Wilkes, E., 1992. Complementary therapy in hospice and palliative care. Sheffield Trent Paliative Care Centre and Help the Hospices.

Wilkinson, S., Aldridge, J., Salmon, I., Cain, E., Wilson, B., 1999. An evaluation of aromatherapy massage in palliative care. Palliat. Med. 13 (5), 409–417.

Wilkinson, S., Love, S.B., Westcombe, A.M., Gambles, M.A., Burgess, C., Cargill, A., et al., 2007. Effectiveness of Aromatherapy Massage in the Management of Anxiety and Depression in Patients with Cancer: A Multicentre Randomised Control Trial. J. Clin. Oncol. 25 (5), 532–539.

Williams, L.R., Stockley, J.K., Yan, W., Home, V.N., 1998. Essential oils with high antimicrobial activity for therapeutic use. Int. J. Aromather. 8 (4), 30–40.

Bereavement

16

Robert Stephen

CHAPTER CONTENTS

Introduction

Aromatherapy, in its simplest definition, is a 'balancing' medicine that affects the whole person. Surveying the literature, it becomes clear that the theme of loss is seldom approached in core aromatherapy texts, yet is something that each of us experiences, not once, but often throughout our lives. It would be rare for a practitioner in any field of care not to be called upon to support a person through this traumatic event.

Bereavement as loss

Bereavement is a fact of life. Talk of bereavement is mostly associated with death, but it is an emotional response that follows many events in life. Unlike many species in the animal kingdom, we take time to grieve after we sustain a loss: it may even be one of the things that make us distinctively human. The experience of grief almost certainly makes us more self-absorbed, grieving over what has been lost and because life has changed. It is 'our' loss and we are at the centre of our feelings and emotions. Loss is something we all have to come to terms with. In some ways the absolute nature of death may be easier to deal with than some of the less definite (even less obvious) happenings that cause grief.

Grief is essentially a product of love: the more we have loved, the greater our experience of loss. A world without grief would be a world without love: that, surely, would be sadder and more difficult to live with than loss. It is essential to recognize that we do not ever bring an end to the experience of loss, although

> excess of grief is madness; for it is an injury to the living and the dead know it not.
>
> (Xenophon)

In normal circumstances it takes around 3 months for a person to accept that a bereavement has taken place: if the circumstances are traumatic or sudden, this period will most probably be extended. Grief takes time to adjust to and will become an important step towards recovery from the immediate trauma – there is no guaranteed formula that can act as an effective anaesthetic. One has to decide to face the pain – and it is not until that decision is made that moving beyond grief becomes possible.

Every change involves loss and gain: arriving; departing; growing; declining; achieving; failing.

The old environment must be given up, the new accepted (Murray-Parkes, 1986: 30).

The grief process

Grief is a process with successive stages, the progression of which is not strictly linear: often a stage will be repeated and emotions apparently dealt with may be rehearsed again. Murray-Parkes (1986) speaks of five stages: alarm – searching – mitigation – anger and guilt – gaining a new identity. Ainsworth-Smith et al. (1988) identifies three stages: shock and disbelief – awareness – resolution. Bradley (1990) speaks of: numbness – pining – depression – recovery.

Whichever scheme is followed, there is much that is common ground, accepting the difference in phraseology. The author suggests that there are five distinct stages in working through grief:

Shock

Shock following bereavement is controlled by the reticular activating system (Fig. 16.1). The reticular formation, a part of it, is a complex neural network in the central core of the brainstem which passes nerve impulses between the brain and the spinal cord, monitoring the state of the body's behaviour and alertness (see Wikipedia). It has a vast number of synaptic links with other parts of the brain that constantly receive 'information', transmitted in ascending and descending tracts (Wilson 1994 p. 253). One of its functions is to pass (or block) selective information to the cerebral cortex. Stimulation of the reticular formation has been shown to produce first, curiosity, then successively (as the intensity of stimulation increases) attention, fear and panic (Murray-Parkes 1986 p. 51). It is because of this that:

- people who are in shock can do strange things that are out of character for them
- sleep patterns, appetite and control of the sympathetic and parasympathetic systems are often disturbed.

Disbelief and denial

Loss is so unwelcome that people often try to pretend it is not happening. This sort of avoidance is a self-protection mechanism as a means of getting through

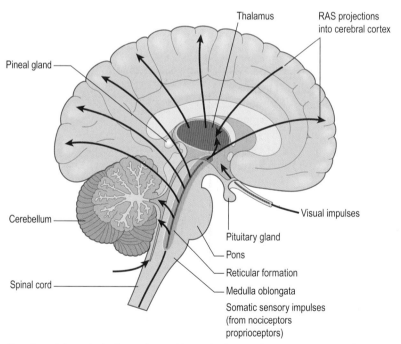

Fig. 16.1 • General location of the reticular formation and its projections to the cerebral cortex. Shown in a single red bar in this figure, the reticular formation consists of numerous brainstem nuclei. www.daviddarling.info/encyclopedia/R/reticular_formation.html

the crisis. Many speak of 'being in a dream', and one common feature to all who cope with loss is a determined unwillingness to plan clearly and to acknowledge that things actually are different and will not change. Some may turn to drugs (mostly prescription medication) or alcohol, with the ever-attendant danger of excess. This stage of grief does not need so much to be challenged as to be encouraged through, as it is unhealthy for an individual to linger in the denial stage.

Acceptance

Attempts currently being made to make people more part of – and involved with – the dying process are to be welcomed, for many are held back from coming to a point of acceptance because they have no real awareness of what has happened (it used to be popularly accepted that children had to be protected from death). As death is a normal part of life, true homoeostasis is brought closer if the loss is accepted and the bereavement embraced.

Anger and remorse

There are some strange reactions to loss. Anger following bereavement comes in many different forms, i.e.

- anger directed against the person who has died: How could they do this to me? This sort of anger is more often thought than expressed: it is an emotive rather than a properly emotional response, not based on reason – and is unsustainable. It is easier to accept when there is a 'reason' to justify anger, for example if a person has been unreasonable, or there are debts. But someone who gets angry simply because they have been left alone, because they have been bereaved, can become very guilty about what appears to be self-indulgence.
- deflected anger: although many experience anger because the situation is not what they would have wanted (we would rather not have experienced loss), it becomes focused on the nearest available target. Doctors are not uncommon targets after a long illness: relatives sometimes find it hard to believe that there really was nothing that could have been done.
- frustration can be expressed as anger. Death is so absolute and immutable. Frustration (and subsequent anger) grows out of a sense of hopelessness and the inability to 'make things better.' Loss cannot be prevented, nor our reaction to it.

To help relieve these situations with essential oils, see below.)

The problem with anger is that it is always self-destructive, even for those who are able to express anger.

Remorse is stronger than regret and can be debilitating. It is to have to let go of someone who was loved while issues between the survivors and the deceased remain unresolved. It is difficult to live with, and the deep feeling of sorrow (and sometimes guilt) at missed opportunities is nigh on impossible to come to terms with. Many who have been hurt as relationships have ended reflect on 'if onlys' concerning what might have been said or done, or how things could have been worked through differently.

Anger and remorse are normal, natural reactions to loss. It is never good for an individual to suppress or attempt to contain these feelings, for they could become harmful. The bereaved person becomes a victim and is often handicapped in life if anger and remorse remain unacknowledged and unresolved.

Adjustment

It is often said that time is a great healer, and there are few exceptions to this, with adjustment from debilitating loss to a new balance taking about 2 years. Adjustment is not living without the pain of loss: it is rather living without it being a constant companion or without being debilitated by it. Memories begin to become a comfort rather than a handicap because remembered good things become bearable again. A new life starts to be created with real interests instead of mere ways of filling time.

Two years is a significant timing for adjustment, for in the natural course of events it means that all the anniversaries have been met twice. If nothing else, the routine of life in a new pattern will have become more familiar and less traumatic.

Holistic grief

The most characteristic feature of grief is not prolonged depression but acute and episodic 'pangs'. Murray-Parkes (1986 p.60) maintains that the most characteristic features of grief are the 'pangs' of severe anxiety and psychological pain, often ending in outbursts of sobbing and crying. This is a release and preferable to bottle it up by 'being brave'. He continues by saying that pangs of grief usually begin a few hours or days after the bereavement and usually reach a peak of severity within 5–14 days.

Lawlis (2001 p. 20), reflecting on the effects of loss, states:

> It is generally believed that with the exception of the loss of a child, no greater or more painful stressor occurs in life than the death of one's spouse.

Mortality after bereavement

Bartrop et al. (1977) set out to explore and establish the behavioural, hormonal and immunological consequences of bereavement. Their study demonstrated that the body responds to grief and loss with a measurable abnormality in immune function, the body's ability to produce T cells being compromised.

Follow-up work revealed that there is a higher than normal mortality among the recently bereaved (Helsing et al. 1981). This is attributable directly to the suppression of mitogen-induced lymphocyte stimulation in the subjects. Recovery of lymphocyte response within the body took between 4 and 14 months. In supporting victims of loss it is important to be mindful of this as part of the treatment regime.

Case 16.1

Shock and anger after bereavement

Assessment

James had been ill and had died unexpectedly. His widow (Pat) was unprepared and had not been with him as much as she had planned, neither was she present at the moment of death. Pat was at the same time in shock and angry with herself (it took her some time to realize that she was also angry with James for dying without her there!). The emotional toll was immediate, and the first response was to aid rest and enable sleep, as the first night after the death was, understandably, very disturbed.

Intervention

A therapist friend suggested she put the following oils on a tissue and place it inside her pillowcase:
- 1 drop of *Lavandula angustifolia* – analgesic, anti-inflammatory, balancing, calming and sedative (helping sleep and calming anger)
- 2 drops of *Boswellia carteri* [frankincense] – analgesic, anti-inflammatory, antidepressive, immunostimulant, and emotionally healing for both grief and anger
- 2 drops *Citrus limon* [lemon] – anti-inflammatory, antispasmodic, calming, immunostimulant.

She was also advised to go to bed at a particular time (with the aromatic tissue) and stay there until it was time to get up. Massage was not considered fitting but, mindful of the need to maintain her wellbeing, the following essential oils were put into Pat's PPA (Penny Price Aromatherapy) moisture cream (50 mL):
- 2 drops *Pelargonium graveolens* [geranium] – analgesic, anti-inflammatory, antispasmodic, cicatrizant, decongestant, relaxant
- 1 drop *Rosa damascena* [rose otto] – anti-inflammatory, neurotonic (as well as adding a touch of luxury – so necessary in true caring)

2 drops *Boswellia carteri* [frankincense] – for the properties above

Crisis management for the day of the funeral was twofold. Pat was shown how to massage the solar plexus reflex on her hand, in the centre of her palm, by applying pressure in a circular movement with her thumb, and a small inhaler was given to her, containing a few drops of *Melissa officinalis* [melissa] – anti-inflammatory, calming to depression and grief.

Outcome

During the funeral Pat was clearly very upset, but from time to time she reached for the inhaler, which helped her regain her composure. The better quality of rest due to the bedtime routine and the pillow tissue helped her to cope from the second night until long after the funeral. The treatment moisturizer was used well beyond the initial stages of bereavement, and Pat did not succumb (as many do) to any cold or flu in the weeks immediately following the death.

Apart from the clear chemical and physiological benefits, using the oils given to her gave Pat things to do during the day, when so much else was out of her control. She was encouraged to put some of James's personal belongings into a sealed bag – things that carried his own odour, as part of the support afterwards; this allowed Pat (via the aroma) to reconnect emotionally, something that was particularly important to her while she worked through the anger she felt.

The therapeutic relationship allowed Pat to talk freely with someone she trusted and progress at her own pace. It was also holistic, in that it drew the physical, emotional and spiritual together.

The use of aromatherapy and essential oils

One of the first approaches in supporting those experiencing loss is to boost the immune system.

Precise statements about the specific interaction between essential oils and the various functions of the immune system are not possible at this time (Schnaubelt 1995 p.119). There have been, in recent years, a number of attempts to develop a study of what Schnaubelt calls aroma-immunology. He suggests that:

- various terpenic alcohols have the ability to correct pathologically elevated or depressed γ-globulin counts to their proper level (1995 p. 119).
- terpenes increase immune system and metabolic activity. To this end they can change the expression of receptors, meaning that they are able to alter the amount of receptors present on a cell surface, either increasing or decreasing them (Schnaubelt 1999 p. 98).

Strengthening the immune system

Addressing the immune system is a truly holistic method of treating grief and supporting a person with loss, and two immunostimulant essential oils particularly useful in assisting the grief process are *Boswellia carteri* [frankincense] and *Melissa officinalis* [melissa]. These have traditionally been associated with coming to terms with loss – the evidence is traditional, not scientific. The particular aroma used at a time of crisis is retained in the olfactory memory and recurrence of that aroma can stimulate the emotional memory – even the pain felt – at that particular time. Therefore care has to be taken to ensure that the sufferer will not be constantly 'tripped up' by association with the loss from which he or she is trying to recover.

Boswellia carteri [frankincense] is perhaps the most obvious oil to use as, along with its immunostimulant properties, it is also a tonic to the heart, decongestant, detoxifying and healing, which properties may help to relieve any guilty feelings (Price 2000 p.152). It is also suitable for treating nervous depression (Scimeau & Tétau 2009) and insomnia (aee Appendix A on the CD-ROM).

These facets of frankincense offer obvious benefits for those who have experienced the trauma of loss. Perhaps there was a good reason in antiquity for loved ones' bodies to be anointed with frankincense, or for the funeral rites in many traditions to have incense used as part of the ceremonial.

Melissa officinalis has long been associated with the treatment of nervous disorders and the emotions. Paracelsus called it 'the elixir of life', and Culpeper said it 'driveth away all troublesome cares and thoughts out of the mind' (*The English Physician* 1652). The Arabs introduced melissa as a medicinal herb specifically for benefit in anxiety or depression, and it has been used as a sedative or tonic tea ever since (Stuart 1989 p. 222).

On an emotional level melissa has traditionally been used as a tonic for the heart and a remedy for the distressed spirit. It is balancing, historically known as an antidepressant, and its calming effects help cope with anxieties and worries felt during the grieving process (Price 2000 p.125).

These two oils are best used by inhalation. A full-body aromatherapy massage may be too much to cope with in the early stages of grief and too intrusive: it is something that may become important as the grief process moves along. The level of contact and response to a bereaved client has to be adjudged afresh at almost every encounter, particularly in the first year. All who are engaged in the study of bereavement speak of the benefit of touch, especially for those who feel isolated through bereavement. It has not been uncommon to sit in silence for as long as half an hour, just holding a hand. The client needs to be treated holistically, and massage may have to be subservient to the emotional needs of an individual in the early stages of grief.

Two other essential oils which may help at this stage are:

- *Syzygium aromaticum* [clove bud] – analgesic, healing and neurotonic
- *Thymus vulgaris* ct. *linalool*, ct. *geraniol* [sweet thyme] – cardiotonic, neurotonic and also aids insomnia.

Schnaubelt (1995 p.119) suggests that the addition of 1.8-cineole to the terpenic alcohols gives a better synergistic approach. Two immunostimulant essential oils with these constituents are:

- *Eucalyptus radiata* [narrow-leaved peppermint] – anti-inflammatory, energizing
- *Melaleuca viridiflora* [niaouli] – analgesic, neurotonic; its anti-inflammatory and antispasmodic properties may also help to relieve anger or resentment (Price 2000 p.132)

Sadness and anger

When so-called negative emotions such as sadness and anger are stifled a person may become depressed and hopeless, which can be harmful to health. Once acknowledged and expressed, this likelihood is lessened (Domar & Dreher 1997). These feelings can be relieved by calming, antispasmodic, anti-inflammatory essential oils, hopefully relaxing the mind enough to be able to forgive – itself a healing aspect for anger, frustration and resentment (Price 2000 p. 131–3). Again, inhalation is the main effective method to be used, taking three full, deep breaths from a tissue onto which 6–8 drops of the following oil/s have been sprinkled:

- *Citrus bergamia* [bergamot] – the calming, refreshing and uplifting action can help soothe anger and hopefully encourage thoughts of forgiveness
- *Citrus limon* [lemon] – anti-inflammatory, antispasmodic and also immunostimulant
- *Mentha* x *piperita* [peppermint] – as well as being uplifting, the anti-inflammatory and antispasmodic properties suggesting an ability to soothe and unblock hidden anger or resentment
- *Pelargonium graveolens* [geranium] – its analgesic, anti-inflammatory, antispasmodic and healing properties suggest it would not only assist with grief, but also help the emotional pain of frustration and inner anger, encouraging acceptance of the painful situation and promoting forgiveness.

Therapist involvement

Being confronted with a bereaved person can be unnerving. What should one say? What ought one to do? It can be difficult to know how to 'break the ice'. Part of the vulnerability of grief is its irrational nature. If someone has made a choice to seek help from a therapist, be encouraged, for they have already made a positive decision to invite the therapist to share their journey. Three simple points of guidance are offered:

- Be yourself – if you act out a part there will be little of yourself that you can give to the client

- Be prepared to listen more than is usual during a consultation, and at the same time do not be frightened of silences
- Avoid the temptation to enter into bereavement counselling unless you are competent in that field. If it becomes clear that more specific help is required, do not hesitate to refer your client to qualified help.

Questions about what has become of the loved one after death must be treated very cautiously: your beliefs and convictions are valid to you, but it would be inappropriate for them to be offered in any professional and therapeutic relationship.

Bereavement – a lifelong process

The bereavement process continues throughout life. The many other experiences of loss have not been explored – the 'little' deaths, as they have become known, which range from amputations and mutilating surgery to moving home away from a community in which one is established; from the unwanted and unwelcome loss of a relationship to the natural progress in life when children leave home; from the rejection of redundancy through to the frustration at the loss of independence. All of these are significant losses and most have a similar response pattern, not always appropriate to the perceived significance of the loss. In these situations aromatherapy works in an excellent synergistic relationship with the talking therapies that exist.

Conclusion

This chapter has sought to give an understanding of the psychology of loss, with some suggestions as to the use of suitable essential oils, using a combination of the scientific and the traditional wisdom available. The emphasis has been on a holistic and synergistic response. One can never be compensated for any loss experienced: all that anyone can do is simply journey with the person as they attempt to find a new balance in life, and using essential oils in a controlled way to deal with physiological symptoms and supporting the emotions is well within the competence of any suitably trained therapist.

References

Ainsworth-Smith, I., Speck, P., 1988. Letting Go: care for the dying and bereaved. SPCK, London.

Bartrop, R.W., Lazarus, L., Luckhurst, E., Kiloh, L.G., Penny, R., 1977. Depressed lymphocyte function after bereavement. Lancet 16 (1977), 834.

Bradley, W., 1990. Mary: a case study through the bereavement of a child. Unpublished Oxford University research paper.

Domar, A.D., Dreher, H., 1997. Healing mind, healthy woman. Thorsons, London.

Helsing, K.J., Szklo, M., 1981. Mortality after bereavement. Am J Epidemiol 114 (1), 41.

Lawlis, F., 2001. Complimentary and Alternative Medicine: a research based approach. Mosby, St Louis.

Murray-Parkes, C., 1986. Bereavement: studies of grief in adult life. Pelican, London.

Price, S., 2000. Aromatherapy and your emotions. Thorsons, London.

Scimeau, D., Tétau, M., 2009. Votre santé par les huiles essentielles. Alpen, Monaco, p. 55.

Schnaubelt, K., 1995. Advanced Aromatherapy. Healing Arts Press, Vermont.

Schnaubelt, K., 1999. Medical Aromatherapy. Frog Ltd, Berkeley.

Stuart, M., 1989. The Encyclopaedia of Herbs and Herbalism. MacDonald & Co., Novara.

Wilson, K., 1994. Anatomy and Physiology. Churchill Livingstone, Edinburgh.

Section 4

Policy and practice

Section contents

Aromatherapy in the UK

17 (Part I)

Carole Preen

CHAPTER CONTENTS

Introduction

Part I of this chapter shows how professional aromatherapy has developed (and is still developing) in the UK, from simple beginnings to being the model for many other countries to follow (see Ch. 18). It reports the current situation in the field of complementary medicine and aromatherapy in particular, giving details of the relevant associations that look after the interests of aromatherapy and the therapists who practise it, especially with respect to standards of education and legislation regarding the use of essential oils. Part II discusses issues relevant to most health professionals – physiotherapists, occupational therapists, those who work in mental health etc. – as well as aromatherapists. A model set of the policies and protocols set up for nurses could be proposed for the professional practice of aromatherapy in UK healthcare settings.

Aromatherapy development

Since arriving in Britain in the late 1960s via the beauty therapy industry, aromatherapy has greatly expanded into health, both in and out of hospitals, doctors' surgeries and complementary health centres. Two people well known throughout the world – and considered by many to be somewhat responsible for its advancement since the 1980s – are Robert Tisserand and Shirley Price, educators and authors of several textbooks on the subject. Both helped instigate the first association purely for aromatherapy in Britain, the International Federation of Aromatherapy (IFA).

By the 1990s, more and more physiotherapists, nurses and midwives were attending accredited courses, and other countries are still keen to follow the 'British way'.

Educational standards have changed considerably over the last decade. The first set of National Occupational Standards (NOS) for Aromatherapy was published in 1998 and has since been revised twice, the latest in 2009. The Aromatherapy Council (AC), lead body for the UK aromatherapy profession, is consulted on revisions of the NOS and on qualifications when awarding bodies are writing professional qualifications. It is now imperative that an aromatherapist, whether in nursing or private practice, is trained to the NOS and AC Core Curriculum (see Education below).

Many aromatherapy associations have been launched over the last 25 years. Most of those that exist today work with the AC to maintain standards and promote and enhance the aromatherapy profession as a whole. Member associations can be viewed on the AC website: www.aromatherapycouncil.co.uk

Aromatherapists are now showing an interest in studying advanced clinical aromatherapy (aromatic medicine/aromatology), first introduced in 1990 by the editors and now offered at two aromatherapy schools in the UK. Although this involves the intensive application of essential oils to the skin and the use of hydrolats by mouth to fight bacterial and viral infections as well as chronic conditions, graduates of advanced clinical aromatherapy courses do not necessarily practise all methods on their clients. Such courses, however, do provide complete and full training in these methods, ensuring that essential oils and hydrolats are used safely and with understanding for intensive skin applications, gargles, pessaries and suppositories. The editors sincerely believe that aromatherapy schools already teaching to a high standard should move with the times, and include a separate course on aromatology in their syllabus (see Ch. 9). Nurses, however, will not be able to integrate these skills into NHS care.

Legal requirements

Practice of aromatherapy

Unlike some other European countries (e.g. France and Germany, see Ch. 18), non-medically qualified practitioners of complementary and alternative therapies in the UK are, at present, free to practise under common law, irrespective of their levels of training or clinical competence.

The UK adopted European Medicines Law in 1994 and in most European countries CAM (complementary and alternative medicine) practitioners are required to be medically qualified before they can practise. There is, however, some temporary easing of the regulations for Member States within Medicines Law, principally in Section 12(1) of the Medicines Act 1968. These regulations are unique to the UK and permit unlicensed herbal remedies to be supplied to individual patients under certain conditions (confirmed by the Medicines and

Healthcare products Regulatory Agency [MHRA] to be applicable to aromatherapists). One such condition allows them to use essential oils only when a personal consultation has been undertaken with the client. However, there is currently no definition in law about who carries out the consultation. As this implies that anyone can carry out this procedure, Section 12(1) is currently undergoing reform by the MHRA and Health Ministers.

There are concerns that aromatherapists may then lose their right to practise under Section 12 (1) and to use essential oils as medicines, including labelling a specifically formulated remedy with health claims – medicinal claims for unlicensed products are not permitted under any circumstances, including product names, advertising and promotional material, and particularly websites, which are regarded as exactly the same as any other advertising media. Details can be viewed on www. mrha.gov.uk.

Aromatherapy products

The retail supply of aromatherapy products may be subject to the amended UK Cosmetic Products (Safety) Regulations 2008, the General Product (Safety) Regulations 2005 or other applicable legislation, such as the Biocides Directive. The Aromatherapy Trade Council (ATC) responds to all Government Consultation Documents that could affect the aromatherapy industry. Further information and guidelines can be found on their web-site: www.a-t-c.org.uk.

The Traditional Herbal Medicinal Products Directive (THMPD) was implemented in the UK in 2005 and states that all herbal products must have a continuous traditional medicinal use of 30 years, including at least 15 years within the European Community. Details are available on the MHRA's website at www.mhra.gov.uk. The MHRA has assured the ATC that any product not classified as a medicine should not be affected by the Directive, and that essential oils and aromatherapy products can continue to be sold under the current regulatory regimes for cosmetics and general products.

Cosmetics legislation requires all cosmetic products to be safety assessed by a suitably qualified person, such as a doctor, chartered biologist or chartered chemist, before being placed on the market. This includes a ban on animal testing as from March 2009, and was extended to include 26 chemical substances identified by the EC as an important cause of contact-allergy reactions; 16 of these occur naturally in essential oils commonly used in aromatherapy. As from 11 March 2005, if a product contains one of the 26 named fragrance chemicals in excess of 0.01% (wash-off) or 0.001% (leave-on), that chemical must be included in the list of ingredients on the label, together with a sell-by date.

The UK Cosmetic Products (Safety) Regulations 2008 can be downloaded from the OPSI Office of Public Sector Information) web site www.opsi.gov.uk/si/si2008/uksi_20081284_en_1, or by simply putting the regulations into Google.

Education/training

Professional training in aromatherapy can be delivered via colleges of further education, adult education colleges, universities and private academies. Not all of these courses offer a qualification that gives the student the possibility of practising afterwards, but those that do have to comply with NOS and the AC core curriculum. The awarding body qualifications are available for funding on the National Qualifications Framework and therefore are most likely to be found in further education or adult education colleges. Some colleges may also have sought accreditation from one of the professional associations to enhance their standing, as have many of the universities. All awarding bodies have to seek approval from the AC prior to submission to Ofqual, the new regulator of qualifications and examinations in England, in order to uphold standards.

A copy of the AC Core Curriculum can be downloaded from their website at www.aromatherapy-council.co.uk, along with information on training and approved courses. From April 2010, the AC has a new school's accreditation scheme where schools can be individually vetted, then entered on a list, ensuring that prospective students receive adequate training, which should include the following:

- anatomy, physiology and pathology
- applied aromatherapy (aromatherapy massage routine and completion of 60 case studies)
- theory and safety aspects of essential oils and hydrolats (including basic botany and chemistry/toxicity) and their possible effects on the human organism

- business studies, professional studies
- understanding of research, reflective practice and therapeutic relationship skills.

Although standards are now set to cover the basics necessary for all complementary medicine approved courses (Skills for Health made this a priority in 2009 when revising the NOS for CAM), it would be helpful for students wishing to study several CAM therapies if more colleges offered the basics, such as anatomy, physiology and pathology; fundamentals of orthodox diagnosis; patient referral guidelines; professional ethics; codes of practice; counselling and organizational skills (including record keeping) to be studied separately, enabling further CAM therapies to be offered and studied without unnecessary repetition – and unwanted expense.

It is unfortunate that herbal medicine and aromatherapy cannot be combined into one subject for a degree course, as the practice of aromatic medicine would then become possible for all aromatherapists. The difficulty may be mainly due to the large percentage of massage content in aromatherapy training, which is not needed by a medical herbalist. However, it seems strange that medical herbalists can legally administer essential oils by mouth when their training in essential oils is less in-depth than that of an aromatherapist. Fortunately, aromatherapists who go on to study aromatic medicine/aromatology are at least able to increase the scope of treatments they can offer clients, by intensive application (see Ch 9).

National occupational standards (NOS)

Aromatherapy and reflexology were the first complementary therapies to have Government-endorsed educational standards, published in 1998. Skills for Health – a government agency – is responsible for NOS, but works with the various lead bodies for complementary therapies to write the content.

The purpose of developing the NOS for healthcare was to continually improve services for all those who receive care. NOS are competence based, covering the practice of aromatherapy and other elements common to all complementary health practitioners. NOS are not qualifications, but are baseline standards – i.e. the minimum requirements needed in order to qualify as an aromatherapist. The core curriculum developed by the Aromatherapy Council is the bridge between NOS and a syllabus, and the two are inextricably linked. Individual schools and professional associations are not limited to the NOS and core curriculum, and are therefore able to include more depth, cover more essential oils, and include other elements of interest relevant to an aromatherapist. Those wishing to undertake a more in-depth training course should send for the syllabus and check the extras against the AC core curriculum.

Beauty therapy qualifications include some basic study of aromatherapy, although these usually use pre-blended oils and there is no study of botany or chemistry, blending or safety data of individual essential oils. The resulting qualifications are not recognized by the AC or the new regulatory body, the Complementary and Natural Healthcare Council (CNHC); beauty therapists are therefore not deemed to be aromatherapists without also obtaining an approved aromatherapy qualification. To register with the CNHC or to work within the NHS, graduation from an AC accredited course is essential.

As more research is done it becomes even more important that aromatherapists understand the chemistry behind essential oils and the relationship (if any) between these and their effects on the body and mind. In addition, holism (the theory that a complex entity, system etc. is more than merely the sum of its parts) has still to play a major part in aromatherapy treatments for the scientific application to be truly successful.

Which course?

There is no excuse for anyone to undertake a course not accredited by the AC, as all the information is available on the AC website. It is up to the student to question the course provider and check the AC website.

The number of training options creates a minefield for potential students, and many schools and institutions still offer substandard training; the AC website allows prospective students to check these out. If a course cannot be accessed via the AC website it is probably not worth the money, unless it is for personal interest only. If the intention is to train as a professional aromatherapist in the UK, the course should be thoroughly checked first. Courses must be at least over one academic year (9 months), with a minimum of 250 hours in class; 60 case studies must be included – those from a previous massage course cannot be counted. Fast-track courses or distance learning courses where attendance is not required will not be recognized.

House of Lords report

In November 2000 the House of Lords Select Committee on Science and Technology published a report on complementary and alternative therapies which called for more evidence-based research, tighter regulation of therapies and practitioners and more reliable information, so that the public could make informed choices regarding their healthcare. The training and qualification of therapists is a key issue in policy development and the House of Lords report identified the need for all complementary therapies to develop a sound system of regulation and accreditation.

In response to this, the government urged the representative bodies for each therapy to unite to form a single body for regulating their profession (DoH 2001) in the best interests of patients and the wider public (Tavares 2003). It also urged CAM regulatory bodies to put in place codes of practice to limit claims made by practitioners, and to ensure that their members recognize and follow them.

One of the principal requirements of modern healthcare provision can be summed up by the term 'evidence based'. It is no longer sufficient for any therapeutic approach simply to rely on a long history of use, or popularity, or widespread availability, to justify its continued acceptance. Evidence of both safety and efficacy of all forms of therapeutic intervention is now required (Field 2003).

The report classified therapies according to their evidence base and level of professional organization in relation to regulation (see Part II and Table 17.1).

Helping the public select therapies and therapists

It has been difficult for a member of the public to have a central point where they can go to obtain information on therapists who have trained to the required standard and are competent, fit to practise and insured. This is because, owing to the popularity of CAM – particularly aromatherapy – over the last 20 years, many new associations and organizations sprang up purporting to represent the profession. Each individual association holds its own register

Table 17.1 Therapies classified according to their evidence base and level of professional organization in relation to regulation

Group 1 Professionally organized alternative therapies	Group 2 Complementary therapies	Group 3 Alternative disciplines
Acupuncture Chiropractic Herbal medicine Homoeopathy Osteopathy	Alexander technique Aromatherapy Bach and other flower remedies Massage Reflexology Healing, including Reiki Hypnotherapy Shiatsu	**3a Long-established and traditional systems of healthcare** Ayurvedic medicine Anthroposophical medicine Chinese herbal medicine Traditional Chinese medicine
		3b Other alternative disciplines Crystal therapy Dowsing Iridology Kinesiology Radionics

Categories of CAM disciplines (House of Lords Report 2000).

of members, but there is no external check on whether or not they hold an appropriate aromatherapy qualification.

Following the House of Lords Report in 2000 and the government's response in 2001, the Prince of Wales's Foundation of Integrated Health (formed in 1993), was given a grant by the Department of Health to help bring therapies together under one lead body and help them to write standards and policies to enable each therapy to regulate itself (the FIH was closed in April 2010).

Aromatherapy was originally governed by the Aromatherapy Organizations Council (AOC), launched in 1991. Prior to the House of Lords report, the AOC was already discussing statutory regulation of aromatherapy with the Department of Health, but after the report the government preferred voluntary self-regulation for complementary therapies, so in 2001 the AOC set up a regulation working party.

In 2003 the AOC was dissolved and the Aromatherapy Consortium was born, working towards voluntary self-regulation of the aromatherapy profession. The Consortium worked closely with the Prince of Wales's Foundation, and the new voluntary self-regulatory body for aromatherapy was launched on schedule in December 2006 at a special reception in the House of Commons under the new name 'Aromatherapy Council'.

Around the same time, Professor Julie Stone published a report via the Prince's Foundation showing the benefits of having one regulatory body for all complementary therapies, rather than an individual body for each therapy. The AOC had presented a similar document to the Foundation in 2000, but at that time it was not thought to be relevant. The aromatherapy profession supported the idea, as the majority of them also practise other therapies and it would be to their advantage not to pay individual regulators. Equally, it would also benefit members of the public, making the finding of a suitable therapist much simpler.

In January 2007, the Federal Working Group (FWG) had its first meeting, hosted by the Foundation as a result of a further government grant. This meeting brought together 12 complementary therapy disciplines hoping to find agreement on the structure of a single regulator to represent all the therapies. The last meeting took place in July 2007, at which time there was not total agreement; this included the Aromatherapy Council, at that time a regulator itself.

Fortunately, the Foundation passed responsibility to a new body, the CNHC, to carry on the work and the AC has collaborated with them to iron out discrepancies (the CNHC aromatherapy regulatory register was launched in May 2009). The AC has selected four Profession Specific Board (PSB) members to advise the CNHC of any aromatherapy issues, and has supplied a list of qualifications which are acceptable for registration. It is likely in the future that any aromatherapist wishing to work in the NHS will need to be CNHC registered, and the Department of Health supports the CNHC.

Use of essential oils in hospices and hospitals

As long ago as 1997 a survey by the University of Exeter revealed that, of the number of members from complementary therapy associations working in the NHS, up to 50% were from aromatherapy, healing and reflexology associations. 'Aromatherapy and reflexology are popular with nurses and this is likely to account for much of their involvement' (University of Exeter 1997 p. 60). This percentage has no doubt increased greatly since then.

Almost 20 years ago Barker (1994) believed himself to be just that, saying he was a trained professional aromatherapist, despite being a nurse. 'It does aromatherapy a great disservice by tagging it on to another discipline to give it credibility when it is already a valid system of medicine. We should be proud of our profession in the use of essential oils and not need to use another profession as a crutch.' Nowadays complementary therapists practise a range of disciplines, professions quite separate from nursing or any other, albeit still allied to medicine, and so aromatherapists can call themselves healthcare professionals in the same way as nurses. In the past, many hospitals have funded nurses on aromatherapy courses, many of these being run specifically for the nursing profession and consultants. A major breakthrough occurred in 1993, when GPs were empowered to refer patients to complementary therapists for treatment on the NHS, provided that the GP concerned remained clinically accountable for the patient. As a result, since the mid-1990s GPs have a much more sympathetic and cooperative attitude towards aromatherapy than when the editors came into the profession in the early 1970s. The medical profession are now more willing to listen seriously to claims of the positive and sometimes dramatic effects that essential oils can have on people's overall health and many private therapists now work in conjunction with their local GP on minor health problems that can be helped by essential oils.

There have been many clinical successes in hospitals where essential oils have been used, and the results of projects and trials (albeit not of rigorous research standard – very difficult in the case of essential oils) have led to a greater willingness to listen and to use aromatherapy in hospitals and community care.

The NHS and Community Care Act Self-Governing Status for NHS hospitals – NHS Trusts – was created in 1990, set up to manage hospitals and other NHS services. This change in status may have been a contributory factor in the increase in complementary therapies being practised in health care.

Aromatherapy associations

Aromatherapy has many professional associations, most of which are multidisciplinary. Most associations are paid members of the lead body, the Aromatherapy Council, where they work together in the interest of the profession as a whole. The Aromatherapy Council advises the CNHC (whose main concern is public safety) on specific aromatherapy matters. The professional associations are more like a trade body, looking after the interest of the therapists who are members. They provide insurance, conferences, magazines/newsletters, continuing professional development (CPD) opportunities and support their members in the event of a complaint. We see similar structures in other professions, such as in nursing, where one of the professional associations is the Royal College of Nursing and the regulatory body is the Nursing and Midwifery Council. The difference in the aromatherapy profession is that there are many professional associations; these are listed below in alphabetical order, those dedicated purely to aromatherapy being at the top. All but the first are Members of the Aromatherapy Council, which is the lead body.

The Institute of Aromatic Medicine (IAM)

The IAM is not a member of the AOC as it is an umbrella group for both aromatherapists and those who practise intensive application of essential oils and/or use essential oils and hydrolats orally. The range of competence covered is unique to the UK, as it has three levels of membership: Associate membership, Membership, Licenciate membership and

Fellowship (FIAM), UK Master's degree level. It offers comprehensive insurance, support and advice to all members and associates.

The International Federation of Aromatherapists (IFA)

The IFA was launched in 1985 and is an aromatherapy association that has spread worldwide. Members receive quarterly editions of the *Aromatherapy Times* magazine, have access to a block insurance scheme, and receive discounts on IFA conferences, offers on CPD courses and exemption from London Borough licensing.

The International Federation of Professional Aromatherapists (IFPA)

The IFPA was launched in 2002 following a merger of the International Society of Professional Aromatherapists (ISPA), originally formed in 1990 by Shirley Price, and the Register of Qualified Aromatherapists (RQA), originally formed in 1991 by Gabriel Mojay. It is the largest aromatherapy-only association in the UK. It offers an insurance scheme, reduced prices at national aromatherapy conferences, a quarterly aromatherapy journal – *In Essence* – CPD opportunities and exemption from London Borough licensing.

The International Holistic Aromatherapy Foundation (IHAF)

IHAF was formed in 1988 by practising therapists. Members can obtain insurance, discounts on CPD workshops and receive articles on aromatherapy.

Multidisciplinary associations

Aromatherapy and Allied Practitioners Association (AAPA)

This AAPA was established in 1994 and is a member of the lead body for massage therapy, the General Council for Massage Therapy (GCMT). It covers all therapies, seeing aromatherapy and massage as its main concern, and offers an insurance scheme, low-cost or free CPD and a regular newsletter. The helpline is staffed by qualified therapists. Members enjoy exemption from London Borough licensing.

Association of Physical and Natural Therapists (APNT)

The APNT was established in 1986 with the aim of representing practitioners of complementary medicine who have reached the required standards of training and education. It is also a member of the GCMT and the British Complementary Medicine Association (BCMA). It offers an insurance scheme and CPD opportunities.

British Register of Complementary Practitioners (BRCP)

This register is part of the Institute for Complementary and Natural Medicine (ICNM). It was formed in 1989 and offers low-cost insurance, CPD opportunities, a regular journal, advertising opportunities, and members enjoy exemption from London Borough licensing.

Complementary Therapies Association (CThA)

This large multidisciplinary association was a merger between the Guild for Complementary Practitioners (GCP) and the International Therapies Examination Council (ITEC) in 2001. Members receive a free copy of the *Embody* magazine, low-cost insurance, CPD opportunities, advertising opportunities, local therapy clubs and exemption from London Borough licensing. Most members are graduates of ITEC, one of the awarding bodies that are invited to AC meetings.

Federation of Holistic Therapists (FHT)

FHT is a large multidisciplinary association that was established in 1965. Membership includes free membership of the *International Therapist* magazine and offers local support groups, a helpline, membership of all lead bodies, seminars and workshops for CPD, low-cost insurance and exemption from London Borough licensing.

The Aromatherapy Trade Council (ATC)

This UK trade association is for the aromatherapy essential oil industry. Founded in 1993, its mission is to promote responsible marketing of genuine aromatherapy products and safe usage of essential oils by consumers. To this end, it has established a code of practice for product labelling and packaging and publishes guidelines on the regulation, labelling, advertising and promotion of aromatherapy products to assist those setting up in business, e.g. it will review labels and promotional material prior to printing to ensure they comply with the complexities of the law. It has a policy for the random testing of its members' oils.

The ATC represents the interests of manufacturers and suppliers in the trade at legislative forums where decisions are made which affect the industry; it advises its membership and the public alike on ever-changing legislation and its likely effects on the industry.

The ATC works closely with the Aromatherapy Council and other organizations to ensure the needs of the profession are served appropriately by the aromatherapy trade.

Research

Research in the UK can be viewed on the links page of the AC website; The Essential Oil Resource website, which provides scientific information about essential oils, is fully searchable and available online by subscription (see Useful addresses, p. 528).

Summary

This part of Chapter 17 has given an overall picture of how aromatherapy developed in the UK and how it stands at the time of writing. Legal requirements regarding the practice of aromatherapy and the sale of products containing essential oils have been covered, with a full discussion on the standards of education required and the importance of thorough training. It shows the growth of essential oil use in hospitals over the last decade, and how both aromatherapists and nurses are professionals in their own right. The most respected associations are listed to help qualifying aromatherapists select one suitable for them.

Aromatherapy within the National Health Service

17

(Part II)

Angela Avis

CHAPTER CONTENTS

Introduction

Part 2 shows how the use of aromatherapy is now being integrated into clinical settings and how codes of professional conduct for nurses can also be applied to aromatherapists. It gives guidelines for administering medicines and outlines how to write a policy, followed by a draft example of a protocol, which aromatherapists will find useful.

Development of complementary therapies

Many healthcare professionals are interested in exploring the potential therapeutic use of a range of complementary therapies, which are maintaining their popularity with the public (Thomas, Nicholl & Coleman 2001).

This continued interest has encouraged the use of CAM therapies in palliative care (Gage et al. 2009), midwifery (Mousley 2005) and nursing (Maddock-Jennings & Wilkinson (2004).

Aromatherapy is a multiple therapy embracing touch, massage and the administration of essential oil remedies – not to mention the accompanying pleasing aroma, which may be partly responsible for its being possibly the most popular complementary therapy nurses wish to study. There have therefore been increasing demands that, in the best interests and safety of patients and clients, complementary therapies should become regulated and observe similar ethical and practical constraints to those of orthodox medicine.

The House of Lords Report (2000) classified therapies according to their evidence base and level of professional organization in relation to regulation (see Part 1 and Table 17.1). with regard to nursing and midwifery, the report identified Group 2 as covering those therapies most often used to complement conventional care. It was felt that the therapies mentioned in this 'comfort' category gave appropriate help and support to patients, in particular in relieving stress and pain and alleviating the side effects of drug regimens.

Although there was concern about the lack of scientific evidence – as measured by random controlled trials (RCTs) – the report recognized that there was a growing body of qualitative research. The therapies most frequently used by nurses and midwives, such as massage, aromatherapy and reflexology, come within the 'comfort' category. The RCN survey in 2003 confirmed that these were the key therapies used in clinical practice.

The House of Lords report also encouraged the regulating and professional bodies – Nursing and

Midwifery Council (NMC) and Royal College of Nursing (RCN) – to collaborate in making familiarization of CAM a part of the pre-registration nursing and midwifery curricula, which would enable nurses and midwives to have some insight into the choices that their patients or clients make and to offer knowledgeable support. The report went on to suggest that these bodies should provide specific guidance on appropriate education and training for nurses and midwives who wish to integrate therapies such as aromatherapy into clinical care.

Integration of aromatherapy is currently threatened on several fronts, involving regulation, financial constraints for both education and the NHS and academic hostility. The regulation process for aromatherapy has stalled because a number of professional bodies have chosen not to align themselves with the newly launched federal regulation body, supported by the Department of Health, the Complementary and Natural Healthcare Council. This will cause problems for nurses and other healthcare professionals who wish to advance the use of aromatherapy, as their employers will expect them to be members of a rigorous and transparent system – still having several 'regulation' bodies is confusing for NHS Trusts and the general public alike (Stone 2010).

The recession has meant that financial constraints on universities have seen many courses facing closure as priorities shift. Within the NHS financial cuts have meant that nurses have even less time to attend to their patients' comfort and emotional needs – an area in which the use of massage and essential oils had demonstrated good possibilities (Hadfield 2001).

Successful regulation depends on increasing the research base of a profession, but recent academic hostility from science faculties has resulted in the closure of many leading complementary therapy degree courses, including degrees or diplomas leading to aromatherapy qualifications, e.g. those at the Universities of Westminster and Central Lancashire. With a diminishing research base, complementary therapies, including aromatherapy, will be less able to maintain the confidence of the public and orthodox healthcare.

Integrating aromatherapy into clinical care

There are key principles of professional practice that must be considered before integrating any complementary therapy into clinical care. These involve

the following and can be found in policies that have already been developed:

- patient-centred care – identifying patients' needs or problems and the subsequent outcome of care
- appropriate choice of therapeutic intervention
- identification of the parameters of practice
- pinpointing the evidence supporting integration
- identification of the appropriate integration model
- ensuring education and training needs that will provide safe and effective practice
- the development of effective evaluation strategies and ongoing development needs that will support a sustainable service.

A policy for integration, based on evidence and a valid audit process (Mousley 2005), is essential, otherwise it is difficult to see how nurses and midwives can argue for integrating CAM into clinical practice, especially as therapies are often used as a result of enthusiasm on the part of one or two nurses or midwives. A number of Trusts have already allocated time and effort to developing policies, and it is by such work that standards are defined and patients are assured of care that is safe, appropriate and effective. The appropriate therapy is often determined by the nature of a particular clinical area. The area of cancer and palliative care is one in which national guidelines on the integration of complementary therapies have been published by the Foundation for Integrated Health (PWFIH 2003) (Tavares 2003) and offer a wealth of information, including models of good practice.

As there is no national strategy to collect data, professionals have to rely on publications in journals that describe the use of complementary therapies within the various health fields. A small proportion of these are based on research projects, but most are anecdotal.

Nursing and Midwifery Council (NMC)

Code of professional conduct

Registered nurses, midwives and health visitors have to follow the NMC Code of Professional Conduct (CPC) (2008a), the Standards for Medicines Management (2008b) and Complementary Alternative Therapies and Homoeopathy (2009) and are personally accountable for their practice. Some of the following points would also be applicable to aromatherapy practitioners; all must:

- respect the patient or client as an individual
- obtain consent before giving any treatment or care
- protect confidential information
- cooperate with others in the team
- be trustworthy
- act to identify and minimize risk to patients and clients.

Aromatherapists and nurses should acknowledge any limitations in their knowledge and competence and decline duties or responsibilities they cannot perform in a safe and skilled manner. Suitable insurance to cover specific use of essential oils is essential. RCN members are covered when working as a nurse; however, when working independently cover can be obtained from one of the professional aromatherapy or aromatic medicine associations on becoming a full member. The International Federation of Professional Aromatherapists (IFPA) and the Institute of Aromatic Medicine (IAM) also insure student aromatherapists during their time of study.

Complementary therapists and nurses should regularly update their knowledge – of paramount importance in a world where ideas and accepted behavioural patterns are changing fast.

Standard for medicines management

Nurses, midwives and health visitors using essential oils, whether for baths, inhalations, topical application (including compresses), suppositories, pessaries and/or massage, should accept that they are administering medicines, and recognize the personal professional accountability they bear for their actions.

Since 1992 medicinal preparations have been prescribed by a physician or nurse, checked and dispensed by a pharmacist and administered by a nurse. An essential oil prescription is prescribed by a competent aromatherapist or aromatologist and administered by that practitioner, or by a nurse suitably trained in its method of administration.

The prescription should:

- be based, whenever possible, on the patient's informed consent and awareness of the purpose of the treatment

- be clearly written, typed or computer-generated and be indelible
- be dated and signed by the authorized prescriber
- not be for a substance to which the patient is known to be allergic or otherwise unable to tolerate
- clearly identify the patient for whom the medication is intended
- clearly specify the substance to be administered, using the generic or brand name (in the case of aromatherapy the scientific plant name/s should be used), together with the strength, dosage, timing, frequency of administration, start and finish dates and route of administration.

Aromatherapists and nurses working in the NHS

Work supporting the regulation of therapies such as aromatherapy, massage and reflexology is presently under way (see Education in Part 1, above), and each healthcare professional must act within the code of conduct of their professional body, for example the NMC Complementary Alternative Therapies and Homeopathy (2009) requires that nurses and midwives ensure that the use of complementary therapies is safe and in the best interest of patients; they should also act in accordance with the policies and protocols set by the particular hospice or hospital in which they work. Collaboration is part of professional practice, hence the need to discuss the use of CAM with members of the multidisciplinary team caring for that particular patient.

In some areas of the NHS services are being developed which include therapies such as massage and aromatherapy, especially in palliative and cancer care, where aromatherapists are either employed or work as volunteers. Patients can be referred by other healthcare professionals or have direct access to aromatherapists – and a full assessment is undertaken to determine an appropriate treatment regime (Gage et al. 2009).

The emphasis is on protocols demonstrating safe and effective clinical decision making, for example where midwives use essential oils to support women in childbirth (Burns, Blamey & Lloyd 2000) at the John Radcliffe Hospital in Oxford.

Two midwives who were also qualified aromatherapists led the initiative in the early 1990s. The reaction of the women who experienced essential oils in the delivery suite was so positive that a decision was made that all women who delivered their babies in the unit would have access to the use of essential oils for symptom management. A basic training programme was set up so that all midwives on the unit could offer women a prescribed range of essential oils under the supervision of trained aromatherapists. The midwives understood that this training did not qualify them as aromatherapists, but provided knowledge to use essential oils appropriately and effectively in their midwifery practice.

The training might or might not be accepted if they moved to another hospital: it would depend on the policy of that hospital and the type and range of care offered on that unit. The midwifery education package continues to be refined and developed.

Polices are framed somewhat differently where independent aromatherapists are employed by the NHS or are volunteers within a service. For example, at St Ann's Hospice in Manchester, emphasis is placed on establishing a register of therapists with specific qualifications and the establishment of a training and supervision programme which supports aromatherapists working with patients who have complex clinical and psychological needs.

Policies and protocols

Written polices and protocols are designed to provide a framework of consistency and continuity, which is particularly important during any change of personnel. Once recorded, policies become the means for providing legal indemnity.

- *Policies* – state clearly what is expected of staff and cover issues the organization considers important for the delivery and management of the integration of complementary therapies.
- *Protocols* – are the step-by-step methods for achieving policy statements. A policy statement records 'what the rule is and to whom it applies' and should indicate clearly 'what must be done and by whom'.

Policies

Operational policies are those for the day-to-day management and practice of individual therapies, including the expectations of therapists.

Developing policy is not an overnight task. The minimum period from planning to ratification is usually 2 years, and many have taken as many as 4½ years...stamina is needed!

Below are some tips from nurses who have been involved in the development of policies:

- Talk to the right people – know who is on your side.
- Know the organizational structure that you are working in.
- Keep up-to-date with national developments.
- Plan the scope of the policy from the beginning, keeping your options open.
- Keep the document simple – detail is more appropriate at the clinical protocol level.
- Be prepared – there will no doubt be compromises, so don't have unrealistic expectations.
- Make sure firm review dates are built into the system to keep the document alive.
- Prepare to become the 'expert'.

It won't happen overnight, so be prepared for the long haul. Nor will it necessarily be a smooth path – there will be times when you think the way has been blocked, which is when you need to be able to think laterally and be flexible about what you want to achieve.

Because organizational cultures differ there is no one template that can be used. However, a review of existing policy documents would suggest that the following headings might be taken as core requirements:

- **Title of policy** – needs to communicate clearly what the policy is about.
- **Identification of aims of the policy** – tells people what the document will cover.
- **Definition of terms used in the policy document** – sometimes presented as an appendix.
- **Identification of objectives that can be evaluated and measured** – will describe the outcomes that are hoped to be achieved.
- **Identification of what will be covered by the policy** – sometimes only a particular aspect or technique of aromatherapy will be used, and this needs to be defined.
- **Reasoning behind the use of aromatherapy** – will include clinical information and any relevant research or evidence of efficacy.
- **Identification of who should deliver the aromatherapy treatment** – may involve setting up a register of available practitioners.
- **Definition of competency to practise** – will include a description of the aromatherapy

knowledge and skills needed to practise in a particular clinical area.

- **Identification of educational criteria to determine competent practitioners within a particular clinical area** – may identify specific aromatherapy training courses.
- **Identification of lines of accountability** – may include medical authorization.
- **Safety issues** – will include contraindications and risk assessment.
- **Informed consent** – clear guidelines about how and when this is obtained.
- **Documentation to be used within the clinical area** – ideally based on multiprofessional collaboration.
- **Equity of access** – do all patients in a particular clinical area have equal access at any one time to suitably trained aromatherapists?
- **Environmental issues** – providing peace and privacy etc.
- **Methods of evaluation** – what tools will be used to audit and evaluate the service?
- **Financial considerations** – a) who should pay for essential oils used? b) will the aromatherapy be carried out within the existing contract of the practitioner or will there be additional hours and payment?
- **A timetable for the review of the policy** – must be stipulated.

This list is not exhaustive and extra ideas can be found in the *Nurses' Handbook of Complementary Therapies* by Denise Rankin-Box and Maxine McVey (2001). Also, Tavares (2004) has produced a comprehensive guide on writing policies, procedures and protocols for complementary therapies in supportive and palliative care. It contains examples of several policies – some relatively simple.

Draft protocol for the use of essential oils

A draft example of a protocol for using essential oils, by nurses at St Gemma's Hospice, Leeds, is included in Tavares' guide and is divided into the following headings:

- **Preamble** – describing situations for using essential oils, e.g. to help mask offensive odours or to help patients enjoy better sleep.

- **Electrical diffusers** – explanation of diffusers and precautions to be observed.
- **Choice of oils** – a limited range of oils is used, under the supervision of a nurse/aromatherapist. These include bergamot, grapefruit, lemongrass, lavender and sandalwood. (NB: Editor's note: Latin names should always be used to ensure the correct variety or chemotype is used).
- **Method of use** – three different methods of application are described: Aromastream, Aromastone, and via a tissue or external dressing. There is detailed instruction on how to proceed, depending on the method used.
- **Storage** – how and where the essential oils should be stored.
- **Advice** – staff are reminded that if they have any queries they must consult the complementary therapy coordinator for the unit, who is a qualified aromatherapist.
- **Accidents and adverse reactions** – instructions about how these should be reported.

At the bottom of the protocol is a section for the date when it will be ratified, a date for review, and the person responsible for the review. An interesting issue that falls within policy development is that of informed consent. Because aromatherapy is not part of mainstream healthcare, explicit consent must be obtained from the patient, who must understand not only the potential benefits but also the limits of a treatment. Any safety issues must also be highlighted. Many units are producing leaflets explaining the services offered, making sure patients have access to the information before they arrive, so that they can raise any concerns during the initial assessment.

Policy development for integrating aromatherapy within the NHS is a complex process. While there is undoubted enthusiasm within many healthcare professions, the development of policy is most often 'guarded' by the medical establishment. Naturally, all healthcare professionals understand the need to base any care on evidence, and wish to provide a service to patients which is responsive to needs, appropriate and effective. For many, the use of essential oils adds another dimension to care, to complement the often harsh orthodox regimes – and to enhance a patient's quality of life. Unfortunately, the preoccupation of the medical establishment with randomized controlled trials means that qualitative research methods which, for example, explore patient outcomes, are denigrated. Winning the support of medical colleagues is part of the complex process.

The practical approach would be for the use of essential oils to be limited to a relatively small range of therapeutic interventions in appropriate clinical settings, which should be fastidiously evaluated. The evaluation should then be published so that success is well documented and will build a foundation from which the use of essential oils can be appropriately spread throughout the health service.

Summary

Part 1 of this chapter showed the great steps that have been taken towards self-regulation of aroma-therapy in the UK and the current legislation situation directed by the European Union. Part 2 has demonstrated how nursing policy and practice guidelines can be put into practice by aromatherapists also, and it is to be hoped that more health provision agencies will follow the lead already made in the UK.

References

Barker, A., 1994. Aromatherapy in a hospital setting. In: Aromatherapy World, Spring, pp. 6–7.

Burns, E., Blamey, C., Lloyd, A., 2000. Aromatherapy in childbirth: an effective approach to care. British Journal of Midwifery 8 (10), 639–643.

Department of Health, 2001. Government Response to the House of Lords Select Committee on Science and Technology's Report on Complementary and Alternative Medicine. CM5124. The Stationery Office, London.

Field, T., 2003. Touch therapy. In: Elsevier, London, p. vii.

House of Lords Select Committee on Science and Technology, 2000. Complementary and Alternative Medicine. HL Paper 123. November. The Stationery Office, London.

Gage, H., Storey, L., McDowell, C., Maguire, G., et al., 2009. Integrated care: Utilisation of complementary medicine within a conventional cancer treatment centre. Complement. Ther. Med. 17, 84–91.

Hadfield, N., 2001. The role of aromatherapy massage in reducing anxiety in patients with malignant brain tumours. Int. J. Palliat. Nurs. 7 (6), 279–285.

Maddocks-Jennings, W., Wilkinson, J., 2004. Aromatherapy practice in nursing: a literature review. J. Adv. Nurs. 48 (1), 93–103.

Mousley, S., 2005. Audit of an aromatherapy service in a maternity unit. Complement. Ther. Clin. Pract. 11, 205–210.

Rankin-Box, D., McVey, M., 2001. Policy development. In: Rankin-Box, D. (Ed.), The nurse's handbook of complementary therapies. Ballière Tindall, London.

Stone, J., 2010. Risk, regulation and the growing marginalization of CAM. Guest Editorial. Complementary Therapies in Clinical Care 16, 1–2.

Tavares, M., 2003. National Guidelines for the Use of Complementary Therapies in Supportive and Palliative Care. The Prince of Wales's Foundation for Integrated Health and National Council for Hospice and Specialist Palliative Care Services, London.

Tavares, M., 2004. Guide for writing policies, procedures and protocols. complementary therapies. In: Supportive and palliative care. Help the Hospices, London.

The Prince of Wales's Foundation for Integrated Health (PWFIH), 2003. Setting the agenda for the future. The Prince of Wales's Foundation for Integrated Health, London.

Thomas, K., Nicholl, J., Coleman, P., 2001. Use and expenditure on complementary medicine in England: a population based survey. Complement. Ther. Med. 9, 2–11.

Nursing and Midwifery Council, 2008a. Code of Professional Conduct. Nursing and Midwifery Council, London.

Nursing and Midwifery Council, 2008b. Standards for Medicines Management. Nursing and Midwifery Council, London.

Nursing and Midwifery Council, 2009. Code of Professional Conduct. Complementary alternative therapies.

University of Exeter, 1997. Professional organization of complementary medicine in the United Kingdom. Cenre for Complementary Health Studies, University of Exeter.

Sources

Avis, A., 1999. When is an aromatherapist not an aromatherapist? Complement. Ther. Med. 7 (2), 116–118.

Corner, J., Cawley, N., Hildebrand, S., 1996. An evaluation of the use of massage and essential oils on the wellbeing of cancer patients. Int. J. Palliat. Nurs. 1, 67–73.

Currie, L., Morrell, C., Scrivener, R., 2003. Clinical Governance: an RCN resource guide. Royal College of Nursing, London.

Department of Health, 1995. The Policy Framework for Commissioning Cancer Services. The Stationery Office, London.

Department of Health, 1997. The New NHS, Modern Dependable. The Stationery Office, London.

Department of Health, 1998. A First Class Service: quality in the new NHS. The Stationery Office, London.

Department of Health, 1999. Clinical Governance: Quality in the new NHS. The Stationery Office, Leeds.

Department of Health, 2000. The NHS Cancer Plan: a plan for investment, a plan for reform. The Stationery Office, London.

Hudson, R., 1996. The value of lavender for rest and activity in the elderly patient. Complement. Ther. Med. 4, 52–57.

Luff, D., Thomas, J., 2000. 'Getting somewhere'. Feeling cared for: perspectives on complementary therapies in the NHS. Complement. Ther. Med. 8, 253–259.

Mackereth, P., 2001. Supervision and complementary therapies. In: Rankin-Box, D. (Ed.), The nurse's handbook of complementary therapies. Ballière Tindall, London.

National Institute for Clinical Excellence, 2004. Guidance on Cancer Services: improving supportive and palliative care for adults with cancer. The Stationery Office, London.

Rankin-Box, D. (Ed.), 2001. The nurse's handbook of complementary therapies. Ballière Tindall, London.

Russo, H., 2000. Integrated healthcare: a guide to good practice. Foundation for Integrated Medicine, London.

Sanderson, H., Harrison, J., Price, S., 1991. Aromatherapy and massage for people with learning difficulties. Hands-On Publishing, Birmingham.

Semple, M., Cable, S., 2003. The new Code of Professional Conduct. Nurs. Stand. 19 (17), No 23, 40–48.

Shuttleworth, A., 2003. Protocol based care. Nursing Times Publication, Emap Healthcare, London.

Tiran, D., Mack, S. (Eds.), 2000. Complementary therapies for pregnancy and childbirth. second ed. Baillière Tindall, London.

Aromatherapy worldwide

Introduction

The practice of and knowledge in aromatherapy vary widely across the globe. In some countries, such as France and Belgium, phytotherapy (which includes aromatic medicine – see Ch. 9) is an established branch of medicine for which essential oils may be prescribed by the doctors concerned and used by application to various parts of the body (usually without massage, and very often orally, per rectum and per vaginam, in compresses and in gargles); or in diffusers. In other countries, such as Croatia, aromatherapy is in its infancy; it is practised in hospices using mainly massage, often on a voluntary basis, by aromatherapists and interested nurses.

This chapter examines aromatherapy use in 19 countries, representing a range of different stages of development, implementation and styles of practice.

The following headings are used for each country:

- The general picture
- Regulations
- Essential oils
- Education
- Use of essential oils in medical establishments
- Aromatherapy associations
- Research/pilot studies

Australia

Ron Guba

The general picture

Aromatherapy is a popular complementary therapy, widely used in nursing practice, with increasing cooperation between complementary and conventional practitioners. Although still having applications in beauty care, use is increasing in care of the elderly, palliative care and midwifery. Some aromatherapists are employed by aged care facilities, although most are in private practice and contract services to individuals or health service providers.

Regulation

Although there is no legislation as yet, there may be some changes affecting aromatherapy education, practitioner regulation and the labelling of products. Chiropractors and osteopaths require some governmental oversight – other complementary therapies do not require this. In most states, therapists are self-regulated through their relevant professional associations, who offer practitioner liability insurance. A number of private health insurance companies will offer some level of rebate for aromatherapy treatments given by qualified practitioners.

Allopathic medicines, complementary medicines and essentials oils are regulated through the Therapeutic Goods Administration (TGA), under either Therapeutic Goods Listing or Registration. Under Listing, whether inhaled, ingested, topical applications etc., one may claim to 'relieve the irritation of eczema' but not 'to cure it' – this would require registration.

Listed products must make a lesser therapeutic claim, do not require a prescription and are considered safe for general use when used according to the directions. However, a supplier of TGA-listed essential oils can provide more in-depth information about the therapeutic properties of essential oils to qualified practitioners, compared to what can be advertised to the public.

Practitioners do create their own preparations for clients, but in this situation TGA requirements do not apply with regard to advertising and for what purpose the preparation is intended – there is greater latitude when practitioners are dealing directly with their clients.

Essential oils

Companies that have a therapeutic goods manufacturing licence must follow good manufacturing practice (GMP) pharmaceutical standards – internationally recognized, including a regular audit by a TGA auditor. In the case of an essential oil they must be able to analyse and demonstrate that it is genuine and meets authentic standards, e.g. those of the British Pharmacopoeia (BP) 2010.

There are a few large suppliers of essential oils and other natural materials with little or no background in aromatherapy that do not follow TGA standards, and if they do not make a therapeutic claim the TGA has no authority over them. Some adulterated oils are promoted as '100% pure and natural', sometimes even 'therapeutic grade', with nursing homes and naive therapists buying them. Hopefully the Australian Competition and Consumer Commission (ACCC) will take an interest and deal with these obvious cases of fraudulent misrepresentation.

Education

There is now an approved standard for a Certificate level 4 aromatherapy training (about 1 year), Diploma (about 2 years) and an Advanced Diploma in Aromatic Medicine (about 3 years). In 2008, aromatherapy training was finalized as a 'training package' by the Community Services and Health Industry Skills Council (CS and HISC). This means that any approved college (registered training organization) must use the full training package courses and demonstrate the competencies gained. The CS and HISC comes under the Department of Education, Employment and Workplace Relations.

Almost all colleges offering aromatherapy training in Australia are approved registered training organizations. There are a few non-approved training courses, but they need to meet the same training standards in order to obtain membership with the lead association, the International Aromatherapy and Aromatic Medicine Association

Education curricula include theoretical and clinical hours as well as home study. Courses are no longer based on hours per se, but on the competencies (or learning outcomes) that are gained.

A plethora of short aromatherapy courses of a few hours, days or a week reflect the growing popularity of aromatherapy. Nurses are major participants in these courses, and although they are important professional development programmes, they are insufficient for autonomous aromatherapy practice.

A number of aromatherapy-specific policies/ guidelines for nursing practice have been developed, and these include position statements by the Royal College of Nursing, Australia, and the Australian Nursing Federation. Nurses are regulated in each state through nursing authorities which issue licences to practise nursing, but not aromatherapy. Nurses have a duty of care under their professional standards and codes to practise at the level of their knowledge and competence – and this includes aromatherapy.

Use of essential oils in medical establishments

Aromatherapy is widely accepted in aged care facilities, largely due to the Federal Government's 1997 policy reforms and subsequent accreditation standards for aged care facilities; in some, 53% of residents have aromatherapy treatments routinely. Aromatherapy is accepted in some coronary care units, maternity and neonatal care, mental health and palliative care.

Essential oils are used in vaporizers, on linen or clothing, compresses and/or massage to promote sleep, reduce wandering behaviour, manage 'sundowner's syndrome', reduce anxiety and stress and care for wounds, especially skin tears. Sometimes the facility purchases the oils; in other cases the aromatherapists or individual patients supply them.

Associations

International Aromatherapy and Aromatic Medicine Association (IAAMA)

This is the only aromatherapy association in Australia. The IAAMA originally began as the IFA Australian branch in 1988. The association had little involvement for a number of years with the IFA UK and became the IAAMA in 2008.

The IAAMA requires Diploma level training to become a full member.

The association holds regular state-based meetings and an annual conference. Comprehensive practitioner liability insurance is offered and a requirement for all practising members.

The IAAMA produces a quarterly magazine, *Simply Essential*. www.iaama.org.au

The International Federation of Professional Aromatherapists (IFPA)

Many Australian aromatherapists are members of this UK association, but there is no branch in Australia.

Australian Traditional Medicine Society (ATMS)

The ATMS is not an independent association, but a non-profit company run primarily by ATMS-accredited colleges. The ATMS is a large umbrella group that covers many complementary therapies, including aromatherapy and especially massage. Comprehensive practitioner liability insurance is offered and a requirement for all practising members.

Continued professional development (CPD) is a requirement of membership.

Nursing associations

A number of nursing complementary therapy associations exist, for example the Complementary Therapy Special Interest Group (CTSIG) and the College of Holistic Nurses (CHN), aromatherapists making up a significant number of their members. These bodies hold regular meetings and national conferences, as does the IAAMA. Attendance at these forums contributes CPD points to both nursing and aromatherapy professional associations.

Research/pilot studies

Since the establishment of the Office of Complementary Medicine much laboratory-based research has been conducted into the chemical constituents and properties of essential oils.

Individual aromatherapists are conducting some clinical pilot studies which can be directly applied to patient care. Examples include Guba's and Casey and Kerr's works in wound care, Bowles et al.'s work in aged care, Dunning's work with people with diabetes and Dunning and James' work in rehabilitation.

In the last few years data are being generated about the chemical composition of a range of unique Australian essential oils, particularly their antibacterial properties, primarily from Charles Stuart University.

Guba is already working with an aged care psychiatrist, O'Connor, with a study on the effects of lavender oil on agitation in those with dementia, for which he has received funding. They are using a significant dose – a 30% concentration in jojoba oil for topical application.

Warnke and Sherry have done work on essential oils for infections, using first the MAC concentrate and then their own mixture.

Belgium

Anny van Branteghem, Sylvie Lenoir, Philippe Gérard

The general picture

Aromatherapy is well known in Belgium and is practised as in France, both externally and internally; it is quite different from the common use of 'aromatherapy' in Britain, where it is more related to massage and external use. Aromatherapy does not exist as a profession on its own, as it does in the UK; as in France, it is a complementary training to medicine, physiotherapy, dentistry, pharmacy and nursing, and has a more scientific and medical approach than in the UK.

Many people practise self-medication with plants and essential oils – unlike in Britain, they have never lost that part of their culture.

Aromatherapy can be divided into two sections:

- external use – mainly for the purpose of *wellness*
- internal use – for the treatment of *disease*

The former is widespread and supported by a vast number of commercial initiatives: products, wellness and health resorts, workshops and courses. The latter is limited, since it is practised by the specialists mentioned above.

Regulations

Internal use is discouraged: it is limited by HACCP (Hazard Analysis of Critical Control Points) – international standards on food and food supplements rules. http://www.haccp-guide.fr/

Non-medical personnel are not allowed to practise internal medicine; medical doctors and pharmacists are allowed to do so with personalized preparations called magistral formulas on prescription.

Several regulations apply, depending on how they are used: raw material for pharmaceutical preparations, cosmetics or food supplements. There is no specific legislation for essential oils, but external use is regulated by cosmetic laws.

After training only in aromatherapy without medical training, alternative therapists are practising 'medicine' illegally – there is no aromatherapist-recognized diploma. A herbalist or phytotherapist,

having knowledge of aromatherapy through their training, is sanctioned by a recognized certification, which allows him to practise.

There has been a regulatory agreement and acceptance of internally used essential oils (in preparations contained in soft gelatine capsules) in products that were already on the market before HACCP and other rules were devised.

Education

Courses are organized by aromatherapists (no official certificate) in the use of essential oils for external use on a regular but small-scale basis. These are attended by enthusiasts, herbalists, nurses, health, wellness and beauty practitioners and paramedics.

Some training centres, often linked to essential oil wholesalers, give quality courses in scientific aromatherapy.

Courses on the use of essential oils for internal use, as well as for external use in pharmaceutical preparations (for the treatment of dermatological ailments or transdermal agents), are organized by:

- **Société Belge de Phytothérapie, d'Aromathérapie et de Nutrithérapie:** philip.antoine@skynet.be
  Courses are organized on the use of essential oils for internal use, as well as for external use in pharmaceutical preparations (for the treatment of dermatological ailments or transdermal agents). These courses offer a general, but qualitative and profound and fundamental knowledge on the therapeutic possibilities of essential oils, their chemistry, their uses, their toxicology and their powers. The lecturers are medical doctors, pharmacists and university professors; the courses can only be attended by dentists, doctors and pharmacists. A diploma can be obtained, after examination, after 3 years of 10 weekends.
- **Primrose Academy: info@primroseacademy.be**
  Courses are organized by aromatherapists (no official certificate) in the use of essential oils for external use on a regular, but small-scale basis. These are attended by enthusiasts, herbalists, nurses, health, wellness and beauty practitioners and paramedics.
- **Institute de Phytothérapie International:** http://www.phytotherapie.be/fr/enseign.htm
- **Centre de Formation en d'Aromathérapie:** http://www.aromamondo.com

- Collège International d'Aromathérapie:
http://www.college-aromatherapie.com

This college provides training for everyone from medical professionals (doctors, pharmacists, dentists, therapists etc.) to laypersons; depending on the type of course, the curriculum and the number of hours can vary.

Hydrolats are always taught and used mostly in paediatrics.

A certificate is given at the end of the course, but has no professional recognition.

Essential oils

Essential oils are available in organic health food shops, pharmacies and online.

The quality varies immensely – as everywhere, the market is full of unscrupulous companies, although genuine oils are available. The only absolute protection for the consumer is to buy essential oils botanically and biochemically defined (EOBBD). EOBBD is a certification guaranteeing the origin and the exact nature of the essential oil by providing:

- the exact Latin botanical name
- the part of the plant from which it is obtained (leaf, petals, bark etc.)
- the location and time of harvest and distillation.

Chromatography is systematically used. Some wholesalers of ethical essential oils test samples of the essential oils they intend to buy by gas chromatography–mass spectrometry (GC-MS) and test the products delivered as well, in case they do not match the samples.

Such oils guarantee good results without the side effects created by solvent-extracted, deterpened, rectified or adulterated products.

Essential oil use

Aromatherapists, massage therapists and other holistic therapists use essential oils regularly; there is limited use in nursing homes, where they are mainly used in palliative care, oncology and comas. They are mostly applied diluted, by massage (professional therapists/nurses/beauty therapists), self-application or diffusion; they are also used in baths (after dissolving in a dispersant), gargles and compresses, but more for wellbeing than for their therapeutic actions.

Sometimes they are used neat; EOBBD essential oils may be used orally. Dentists, pharmacists and GPs trained in aromatherapy or herbal medicine can prescribe them for internal use, but are not paid by the state.

Use of essential oils in medical establishments

Hospitals do not offer aromatherapy training, although this is beginning to change. Hospitals offer aromatherapy massages in palliative care, neonatology, oncology and comas, mostly for wellbeing rather than for their therapeutic purposes.

Associations

Because the profession of aromatherapist does not really exist as in the UK, there is no professional association or society.

Research and/or pilot studies

Research is limited; Philippe Gerard is working on a project with Leuven University concerning plants for the treatment of neurodegenerative diseases.

Brazil

Vera L G O'Neill

The general picture

Aromatherapy became known in Brazil in the late 1980s, when some books were translated from English into Portuguese: first, in 1989, *Practical Aromatherapy – How to use essential oils to restore health and vitality* by Shirley Price, shortly followed by *Aromatherapy Workbook* by Marcel Lavabre.

Interest in aromatherapy gradually increased during the 1990s, and in 1993 the first aromatherapy seminar took place, when, for the first time, a professional aromatherapist from England came to Brazil to speak. During this period, more books became available in Portuguese, such as *The Art of Aromatherapy* (Robert Tisserand 1992), *The*

Aromatherapy Book (Jeanne Rose 1995), *Aromatherapy* (Patricia Davis 1998), *Aromatherapy and your Emotions* (Shirley Price 1997) and *Aromatherapy for Common Ailments* (Shirley Price 1999). This prompted the publishing of aromatherapy books by Brazilian authors too.

By the mid-1990s essential oils could be found in beauty salons, spas and shops and the home in general; aromatherapy had become synonymous with natural. There are now a growing number of people working as aromatherapists or who offer aromatherapy treatments as part of their practice. Few people have studied aromatherapy abroad, and often those who describe themselves as 'aromatherapists' have only attended a short weekend course. The same situation exists in most complementary therapies.

Regulations

The Brazilian government does not recognize aromatherapy as a treatment or as a profession, so it is not regulated. Some academic institutions are attempting to build greater awareness and acceptance by incorporating the therapy into naturopathy, whereby aromatherapy is given equal importance alongside other complementary therapies such as reflexology and Bach flower essences. At present, only homoeopathy and acupuncture are officially recognized as complementary therapies.

Complementary therapies or 'integrative practices' as they are known, include aromatherapy, homoeopathy, flower essences, phytotherapy and acupuncture. They are also part of the Unique Health System (SUS) contained within the National Policy of Complementary and Integrative Practices (PNPIC), which has only a partial presence in Brazil.

Essential oils

Although the sale of essential oils is not regulated, there are licences for homoeopathic and phytotherapy products.

Education, including standards of training

Formal teaching of aromatherapy started in the early 1990s and is now available at different levels, from basic 1-day courses up to courses of 50 hours or more. More advanced courses (100 hours) are taught at two private universities, which although approved by the Ministry of Education, are not endorsed by the Ministry of Health.

Unfortunately, a number of aromatherapy teachers who have little or no formal training give courses, which does not help the general level of quality of training that exists in the country.

In 2010, the Penny Price Academy arrived in Brazil, bringing with it an internationally certified course, the Associate Diploma in Clinical Aromatherapy. This responds to a growing demand for quality training which carries global value and recognition and which gives the practice, teaching and study of aromatherapy a much-needed credibility alongside the other more established complementary therapies.

Education

Universities

UNISUL Florianópolis (SC) – Bachelor Degree in Naturology

The University of South Santa Catarina is a Brazilian Educational Foundation. This complementary therapy degree at UNISUL carries a 60-hour component of aromatherapy, with four assessments (written and oral).

Universidade Anhembi Morumbi, São Paulo (SP) – Bachelor Degree in Naturology (this university has a partnership with the Penny Price Academy in Brazil).

The aromatherapy component of this 260-hour course is 100 hours; the naturology course here considers aromatherapy a complementary and integrative therapy, which allows study leading to an understanding of how aromatherapy integrates with other complementary health disciplines – Bach flower essences, massage, reflexology and others.

Other centres

Athaman Naturology – Health and Beauty Clinic

This is a specialized clinic in aromatherapy; they have trained over 25 people and have offered treatment to over 6000 people over the last 7 years. It is run by teachers at UNISUL.

NovaFloressencia – (Penny Price Academy, Brazil)

This company has been involved with aromatherapy education for over 16 years. The proprietor graduated in 2006 at the Penny Price Academy in the UK and it is now a satellite PPA school – it is the only school which offers a course with an internationally recognized qualification.

Several private companies run a variety of training courses with qualifications validated by themselves.

Availability and quality of essential oils

Essential oils are generally found only in some homoeopathic pharmacies and health food stores. Unfortunately, much of what is available is of low quality, but those who know the importance of having genuine essential oils can find quality products from a small number of reliable suppliers. It is also possible to buy essential oils from an aromatherapist, although it is not easy to verify their origin. Therefore, much care has to be taken by the consumer when purchasing essential oils – only a few brands are of a high grade.

Use of essential oils

Naturopaths, aromatherapists, massage therapists, holistic therapists, and some physicians, dentists, psychologists and physiotherapists use essential oils in their practices – and some veterinarians use them to treat pets and large animals.

Hydrolats are not used to any great extent at present, but hopefully this will change as training progresses.

Methods of using essential oils

Essential oils are used in various ways:

- self-application in vegetable oil or white lotion, or added to skin creams, gels, shampoos, conditioners
- massage via a professional therapist
- compresses and gargles.

Internal application is limited to a small number of experts, there being no proper training for this method of use at present.

Associations

ABRAROMA

Brazilian Association of Aromatherapy and Aromatology. ABRAROMA was created in 1997 by a group of professionals driven by idealism and love of essential oil therapy.

AROMAFLORA

Brazilian Association for Studies and Research in Aromatherapy. This is a non-profit organization whose purpose is to expand the level of public awareness of the benefits of aromatherapy. It endeavours to promote and raise educational standards and professional practice, enhance the awareness and knowledge of aromatherapy, and educate people in the safe, effective and responsible application of essential oils in daily life.

Research

Some research has been carried out at UNISUL University and also at Anhembi Morumbi University on the following:

- Concentration – focus and increase performance of dancers, using *Citrus limon*
- Loss of weight and release of sciatic pain, using *Mentha* x *piperita*
- Backache in pregnant women, using *Lavandula officinalis*
- Women who have suffered domestic violence (students of Anhembi Morumbi university above).

This research was carried out in 2009 and coordinated by Professor Marcia Fernandes. The results are yet to be made available.

Canada

Marlene M Mitchell, Tricia Eagle

Aromatherapy development

Although it is not known exactly when aromatherapy first appeared in Canada, essential oils have been available in health stores – and one or two schools have been teaching aromatherapy for several years.

Regulations

There are no regulations for the practice of aromatherapy in Canada.

The provincial government of British Columbia recognizes aromatherapy as a distinct profession, granting Occupational Title Protection to the members of the British Columbia Alliance of Aromatherapy (BCAOA – see Associations, below), enabling its members to call themselves Registered Aromatherapists (RA).

In 1996, the Canadian Cosmetic, Toiletry and Fragrance Association (CCTFA) started working with Health Canada officials to develop and implement mandatory ingredient labelling for cosmetics and personal care products, including aromatherapy products.

Education

The Canadian Federation of Aromatherapy (CFA) formed an Education Committee in 1999 and over the years has set standards for certification (updated in 2009), safety and professional conduct for its members. A core curriculum that the schools must follow has been established, and passing the CFA National Exam is a requirement for membership. Members are entitled to use the legal designation CAHP (Certified Aromatherapy Health Professional), which is only available and applicable to CFA members.

To graduate from a CFA-approved programme, students must complete 400 educational hours and pass the standardized national CFA examination.

Approved diplomas are licensed through the Ministry of Education in Ontario, Canada, entitling the successful therapist to use the letters RAHP (Registered Aromatherapy Health Practitioner) after their name.

Aromatherapists can apply for a business licence, allowing them to practise in their own area – depending on the Government bylaws of that area. To receive this holistic business licence and practise as an alternative healthcare provider, aromatherapists must prove that they belong to a complementary healthcare organization, which can then supply them with an Errors and Omissions/ Malpractice insurance.

Essential oils

Essential oils are available in stores and health shops, some being therapeutic grade, some poor grade. People wanting to be sure of quality buy their essential oils from an aromatherapist. The general public use essential oils for beauty and health and in vaporizers.

Essential oils are used in all the usual ways except internally, as no school teaches the ingestion of essential oils.

Hydrolats are used in baths, compresses, gargles, sprays and cooking, but not internally as there is no education as yet on this practice.

Use of essential oils in medical establishments

Although doctors are wary about using alternative medicine, nurses are leading the movement towards incorporating essential oils into medical practice. Two hospitals in British Columbia are known to accept aromatherapy at present, although it is offered in many private clinics, but there is no knowledge of aromatherapy being practised in hospices.

Associations

The Canadian Federation of Aromatherapists (CFA)
www.cfacanada.com

This federation was formed in early 1993 by a group of individuals from varying backgrounds who recognized that there was no governing body or organization that the public could contact for information, or to verify that those claiming to be aromatherapists were indeed qualified.

It is a non-profit association, sponsored by contributions, donations, fund-raising events and membership fees.

It aims to foster continuing growth, quality and high standards of education and practice within the aromatherapy profession, and provide ongoing information about the quality of aromatherapy products and services to the public.

To maintain membership, all members must complete ongoing educational programmes and be active in aromatherapy work. Credit Education Units (CEUs) are applied to a large variety of courses, retreats, workshops and lectures across Canada, and ensure that CFA members are continually increasing their breadth of knowledge.

The British Columbia Alliance of Aromatherapy (BCAOA)

The BCAOA was registered in February 1999, under the Society Act of the province of British Columbia, Canada. It was formed by representatives of 16 different associations which had concerns that the practice of aromatherapy/essential oil therapy was being threatened by changes to laws and regulations at both provincial and federal level. In December 1999, BCAOA applied for registration as a professional association under the Health Act of British Columbia. The application is pending hearings.

Its mission is to provide educational and professional standards and ethics for aromatherapy/essential oil therapy in British Columbia, and to support ongoing education. It encourages a sense of community and exchange among aromatherapists, essential oil therapists, healthcare practitioners and associations.

The British Columbia Association of Practicing Aromatherapists in British Columbia (BCAPA)

This association was formed in 1994; it encourages networking, holds conferences and issues regular newsletters. There are four categories of membership, plus corporate membership.

It supports practising aromatherapists, as well as educating the public in the benefits of aromatherapy. The BCAPA has a stringent code of ethics and a high standard in professionalism and continuing education.

Research

There is no known research on aspects of essential oil properties and/or their effects.

China

Shaohua Lu

The general picture

Around 1990, the concept of aromatherapy began to be accepted in China. It was first introduced to mainland China by the family of a Taiwanese businessman, when the basic application of essential oils and the promotion of its possibilities began to spread. Having first appeared as skin care, beauty salons then began using essential oils in face and body massage – now the most common forms of use. Although essential oils are now used in every beauty salon and spa, their quality is a concern, as they are probably adulterated.

Young women aged 18–25 went to Europe and America to study and experience essential oils, returning to spread their knowledge to others via forums and websites etc. As herbalism was already well known, aromatherapy was readily accepted. Most buyers of essential oils are over the age of 25, as they can more easily afford them: they are used mostly in vaporizers. Although essential oil use is widespread, there is a shortage of correct aromatherapy information and training in the Chinese language, making aromatherapy less easily available to people generally.

Around the beginning of the 21st century two books, P Davies' *Aromatherapy A–Z* and M Maury's *Guide to Aromatherapy* were imported – in English, which naturally limited the number of readers. Both books are now translated into Chinese, as are S Price's *Aromatherapy and your Emotions* and L Price's *Carrier Oils for Aromatherapy and Massage*. By 2010 there were over 15 aromatherapy books in Chinese, and information was also available via newspapers, magazines and the Internet. Some large aromatherapy websites have been established which include the translation into Chinese of information written in English.

Aromatherapy has been identified by the Shanghai Vocational Training Orientation Centre (SVTOC) as an area for growth, an agreement being made recently with the International Federation of Professional Aromatherapists (IFPA) to develop British-style aromatherapy training.

Regulations

Many people – including the government – class aromatherapy with beauty and hairdressing, and as most practitioners were without any professional training, many mistakes occurred using essential oils, adversely affecting some clients' health. Because of this, the government introduced an 'Aromatic Masseurs Qualification Standard', which came into force at the end of 2004. Aromatic masseurs have to follow these government recommendations, which will ensure that aromatherapy progresses in the right direction.

Education

The basis for all professional courses follows the syllabi of two British and one American associations:

The International Federation of Aromatherapy (IFA)

Training in China was originally carried out by an English aromatherapist, one of her trainees from Taiwan now training by distance learning. However, the training is expensive, and since little time was spent on essential oils, many graduates were found incapable of practising aromatherapy correctly. However, this lady caused an increase of interest in essential oils and aromatherapy, as she has published two introductory books on aromatherapy and appeared in many TV shows.

The International Federation of Professional Aromatherapists (IFPA)

This organization now has an agreement (see above) with the SVTOC in Shanghai, which was the result of 3 years' work by an IFPA-accredited school based in Singapore.

The Penny Price Academy (PPA), accredited by both the above associations, began distance learning courses in mainland China and now has a school there, which Penny Price and her husband visit to lecture. PPA tutors come to China from Taiwan and Japan to run courses that emphasize the UK training standards, but there will not be any IFPA-accredited Chinese tutors until 2012.

There are also a few schools which run short-term training.

The National Association of Holistic Aromatherapy (NAHA)

This organization is based in the USA but does not have much influence in China.

Associations

At the time of writing, there is no Chinese professional association for aromatherapy.

Research

In January 2004, Shanghai JiaoTong University and the XinJiang Plant Technology Development Company together established the Shanghai JiaoTong University – XinJiang Aroma Technology Universal Research Center to improve research into aromatic materials – at present it is based more on raw materials used in perfumes, with very little on aromatherapy. The research is on a very small scale and not related to aromatherapy. The real research into and development of herbs and commercial essential oils is done by the Botanical Institute of China Science Academy; the man in charge has been appointed to promote the growth of herbs in Xinjiang – mainly *Lavandula angustifolia*, which has been grown non-commercially in China since the 1950s.

Croatia

Zrinka Jezdić

The general picture

Essential oils have been used in Croatia for many years as part of herbal and traditional medicine and the making of candles and aromatic substances. They are sold in speciality shops, people using them in their homes as well as for massage by an aromatherapist. The word aromatherapy was first used in 1990, after a firm began to use and sell oils. Some informal lectures are given to the public.

A small number of nurses, doctors and therapists use essential oils in clinical practice. After training with Shirley Price in England, the first aromatherapy school was opened in 2000, followed by Aromara (the Aroma Academy) in 2002, and the Citizen Open College in 2004.

Regulations

There are no regulations in Croatia concerning the application of essential oils in clinical practice.

Essential oils

Sales of essential oils have expanded over the last 10 years, people using them as a form of self-help. They are imported mainly from France and Germany, some shops putting their own label on them. Although the Institute for Public Health checks the quality of essential oils, there are no regulations regarding quality.

A few essential oils are produced in Croatia, namely: *Laurus nobilis*, *Lavandula* x *intermedia*, *Rosmarinus officinalis* ct. *camphor*, *Salvia officinalis* and *Thymus vulgaris* ct. *thymol*, All essential oils have to pass safety controls for food and cosmetic use.

Education

Three schools in Croatia are licensed by the Ministry of Education, Sports and Science to teach aromatherapy. Although aromatherapy is not recognized by the Ministry of Health as a complementary therapy, and treatment of disease is not permitted, it can be used to support treatment with the personal consent of the patient and/or his/her doctor. The diploma of the author's school, AromaVita, has received a licence from the Ministry of Health to practise aromatherapy in this way. The training offered by the other two schools is quite similar to that offered by AromaVita.

AromaVita concentrates on preventive measures and conditions such as stress management, emotional blockage, anxiety, neuroses, and support for personal and spiritual development.

When aromatherapists finish the course they can obtain a work permit, which allows them to practise legally.

AromaVita cooperates with the Penny Price Academy (PPA) in the UK, through workshops and counselling for their students. The principal of Aromavita lectures in Croatian hospitals to inform and educate nurses, physiotherapists and doctors about the clinical application of essential oils and aromatherapy techniques. Students who finish both aromatherapy courses below can take an examination at PPA to obtain an international certificate.

The training schedule is as follows:

1. Basic aromatherapy training is 6 months – 280 hours.

   Students are taught about 40 essential oils and 15 fixed vegetable oils. After completing this, students are trained in the application of essential oils, including massage techniques to reduce/eliminate stress, and improve health and body care.
2. An advanced aromatherapy diploma training takes 16 months – 460 hours.

   Practical classes are conducted in homes for the elderly and disabled, to learn the clinical application of essential oils and massage. Students have to carry out 10 client case studies with five treatments on each. After completion of training students are qualified in the application of essential oils, massage and consultation for the purpose of maintaining good health, psychological support and help in self-development.

Use of essential oils in hospices and hospitals

AromaVita collaborates with social health institutions (homes for the elderly and infirm) for student practical training.

Research/pilot studies

No research has as yet been carried out on essential oils. However, pilot studies have been carried out in the following areas:

- **Stress management** – Results show a reduction in stress and a better attitude towards work; managers take time for aromatherapy, having learned to use essential oils to keep their psychophysical balance and growth of creativity. The most successful oils used are *Lavandula angustifolia*, *Citrus sinensis*, *Melissa officinalis*, *Citrus bergamia*, *Citrus limon*, *Rosmarinus officinalis* ct. 1,8 cineole and *Cedrus atlantica*.
- **Emotional cleansing** – Essential oils and aromatherapy techniques have helped to open up emotional expressions and their awareness, helping people to achieve a better relationship with themselves as well as with other relationships. The best results were with *Citrus bergamia*, *Melissa officinalis*, *Juniperus communis*, *Hyssopus officinalis*, *Salvia sclarea*, *Eucalyptus globulus* and *Boswellia carteri*.
- **Pain** – Back pain, aching muscles and headaches. Oils that showed the best results were *Citrus limon*, *Lavandula angustifolia*, *Matricaria recutita*, *Mentha piperita*, *Zinziber officinalis*, *Juniperus communis*, *Rosmarinus officinalis* ct. 1,8 cineole, *Salvia sclarea* and *Pinus sylvestris*.
- **Energy/psychological support in crises** – divorce, death of someone close, losing a job, etc. Aromatherapy massage, breathing techniques and creative visualization were used. Oils used were *Melissa officinalis*, *Boswellia carteri*, *Thymus vulgaris* ct. *thymol*, *Lavandula angustifolia* and *Origanum majorana*.

Finland

Ulla-Maija Grace

The general picture

Aromatherapy came to Finland with the general surge of interest in complementary medicine at the beginning of the 1980s. Beauty therapists led the way by inviting an English aromatherapist to teach the use of essential oils in skin care. In 1984 a beauty/aromatherapist returning from the USA started teaching aromatherapeutic massage with ready blended oils. Holistic aromatherapy using individual essential oils was started by a Finnish aromatherapist trained in England. By the middle of the 1990s, several natural medicine institutions offered aromatherapy training.

Regulations

The laws concerning the whole field of complementary medicine are in the process of being finalized, based on a working group set up in 2000 (see below). Currently there are several laws covering cosmetics, medicine and malpractice, which apply indirectly to the use of essential oils. This means that the use of essential oils and products containing them come under cosmetics legislation and that claims of medical benefits cannot be made.

General use of essential oils

The public is now becoming aware of aromatherapy through aromatherapists, beauty and massage therapists, magazines, books and courses. As a result, the use of essential oils and aromatherapy products containing them is steadily growing with the increase in natural self-care.

As a rule, aromatherapists work as private practitioners in their own businesses or in spas. There is a wide range of essential oils available in Finland, some organic or natural, and some of unspecified quality, as well as some synthetic aromatics; unfortunately, the general public is not sufficiently informed to discriminate between them.

Education

The umbrella association Luonnonlääketieteen Keskusliitto (LKL, The Central Association of Natural Medicine) is the accreditation body for all natural medicine training. The LKL gives recommendations concerning minimum teaching requirements for the different complementary medicine disciplines. To become a member a therapist's training has to conform to the standards set by them. In aromatherapy these recommendations cover the in-class training in essential oils and full-body massage with a large number of documented case studies, clinical practice, exams, essays, and a final thesis requiring some original research. The thesis has to cover a medical problem from an allopathic point of view, and a treatment plan with an aromatherapy case study has to be completed, with a report on the results. Some students make several case studies within the thesis and then collect the information to report on how the different cases compared with each other.

Curriculum. A basic curriculum is mandatory for all; the non-medical students take courses in anatomy, physiology, pathology, neurology and psychology. In addition, all students are required to take two or more modules of natural medicine subjects, e.g. phytotherapy, nutrition or other natural remedies.

Currently there are two schools in Finland registered with the LKL, one of which is also a member of the International Federation of Aromatherapy (IFA).

At the beginning of 2000 a working group was set up by the Ministry of Education comprising representatives of orthodox medicine and a few leading aromatherapists. Basic guidelines have been agreed for teaching aromatherapy to massage therapists, foot specialists and beauty therapists at the level of professional further education. The guidelines include treatment protocols and lists of recommended essential oils according to the needs of the different treatment areas and clients.

Use of essential oils in hospitals

Aromatherapy training at basic nursing level in the mainstream medical schools is limited to short courses, which are not obligatory but are part of a free choice selection of study subjects.

Nevertheless, although aromatherapy is not accepted in hospitals, the use of aromatherapy treatments in hospices and handicapped care is increasing. The method of application in hospices varies, with massage being the most popular form; full or part body treatments are carried out with the permission of the clients and senior staff on the ward.

There are many residential homes, both private and local government run, which actively use aromatherapy for the benefit of the residents.

Aromatherapy associations

There are two aromatherapy associations in Finland, **Suomen Aromaterapeutitry (SA)**, with membership which is independent of the training establishments, and **UMG-Aromaterapiayhdistysry**, which is the association for students qualified by the Finnish College of Aromatherapy.

Public, product and malpractice insurances are available from LKL for those trained to the required standard, and IFA insurance is available through the Finnish College of Aromatherapy for students who have taken the IFA examination.

Research

Currently there is no scientific research on essential oils or their systematic use in the mainstream allopathic healthcare in Finland.

France

Rhiannon Harris, Kuniko M Hadji-Minaglou, Christian Busser

The general picture

Among the most common natural therapies in France, only acupuncture and homoeopathy are officially recognized, and then only if practised by doctors. Many doctors practise other therapies, such as osteopathy and phyto-aromatherapy, but these are 'unofficial' therapies as they are not covered by French law. Essential oils are used more and more by masseurs/ physical therapists, osteopaths and physical therapists, but non-medical persons can use essential oils on condition that they do not claim therapeutic effects.

Aromatherapy, massage and the law

Any non-medical person using a therapy designated as having a therapeutic effect is in effect practising medicine without a licence and thus illegally, even if they are working alongside – and with the support of – a medically trained person.

Difficulties facing non-medical aromatherapists:

a) use of essential oils and related products having health benefits, putting them at risk of practising medicine and/or pharmacy illegally

b) practice of 'Anglosaxon'-style aromatherapy, involving touch or massage; since 1946 this has been the exclusive remit of the masseur-kinésithérapeute.

The Syndicat National des Masseurs-Kinésithérapeute Rééducateurs (SNMKR) protects its members' rights, particularly kinésithérapeutes (physiotherapists), by challenging practitioners through legal proceedings. Similar organizations include the Confédération Nationale des Masseurs Kinésithérapeutes Libéraux and Action Kiné-Massage (which promotes massage exclusively through kinésithérapeutes).

French law (2000) clearly states that only those who have a State-recognized diploma as a Masseur-Kinésithérapeute may practise massage or medical gymnastics. The exclusion also includes the practice of manual lymph drainage (MLD). A German-trained MLD practitioner (Vodder technique) was taken to court in 1996 for illegal practice, despite receiving direct referrals from a French medical doctor. She was found guilty, ordered to pay damages and banned from practising.

Even though aestheticians learn body massage techniques during their state-approved training, they are not legally permitted to practise them. Only light effleurage of the face for beauty purposes can be practised.

Numerous practitioners have attempted to continue their work, calling themselves 'praticien de toucher' (touch practitioner), 'modelage', 'technique manuelle anti-stress' etc., but even then they are skating on thin ice.

The Association Soutien Massage Bien-Etre (www.asmbe.com) was recently formed in response to the case against Joel Savatofski, taken to court for illegal practice of massage. Both he and some of his students (www.toucher-massage.com) were prosecuted for giving seated massage to drivers in an autoroute stop, to refresh and relieve tension.

This case was one of the few success stories, and despite an appeal by the SNMKR it was upheld that on-site massage did not come under the monopoly above.

In spite of this, there are hundreds of non-medical practitioners of natural therapies in France, reflecting the enormous public demand. It is hoped that with increasing collaboration between countries in the European Union, the French legal system will permit the practice of aromatherapy and other forms of CAM.

Education

Complementary/alternative training for doctors, pharmacists and other healthcare professionals varies in depth and duration. As aromatherapy is recognized as a branch of phytotherapy/herbal medicine, studies usually include herbal extracts, not just essential oils.

One main centre is the Faculty of Medicine at the University of Bobigny, Paris.

Two of the university diplomas offered relevant to essential oils are:

- a 3-year diploma in medical herbal practice (252 hours – open only to doctors, veterinarians, pharmacists and dentists)
- a 2-year diploma in herbal advice and information (196 hours – open to a wider audience including osteopaths, kinésithérapeutes, midwives, nurses, pharmacy assistants etc.).

Montpellier University has a more liberal view – phyto-aromatherapy can be studied by doctors, pharmacists, dental surgeons, kinésithérapeutes, veterinarians, midwives, nurses, pharmacy assistants and healthcare students at the end of their studies. The period of study is over 2 years during six weekends, or 1 year with two blocks of study, each of 10 days. Successful participants are awarded a university diploma in phyto-aromatherapy from the Faculty Pharmacy of Montpellier University.

Aromatherapy training is offered for non-medical personnel by the Institut Méditerranéen de Documentation d'Enseignement et de Recherche sur les Plantes Médicinales (IMDERPLAM) (www.imderplam.net), where the study is over 3 years and includes three weekends (24 hours) on aromatherapy.

The Lyonnaise School of Medicinal Plants (www.ecoledeplantesmedicinales.com) also offers training

in applied aromatherapy over three weekends and is open to all, the principal teachers being doctors in pharmacy.

The Plantasanté school, located in Obernai in Alsace and in the Drôme, offers a certificate in medicinal and aromatic plants (phyto-aromatherapy) over 2 years (weekends or weeks), developing all aspects of herbal medicine and aromatherapy. It also offers training in intensive aromatherapy over 24 hours.

The Faculty of Medicine in Paris not only offers several options of natural and ethno-medicinal training (mostly to doctors and paramedic personnel) but also weekend courses for families and herbal shops, some including aromatherapy, some only aromatherapy.

Learning via correspondence is well established and accepted within France; training in phyto-aromatherapy by e-learning is now available, principally open to medical personnel. A leading college offering this form of learning and awarding a diploma in phyto-aromatherapy (300 hours over 2 years) is Hippocratus (www.hippocratus.com).

Essential oils

Most essential oils are freely available, except those with a risk of toxicity, which can be issued only on prescription. They used to be largely obtainable only from pharmacies (behind the counter). Recently, there has been an increasing trend for pure essential oils to be sold in parapharmacies, health and beauty stores and numerous markets in the south of France; the range is limited, blends for massage, diffusion, skin care etc. being more commonly available. Occasionally, essential oils can be found in supermarket chains.

Most practitioners in France obtain their essential oils direct from French laboratories, thereby having access to GC/MS analyses. The idea that it is easier to access good-quality essential oils in France than other countries is not necessarily true, particularly in the north.

Since 2007, essential oils (common and botanical names) restricted to pharmacies include:

- *Artemisia absinthium* [wormwood], *A. arborescens* [shrubby wormwood], *A. herba alba* [white wormwood], *A. pontica* [Roman wormwood], *A. vulgaris* [common wormwood]
- *Brassica juncea* [brown mustard]
- *Chenopodium ambrosioides*/*C. anthelminthicum* [American wormseed]
- *Hyssopus officinalis* [hyssop]

- *Juniperus sabina* [savin]
- *Ruta graveolens* [common rue]
- *Salvia officinalis* [sage]
- *Sassafras albidum* [white sassafras]
- *Tanacetum vulgare* [tansy]
- *Thuja koraiensis* fol. [Korean arborvitae], *Thuja occidentalis* [Canadian white cedarwood], *Thuja plicata* [Western red cedar]

Fennel, star anise and aniseed oils are also restricted by Customs law to avoid the illegal fabrication of alcoholic drinks such as pastis.

Aromatherapy in medical establishments

The use of aromatherapy by medical personnel is largely conducted in general practice. The aromatherapeutic approach varies, from a rigorous 'allopathic' approach, using essential oils as medicaments in much the same way as drugs to a more holistic methodology.

Formulations often consist of capsules or solutions for oral use, suppositories or pessaries for rectal or vaginal application, and lotions or preparations for application to the skin. The percentage of essential oil in these is generally significantly higher than those used in the UK.

The cost for a visit/consultation (about 40 minutes) with a doctor/aromathérapeute varies from approximately 60 to 90 euros, and in most cases part of the expense (excluding an essential oil prescription) can be reimbursed by French health insurance.

The majority of illnesses successfully treated with essential oils are infectious or inflammatory in nature, with an increasing tendency to treat children (ear, nose and throat), thereby reducing recourse to antibiotic therapy. Much attention is paid to the health of the liver, so the prescription is often accompanied by measures (dietary or otherwise) to drain and decongest it.

Occasionally an aromatogram is used to discover the most effective oil for an infectious illness. Aromatograms have been used since the 1970s by medical aromatherapists such as Valnet, Belaiche, Lapraz and Duraffourd to identify the most appropriate essential oils for individual client needs. The pioneer of this technique (and the person who named it) was Doctor Maurice Girault, whose work was particularly recognized in the field of gynaecology. He was the first clinician to use the aromatogram to test the antimicrobial powers of essential oils with a view to treating patients from his surgery.

Aromatherapy research in France

There is a considerable amount of essential oil research conducted, but not all is published in the international scientific press; more and more is found only in the French scientific magazine *Herbal Medicine*, which is then issued in universities throughout the world. Most of the research concerns antimicrobial effects, anti-inflammatory and dermocosmetic aspects or other essential oil activities.

The way ahead

Since the 1980s there has been an enormous shift in public awareness as people become more informed and more prepared to exercise their rights to all forms of health provision. There is a clear need for clarification of roles between kinésithérapeutes and other professionals who use touch in their work. The current situation with regard to the law needs to evolve in parallel with public demand and other European countries.

Germany

Anna Maria Hoch

The general picture

Aromatherapy became known in Germany in the 1980s and has grown rapidly, with increasing support from the general public, as well as nurses and alternative practitioners, some of whom also use essential oils.

Regulations

Aromatherapy can only be practised legally by doctors and alternative practitioners. A few doctors use essential oils in their own practices; nurses and occupational therapists working as aroma-care therapists offer 'wellness' and preventative treatments.

Essential oils are considered to be covered by domestic regulations as 'objects for improving the odour of rooms' and not as medicines, which come under pharmaceutical legislation.

No medicinal claims can be made on essential oil labels and the European Union has introduced many restrictions regarding their use, with special labels for oils containing more than 10% hydrocarbons; these carry the warnings: 'Harmful to health, 'Causes lung defects', 'Keep away from children', 'Take medical advice'. Cosmetic companies have to show the contents of so-called sensitizers on the label. Estragol and safrol are not allowed as ingredients of cosmetic products, the content of methyl eugenol having been reduced to 0.0002% in leave-on products. Except for personal use only pharmacists are permitted to mix and label essential oils for hospitals and medical practices etc.

Essential oils

Essential oils are available in all pharmacies, although most stock only those standardized according to the German pharmacopoeia (DAB). However, some pharmacies, essential oil companies and many health shops, tea shops and markets usually stock high-quality, authentic, genuine oils and blends.

Lay people are not aware of the possible hazards of using the cheap adulterated tea tree oil available in supermarkets, which has been responsible for both minor and severe irritation.

Education

There are many professional qualifications available in aromatherapy. The syllabi of the nursing schools include the subject 'aroma-care'.

The following institutions offer aromatherapy training:

- AIDA (Aromatherapy International) follows a British curriculum, offering a certificate after examination and holding courses for care workers, doctors and midwives.
- The Augustinum clinic in Munich offers training for employees from the health professions, which includes aromatherapy basics and advanced seminars, which contain practical cases of the clinic's health care.

- The Bavarian Care Academy in Munich offers a qualification in aromatherapy and health care in cooperation with Maria and Wolfgang Hoch for doctors, midwifes, nurses and therapists. The training includes 168 theory lessons, practical exercise with a large amount of self-study. There are written and oral examinations and a project report.
- The Technical University of Munich, with NORA-International, provides a weekly 2-hour lecture over two semesters for medical and science students.

Many aroma companies and private persons offer courses in aromatherapy for everyone, especially for pharmacists and cosmeticians.

Use of essential oils in medical establishments

From Hamburg to Munich, essential oils are in regular use in around 10% of hospitals and hospices by enthusiastic well-trained nurses. However, most doctors, not conversant with their healing properties, gain information about their curative effects from unscientific press articles, which makes it difficult for nurses to convince them of their pharmaceutically active components.

Many freelance midwives use essential oils in their work outside hospital; nurses within a hospital are allowed to use them to alleviate minor conditions such as dry skin or headaches, but must have permission from the doctor in charge if they wish to use them for more serious conditions. They must keep an up-to-date written progress report of the essential oils used – number of drops, how often, changes in treatment and any improvement.

Conditions treated include anxiety, depression, difficulty breathing, headaches, pneumonia, digestive problems, all kinds of infections, insomnia, burns, scars, wounds, ulcers, postoperative intestinal atony and *Candida albicans*. Essential oils are also used in terminal illness, pregnancy and birth, endocrinology and psychocancer therapy, and with patients in psychosomatic wards.

Since 1995, essential oils have become a fundamental part of nursing and healthcare in Stiftsklinik Augustinium – a hospital with departments for cardiology, pneumology, angiology, nephrology and metabolic diseases. Aromatherapy intervention is carried out with the doctors' cooperation; it is documented and standards and protocols must be followed.

Nurses trained in aroma-care can apply essential oils using gentle stroking (effleurage) without having a recognized qualification in massage. Other methods include inhalation, sponge baths (in cases of fever), compresses, foot and hand massage and foot baths for pain control. High concentration of oils and mixtures are used for wounds and after an operation, sprays being used for decubitus ulcers (bedsores).

Associations

Aroma Forum International e.V.

Established in 2008, this is an association for the national and international support of aromatherapy, aroma-care and aroma culture generally. The focus is to integrate traditional and natural science into the modern use of essential oils.

NORA–International (a branch of the Natural Oils Research Association, UK)

Founded in 1996 in Germany, NORA-International encourages scientific research and development concerning natural essential oils, with the ability to use them for medical therapies, aroma-care and dermatological cosmetics.

Forum Essenzia

Set up in 1991, Forum Essenzia supports aromatherapists and aroma-care workers by publicizing the use of essential oils for healing.

Research

Research has been carried out into many projects, for example at Kiel University in 1996 to compare the analgesic effects of *Mentha* x *piperita* versus paracetamol (acetaminophen) on people with tension headaches. It was found that 10% of peppermint oil in ethanol had the same effect as 1000 mg of paracetamol, leading to the development of Euminz, a commercial roll-on for the forehead and neck.

Another interesting study was published in April 2009: Essential oils of aromatic plants with antibacterial, antifungal, antiviral, and cytotoxic properties. (See: www.pranamonde.co.za/publication.pdf)

At Munich Technical University Prof. Dietrich Wabner is working in cooperation with the dermatological department at Biederstein clinics and NORA-International on several aspects of essential oils, including quality control, physiology of essential oil producing plants, use of essential oils against the hazards of hospitalization, and oil mixtures possible for use against neurodermatitis in children.

Greece

Maria G Zorzou

Aromatherapy development

Aromatherapy arrived in Greece in the early 1990s with the first aromatherapy book, which was translated into Greek – *Practical Aromatherapy* by Shirley Price. The publishers promoted essential oils together with the book to make them and their properties known, and the book has sold over 20,000 copies to date. This was followed by three other books in 1998 and several more over the years.

Today the term aromatherapy is heard not only in terms of alternative therapeutics, but also in cosmetic care. People use it in different ways (massage, hydrolats, vaporizers) to improve their daily lives: as modern life becomes busier an increasing number of people are turning to natural remedies.

Although aromatherapy is not yet used in hospitals, it is employed widely by therapists, beauticians, some hairdressers and spas to enhance their sessions. Some veterinarians and pet owners use essential oils to treat their pets, including horses.

Following the trend in most Western countries, Greece has begun to acknowledge alternative and complementary therapies in the last few years, thus enabling many physical disorders to be treated with natural methods, often with excellent results.

Aura Vitae (the author's company) has been using aromatherapy as an alternative and complementary therapy for about 20 years, helping older people with various conditions, children with atopic dermatitis and eczema, and younger people with psoriasis, skin conditions etc.

Regulations

There is no legislation specific to essential oils. They are subject to laws according to their use, i.e. one for use in perfumery, another for use in medicinal products etc. In general, aromatherapy is considered to be neither legal nor illegal.

Essential oils

Essential oils are imported mainly from Europe (England, France and Germany); most companies guarantee the composition and purity of their products, but there are varying qualities on the market, some of which are adulterated. Essential oils are available in health stores, pharmacies and spas.

Since 2004, the author has been importing essential oils, carrier oils and hydrolats from Penny Price Aromatherapy and distributing them throughout Greece through aromatherapy outlets and those of the public who believe good oils are helpful to their wellbeing. Essential oils are used in everyday life, for relaxing after the pressure of the day – in a bath, to help sleep, to treat conditions such as dermatitis, cellulite, hair loss, weight loss etc. The public use everything: essential oils, carriers and hydrolats.

Education

Several schools teach the theory and practice of aromatherapy, how to use essential oils for common ailments, massage and everyday life. It is difficult to find the right school because aromatherapy has become 'fashionable' and there is a lack of consistency and integrity in training, not intentionally, but due to lack of knowledge:

- The Oriental Medicine and Shiatsu Training Centre (OM) is a specialized centre for physical therapy and traditional oriental medicine. Founded in 1994, it provides a comprehensive knowledge of theory and practice, including some knowledge of aromatherapy.
- The Academy of Ancient Greek and Traditional Chinese Medicine is a multifaceted school. As well as ancient Greek and Chinese medicine and traditional systems such as Ayurveda etc., the school teaches current western medical systems, including some aromatherapy.
- The Medicum College contributes to the development of alternative treatments in Greece, providing reliable and validated studies which include some aromatherapy.
- Aura Vitae (www.auravitae.eu) holds introductory weekend courses on aromatherapy and Penny Price and Dr Robert Stephen give lectures in Greece each year. The school has just become a branch of the Penny Price Academy UK and training now follows the UK guidelines set by the Aromatherapy Consortium. All students will go through the International Federation of Professional Aromatherapists UK.
- The Association of Schools of Alternative Health Sciences (Natural Health Science) was founded in 1992 and offers general and in-depth training and continuous updating in the scientific field of natural therapies – use of essential oils is taught on the massage session.
- The Life Therapy Academy (founded in 2000) is a centre of learning for alternative and complementary holistic healing methods, and includes aromatherapy.

Use of essential oils in medical establishments

There is no aromatherapy training in medical establishments; nurses may study the subject privately, but can only use their aromatherapy skills outside the hospital in their private practice.

Research/pilot studies/cases

No research or pilot studies have yet been carried out in Greece, but two unusual cases have had success using products from PPA, UK.

Case 1: Chalazion (meibomian cyst – swelling of a sebaceous gland in the eyelid)

The man had the cyst for 15 years, having surgery twice, but it recurred often. He visited Aura Vitae, where he was treated with compresses using hydrolat of *Thymus vulgaris* and Nurture Vision Eyedrops (a product of PPA). In 7 days the cyst opened up and by the 11th day it had completely healed – it has not returned.

Case 2: A deep, open wound

The woman came to Aura Vitae with a deep wound, approximately 1 cm in width, left after a caesarean operation and it had become infected with *Staphylococcus*. The treatment was as follows:

The hydrolat of *Thymus vulgaris* was sprayed constantly on the wound; a blend was made with the following and applied directly onto the wound two or three times a day:

○ 5 mL each of aloe vera gel and macerated hypericum oil
○ 2 drops each of *Pelargonium graveolens* [geranium], *Lavandula angustifolia* and *Melaleuca alternifolia* [tea tree] essential oils.

Two drops of each of the same essential oils was taken internally on a piece of bread three times a day. The wound began to shrink within a week and is recovering well.

Iceland

Margrét Alice Birgisdóttir

Aromatherapy development

Unlike most countries, aromatherapy was not introduced to Iceland by the beauty therapy profession, although it is now starting to be included in beauty therapy syllabi. Its use began in 1989, and as the number of practitioners increases, essential oils are used more and more in people's daily life. The introduction of more advanced courses enabled a faster growth, especially in areas of nursing. Most aromatherapists either have their own practice or join complementary health centres, those who are midwives and nurses using their new-found therapy in hospitals. Although insurance is available for clinical work, there is none especially for aromatherapy.

Regulations

There are no laws governing the use of essential oils or aromatherapy practice at present, but the Ministry of Health has assured the profession that this is in progress. In the meantime, people trading essential oils have to fulfil the same requirements as those for other oils used externally, such as sun oils etc.

Essential oils

Essential oils from many different sources are on offer from various importers and private bodies importing small quantities; also, therapists bring them from the UK when visiting.

Education

Most of the aromatherapists are qualified from the Comprehensive College at Ármúli, where aromatherapy is part of a 96-unit massage education. The aromatherapy part is three units (a unit is 25 teaching hours, made up of 40-minute sessions). The students learn how essential oils enter the body, blending, carrier oils, safety, history of aromatherapy and client assessment prior to treatment as part of this prequalification course.

Next, the students have to complete 25 units of clinical work before receiving their massage and aromatherapy degree. The author of this text used her teaching and CPD diploma from the Shirley Price International College of Aromatherapy to give courses to health professionals such as nurses, midwives, massage therapists and reflexologists at her clinic, Fyrir Fólk, www.fyrirfolk.is.

The Lífsskólinn School began teaching aromatherapy in the late 1990s, with professional aromatherapy lecturers. It teaches anatomy, physiology and pathology as well as aromatherapy massage.

Use of essential oils in medical establishments

Nurses caring for elderly people have shown great interest in aromatherapy, taking it into their hospital work. At the University Hospital of Iceland aromatherapy and massage is accepted as a complementary therapy, to be given only if requested by nurses or doctors. It is used for people with all kinds of dementia, particularly those who are very agitated or difficult to communicate with. These patients receive massage with essential oils on their shoulders, feet and hands, with positive results. Patients in the geriatric area are also treated. Icelandic midwifes have shown a great interest in using aromatherapy before, after and during birth.

Associations

The Icelandic Aromatherapy Association

As this association does not give insurance, its members also join the Massage Association in order to obtain this.

Research

Although the existence of research on essential oils is not well known, Sagamedica have been doing research on Icelandic plants for therapeutic use.

Ireland

Christine Courtney

The general picture

Complementary therapies are very popular in Ireland, aromatherapy being introduced not long after it came to the UK. It is becoming more common for GPs to recommend aromatherapy treatments for stress-related illnesses even though such recommendations are normally made on a personal level, where the GP knows the therapist and/or the therapy.

Public health nurses (the equivalent of health visitors) and specialty nurses are showing a great interest in training, although the majority of aromatherapy is carried out in private practice at present.

Aromatherapists rarely use hydrolats as yet, as sadly, most training courses do not include their use. They are rarely sold in health stores or pharmacies, as the general public does not use them.

Regulations

Because there is now such a huge interest from the general public, the Minister for Health at the Irish Department of Health and Children started a process to regulate complementary therapies. In 2003 a working group was set up to look at ways in which complementary therapists could be self-regulated, as this would benefit the general public. The report which was produced by this working group has created two categories of therapy, based on the risk to the public. They are:

• Category 1 – includes herbalism, acupuncture, aromatic medicine, homeopathy and traditional Chinese medicine (TCM)
• Category 2 – all other therapies.

Aromatherapy, because of the power of the essential oils, is included in category 1 under Aromatic Medicine. It was suggested by the Department that professional bodies federate so that their therapies would speak with one voice. As a result of this the

Aromatherapy Council of Ireland was formed. The founding member bodies are the IFPA (International Federation of Professional Aromatherapists), IMTA (the Irish Massage Therapy Association) and CThA (Complementary Therapy Association). To contact the ACI visit: www.aromatherapycouncil.ie.

Essential oils

Essential oils and aromatherapy products of generally good quality are readily available in health shops and pharmacies throughout Ireland.

Although essential oils are used mostly by aromatherapists, the general public purchase a small range, mainly for specific conditions or effects, e.g. PMT, insomnia, acne, and to brighten up their homes. A small selection is also used by massage therapists.

Most people, including aromatherapists, dilute essential oils in vegetable oils or lotion, the most popular forms of application being from a professional aromatherapist or self-application as a body cream/oil.

Education

The accredited training offered in Ireland is either from the UK International Federation of Professional Aromatherapists (IFPA) or from the International Therapy Examination Council (ITEC). No special training is offered by hospitals to nurses, who train privately, bringing their skill to the hospital. On occasions hospitals will pay for their training.

There are two IFPA-accredited schools in Ireland, the Obus School of Healing Therapies, Dublin, and the Body Wisdom School, Sligo. Both principals were trained by Shirley Price.

The internal and external use of hydrolats is covered on the Obus School syllabus.

There is good attendance on 'introduction to aromatherapy' courses run as night classes throughout the country, which encourage some to take an accredited course.

Use of essential oils in medical establishments

The situation is comparable to the UK in that each hospital discusses the introduction of aromatherapy with its Board of Management and Department of Nursing.

Aromatherapy is used and recommended in maternity hospitals, hospice care, nursing homes, cancer support units and some AIDS clinics, as well as in some hospitals for learning difficulties. Many hospices and hospitals are offering posts (called Clinical Nurse Specialists) to nurses who are trained in aromatherapy, making the latter available to patients in long-term and terminal care. This move is an acknowledgement of the benefits of aromatherapy in general healthcare, and together with self-regulation will see it more widely available through the health service. Positive feedback is coming from the patients themselves and their families of the tremendous benefits these treatments are having.

Teaching has been carried out throughout the country within the North Eastern Health Board, with particular emphasis on the Disability and Psychiatric Services. The calming effects of essential oils have been particularly noticed in clients with aggressive behaviour, and tea tree oil has been used to good effect to irrigate wounds that were MRSA (methicillin-resistant *Staphylococcus aureus*) positive, all swabs being negative to MRSA after treatment.

Associations

The Republic of Ireland has no aromatherapy associations of its own, aromatherapists joining UK associations on qualifying or multidisciplinary associations in Ireland.

Research

The subject of research has now been added to training courses run by IFPA schools, as it is an area that aromatherapy needs to address. Therapists now leave courses knowing how to carry out research, how to record findings, and most of all, with a commitment to research.

Scientists based at Sligo Institute of Technology have discovered that some essential oils are 'highly efficient' in the treatment of so-called hospital 'superbugs'. The research team from the Department of Microbiology at Sligo General Hospital have found them capable of killing the most resistant bacteria, including MRSA, vancomycin-resistant *Enterococcus* (VRE) and extended-spectrum β-lactamase (ESBL). They are also effective against bacteria resistant to conventional antibiotics: considered by some to be

'useless' in the fight against superbugs, those that do have an effect are so toxic that they are administered as a last resort because of risks to other organs such as the liver and kidneys. The researchers tested a large range of oils and their components and found that among the most effective at killing strains of MRSA, VRE and ESBL were clove, lemongrass, citronella, thyme, oregano and cinnamon; tea tree oil was also found be 'quite effective'. The list is not exhaustive – a large majority of the oils tested showed activity at relatively low concentrations. Although the results were deemed to be promising, Sligo IT hopes to carry out further research to provide viable alternatives to patients, caution always being needed when using essential oils (McDonagh 2009) http://www.irishtimes.com/newspaper/health/2009/1215/1224260710594.html

Japan

Chieko Shiota

The general picture

Aromatherapy is now becoming well known in Japan, the word 'aroma' increasing its popularity. Since 2000 there has been a campaign to protect the environment and products that are nature friendly have become more common than those containing chemical compounds, which has increased the number of people conscious of the environment and using essential oils as part of their lifestyle.

Regulations

There are no regulations for aromatherapy. When essential oils are mixed with other cosmetics they are treated as synthetic aromatic substances, so it is necessary to trade with trustworthy and knowledgeable companies. Massage for relaxation is not considered to be a medical treatment: it is classed as an aesthetic one and therefore is not against the law. Medical establishments have started to take various therapies on board, even though the national health insurance does not cover them, employing qualified therapists belonging to an aromatherapy organization. Nurses are studying aromatherapy in order to practise in their hospitals.

Education

In the 1990s most students went overseas to countries such as the UK, as there were no organizations to give aromatherapy training in Japan. Later some aromatherapy schools were founded to give training in Japanese methods. At that time, some schools authorized by the International Federation of Aromatherapy (IFA) and/or the International Federation of Professional Aromatherapists (IFPA) started putting on courses, and the number of students who wanted to study British aromatherapy increased. Today (2010), there are 31 schools accredited by the IFA and six by the IFPA.

Essential oils

Essential oils can be purchased from department stores, health shops and drug stores. As most shops have been selling them without distinguishing between individual products, for example for medical purposes or simply for potpourris, we must take responsibility ourselves for using them. Some shops employ an assistant who is qualified as an aromatherapy instructor in Japan. Although the AEAJ has established its own standard of safety and quality, evaluating the quality of products on this basis, there is no government regulation.

Use of essential oils in medical establishments

Introducing aromatherapy in clinics and hospitals has caused dramatic changes to the way in which their profits are made, owing to revisions to the health insurance system. Various treatment options have now become available to both doctors and patients, especially for childbirth. Obstetrics and gynaecology are excluded from national health insurance-funded treatments, but aromatherapy treatments are now used by them. At the Angel clinic in Fukuoka most postpartum patients – approximately 1200 a year – wish to have aromatherapy, and placing aroma diffusers in their wards has resulted in less use of allopathic medicines.

At the Obitsu Sankei clinic, the chair of Japan Holistic Medical Society is offering patients aromatherapy treatments as a part of their overall treatment, thus combining modern medicine with a natural cure.

Associations

The Aroma Environment Association of Japan was established in 1996, and now has 45,000 individual members and 230 corporate members. They have a three-tier system of qualifications:

1. Aromatherapy Advisor – a person who is trained to work as a shop assistant selling aromatherapy products
2. Aromatherapy Instructor – a person who is able to provide home-care advice
3. Practising Aromatherapist – a person who has been approved by members of this association.

The Japanese Society of Aromatherapy is a research body that uses aromatherapy correctly in clinics and is organized mainly by medical doctors.

The Japanese Aromacoodinator Association has been developed throughout Japan mainly by correspondence courses, and has 30,000 members and approximately 800 small private schools.

Research

Today a few Japanese essential oils are being developed, such as yuzu, a citrus fruit originating in East Asia (used mainly for bath products and scented candles), and *Alpinia zerumbet* [shell ginger], an exotic perennial, the leaves of which make a tea with hypotensive, diuretic and antiulcerogenic properties. The universities that grow these plant materials have been researching and developing these oils.

Netherlands

Anneke Weigel-van der Maas

Aromatherapy development

Aromatherapy appeared around the late 1970s, and is now found in gyms, treatment centres and beauty parlours. More and more, aromatherapists are offering massage as a complementary therapy. It is used by nursing staff in hospitals, hospices, nursing homes and care homes, and it is also possible to have a therapist visit at home.

Regulations

In 1973, alternative practitioners were permitted to practise without formal regulation.

Since 1993, only approved professionals may provide medical care, and alternative therapists are able to join a professional organization to take care of any complaints, which in turn can belong to the Natural Health Care Professions Disciplinary Law Foundation (TBNG).

As an aromatherapist cannot give a medical diagnosis, clients are referred to a doctor where necessary, when a holistic treatment plan can then be set out.

Essential oils

Essential oils can be bought in all health-food shops and they are used personally, in health and beauty salons and in public saunas.

Education

There are many good aromatherapy schools in The Netherlands and students are taught many subjects, including:

- how to deal with special complaints, e.g. epilepsy, attention deficit hyperactivity disorder, high blood pressure, maternity complaints etc.
- how to use essential oils safely internally
- additional massage techniques such as pressure point massage
- anatomy, physiology, pathology and psychology
- client consultation, i.e. medical history, diet, lifestyle and health problems.

Initial study at the Mediator school (www.mediator-aromatherapie.nl) comprises 150 hours' theory and 101 hours of practice. The training includes insurance, ethics and business studies, and there are advanced practical and theoretical training modules available after qualification.

Toxicity is covered plus detailed discussion on essential oil properties, for use both internally and externally.

In Breda, there are courses and workshops in aromatherapy. Chi International (www.chi.nl and www.chi.nl/english/homeng/homeng.html) began in 1979 and works nationally and internationally with institutes and/or businesses active in the field of education and aromatherapy.

Trade Fair Manager Jeffrey Go is also responsible for contacts with the healthcare sector at nursing homes and hospitals, where aromatherapy is regarded as complementary to orthodox treatment.

Use of essential oils in hospitals

Although this branch of natural medicine in The Netherlands is just beginning in hospitals etc., Leiden and Utrecht universities are showing huge interest and have active study groups, with the results of scientific research on essential oils being published regularly.

In 2004 there was a symposium at St Elisabeth's Hospital in Tilburg on the care of children, where aromatherapy was referred to as 'smell therapy'. Anneke Huisman of the cancer section at the Erasmus Medical Centre, Rotterdam, related her experience of using essential oils on various complaints, including the support of people with mental health problems.

When challenged whether she used scientific research or traditional/empirical knowledge, her reply was that responsible use of essential oils, with knowledge, could be a new area of expertise for nurses, as an addition to standard care: it is not a case of 'one or the other'. Aromatherapy does not claim to cure, though it may benefit the quality of life.

In complementary care the patient is looked at from a holistic point of view: fighting the pain with medicine (drugs) is not enough – the patient is under a great deal of stress, sometimes with nausea and vomiting despite the use of emetics. It is impossible for them to sleep after being given bad news about their lifespan, and there are also unpleasant side effects from anaesthetics. Under such circumstances complementary care, including aromatherapy, can be used:

- peppermint herbal tea (in the cancer centre in Rotterdam) in cases of nausea and vomiting after a cystoscopy; herbal teas inducing sleep are also used at bedtime
- calendula cream, for skin problems such as AraC syndrome and the after-effects of irradiation
- a few drops of lavender or orange oil on a handkerchief, pillow or stone to help sleeping problems
- a warm towel impregnated with lavender to ease gripe or stomach ache resulting from chemotherapy
- lavender after removing sutures after an operation, especially after a limb amputation

- cajuput, for tension in the neck, shoulders and back, due to stress, supplemented with lavender and juniper berry.

The next speaker, Dr Harmen Rijpkema, one of the leading aromatherapists in The Netherlands, explained that although aromatherapy has still a long way to go, it is expected that essential oils will eventually be given more priority. The oils he talked about included *Lavandula angustifolia* [lavender], *Citrus reticulata* [mandarin] and *Citrus bergamia* [bergamot] etc. as well as almond carrier oil.

He explained how essential oils can:

- be used on children
- aid relaxation in patients and carers
- kill microbes
- relieve muscle pain and mental tension
- open up the bronchial tubes (eucalyptus oils, *Melaleuca cajuputi* [cajuput] and *Myrtus communis* [myrtle])
- cool burning sensations on the skin (*Mentha* x *piperita* [peppermint]
- relieve itchy and/or inflamed skin (*Matricaria recutita* [German chamomile] and *Chamaemelum nobile* [Roman chamomile].

In July 2009, the fifth edition of his book, *Aromecum*, was published, containing the most recent findings on aromatherapy and descriptions of more than 200 essential oils.

Associations

The Federatie voor Additief Geneeskundig Therapeuten (FAGT) (www.fagt.org) is a professional association representing many complementary therapies and is the largest in The Netherlands. The public can source a therapist through them.

FAGT therapists are covered by law for the protection of therapists and clients.

Adequately trained therapists may join the FAGT, giving them the benefits of insurance.

Research/pilot studies

Research by Koot and de Lange indicated that the use of essential oils has a positive effect on rebellious and fearful behaviour in elderly people (Koot A 1979 Activities with the Elderly, HB publishers). People suffering from dementia enjoy aromas, which bring memories of the past and calm down the restless; they were found also to have a positive effect on gloomy elderly people.

Norway

Gry Fosstvedt, Päivi Renaa

The general picture

Aromatherapy was introduced in the late 1970s by Arnould Taylor, Eve Taylor and Shirley Price, becoming known by the 1980s as an effective way of treating stress-related problems, with lay people as well as professionals attending courses.

According to the NIFAB (www.nifab.no) study in 2007, 48.7% of the population had tried alternative treatments. According to the study, more women than men had tried it and the majority had seen their doctor prior to the treatment.

Regulations

Persons providing alternative treatment may in marketing their activity only give an objective and factual description of the nature of it (Norwegian Act No. 64, June 2003). The Act states that serious diseases must not be treated by non-health personnel, although they may administer treatment in cases where the sole purpose is to alleviate or moderate symptoms or consequences of the disease, e.g. side effects, or to strengthen the body's immune system or its ability to heal itself.

Complementary practitioners are encouraged to obtain the doctor's written permission/acceptance and to communicate with him/her when necessary, the aim being to support conventional medical treatment, to stimulate the immune system, encourage the body to heal itself and to enhance wellbeing and quality of life.

In January 2011 new VAT regulations for natural therapies came into force. Those who are not to a standard of education approved by the Norwegian authorities will not be able to register with the national voluntary registry for practitioners of natural medicine (Bronnoysundregistrene) and will have to pay the new VAT. Those who are registered will be exempt.

Education

The Norsk Aromaterapiskole (NAS) was the first school to specialize in aromatherapy (1982), followed by the Norwegian branch of the Shirley Price International College; later, several others appeared and lectures were also given to midwives and children's nurses. In 2010 there were more than 150 practising aromatherapists recorded in the NNH system (see Associations, below). Training varies from short 2–3-day workshops to full diploma courses.

Currently, schools following the new regulations of the Norwegian Association of Natural Medicine give 772 compulsory hours of theoretical and practical training. Practical and theory examinations in aromatherapy plus courses in anatomy, physiology and pathology have to be taken before a certificate is awarded.

Some schools offer advanced short courses in medical aromatherapy, psycho-aromatherapy, aromatherapy for women's health, aromatherapy for babies and children, aromatherapy and cancer care – to mention but a few. From January 2010 a 50-hour course on VEKS (science, ethics, communication and social studies) is compulsory. A basic education in natural medicine (110 hours) is also compulsory, and includes an introduction to the history and philosophy of natural medicine, traditional Chinese medicine, anthroposophy and nutritional studies.

A few teachers teach the oral use of essential oils and hydrolats, which is a valuable (and in many cases, indispensable) method, although therapists cannot prescribe this to patients.

Use of essential oils in medical establishments

Aromatherapy is not officially organized in hospitals, but some will allow (and often encourage) patients to have it if they wish.

Several institutions for multi-handicapped children, youths and adults use essential oils beneficially in diffusers, massage and baths.

Outside hospital settings, a number of medical doctors encourage their patients to consult aromatherapists for problems such as fibromyalgia, headaches, rheumatism, muscular pain and stiffness. Although the majority are still sceptical, there is a growing interest in less harmful medications, especially for nervous and hormonal problems.

Associations

The Norwegian Association of Natural Medicine (Norske Naturterapeuters Hovedorganisasjon – NNH (*www.nnh.no* – information in English also available) was formed in late 1994 to cater for complementary therapies, e.g. reflexology, aromatherapy and kinesiology, the largest professional group being aromatherapy – the Aromaterapifaggruppen.

In cooperation with the health authorities the NNH is currently establishing a common curriculum and examination so that all complementary schools can gain official recognition. The NNH is also working to establish a distinction between *aromatherapy* (Aromatic Natural Medicine) as a serious complementary treatment system with genuine essential oils, and *aroma massage*, as practised by beauty therapists using ready-made blends and commercial products.

Research

In 2000 the National Centre of Research of Complementary Medicine (NAFKAM) was formed at the University of Tromsø for the scientific study of natural medicine, from homoeopathy to healing, including essential oils and aromatherapy.

There are currently few published studies available on aromatherapy. A thesis (Hansen Tore Magne 2000*) evaluated the psychological effects of aromatherapy, but more research is needed. Other studies have been looking into the effects of aromatherapy in various settings in workplaces, but no published reports are currently available.

Portugal

Denise Raines

The general picture

Aromatherapy arrived in Portugal during the 1990s, mainly through its use in beauty salons and spas. The majority of these practitioners have trained outside the

---

*Hansen, T.M., 2000. En psykologisk evaluering av aromaterapi. Hovedoppgave. Norges teknisk-naturvitenskapelig universitet.

country, as aromatherapy is not taught as part of the beauty therapy curriculum in colleges. Unfortunately, Portugal still uses the word 'alternative' when referring to therapies which are complementary in the UK.

Although there is much interest from the Portuguese public, as yet there is no real acknowledgement from the powers that be regarding its efficacy.

It is very difficult for practitioners of aromatherapy to obtain insurance, as most UK associations do not insure those members practising and residing outside the UK. An exception is the International Federation of Aromatherapists (IFA) www.ifaroma .org, which can offer this service. The only way forward would be to try to set up a Portuguese branch of a UK aromatherapy association and have it accredited in Portugal, although the process would be slow and costly. This was attempted in reflexology, but it seems the entire process has collapsed after many years' hard work and huge financial cost.

Regulations

Aromatherapy is still considered to be neither legal nor illegal. Essentially, no one minds what an aromatherapist does, as long as there are no complaints. Health shops are allowed to sell essential oils because they are seen to be for external use only. There appears to be no legislation regarding their sale or quality.

Many of the bureaucratic problems and narrow mindedness in government relate back to the dictatorial regime, which lasted 46 years and only ended in 1974. During this time, the health service was only available to those who could pay. The poor masses were kept in check while the wealthy were kept happy. As a result, it would suffice to say that Portugal is behind Britain by about 20 years.

Education

Aromatherapy training for both non-medical people and nurses is slowly improving. Although it has no proper structure because its not legally recognized, there is a 3-month, 36-hour course run in Lisbon and Porto that is accredited by three associations in Portugal, the Associação Nacional de Terapeutas de Recuperação, Massoterapeutas e Auxiliares de Fisioterapia (ANAFIS); Associação Portuguesa de Naturopatia (APNA); and Conselho Federativo – Federação das Medicinas não Convencionais (CF-FMNC).

Use of essential oils in medical establishments

Aromatherapy is not generally accepted in hospitals because it is seen as an alternative form of medicine, although some hospitals and doctors are open to most things if they can ease someone's suffering. There may be occasional use of essential oils, especially in terminal illness, where alternative methods are acceptable.

Aromatherapy is offered in some private clinics and the occasional single unit in palliative care, although hospices as such do not exist at present. In the south there are outpatient oncology units, where people simply sit on a chair while receiving a treatment.

Oncology hospitals, mainly in the north, are using a few complementary therapies as part of the voluntary sector, but unfortunately aromatherapy is not yet one of them.

Associations

There are no aromatherapy associations. However, there are many foreigners living in the country who have trained abroad and are affiliated to their own associations – for example the International Federation of Professional Aromatherapists (IFPA) and the IFA mentioned earlier.

Research

There is no research being carried out in Portugal at present regarding any alternative therapy.

Switzerland

Eliane Zimmermann

Aromatherapy development

Aromatherapy first became known in 1985/6, when aromatherapists from other countries – Valerie Worwood, Shirley Price, Martin Henglein and Suzanne Fischer-Rizzi – were asked to teach the subject.

Switzerland is a four-language country (in the southeast they mainly speak Romansh), and has 26 cantons (counties), each having its own constitution, so the Federal Government is struggling to find a common jurisdiction. As far as aromatherapy practice is concerned, the German-speaking sector is comparable to Germany, the French to France – more medical (it is common there to use essential oils internally); the Italian part has only one canton (Ticino/Tessin), where the rules of practice are moderate, only registration being necessary. The practice of aromatherapy also depends on each canton's jurisdiction in all parts of Switzerland.

The word therapy is very restricted in the German sector and only those who are legally allowed to heal somebody can use it. The most liberal canton is Appenzell, where most therapeutic activities are allowed to be practised without strict restrictions.

There are two distinct professions concerning aromatherapy, doctors and naturopaths being called 'aromatherapists' and those without medical training 'aromatologists', despite the fact that both may have received the same training in the subject.

Regulations

In most parts of Switzerland the term therapist is reserved for those in a profession approved by the Federal Government, i.e. medical doctors and certified naturopaths (Naturheilarzt); only medically trained people are legally allowed to heal and practise therapeutically (in Jura and Zürich no CAM practitioners at all can practise legally). Non-medical aromatherapists without naturopathic training are allowed neither to practise therapy nor to give any kind of massage commercially. In Appenzell, Basel and Schaffhausen naturopaths/practitioners of CAM can work without regulations from the authorities, but they must register and need to pass a 'cantonal test'; in Luzern and Nidwalden no test is needed for this; in others (Tessin, Zug) they only need to be registered, and in two French cantons (Genf, Vaud) they are merely 'tolerated'. It is expected to be a long time before State approval of aromatherapy practice is granted.

Recommending the internal intake of essential oils is officially permitted only by naturopaths. Unofficially, in the German and French sectors people do practise aromatherapy, declaring it as some kind of 'wellness measure', or 'wellbeing touch', or any other word their fantasy creates.

The legal use of essential oils depends on what they are to be used for and how they are used. They are allowed to be used in general nursing for caring purposes – following necessary guidelines, but if a nurse wishes to use essential oils to cure – or to heal – then he or she needs authorization from a doctor or the leading nurse of the station.

The law regulating pharmaceutical/medicinal products is the Bundesgesetz über Arzneimittel und Medizinprodukte (similar to the American FDA).

Essential oils

Essential oils of a very high quality have been sold in Zürich since 1985, although among the reputable retailers there are, as in most countries, many who sell low-quality, adulterated oils.

Essential oils are used by the general public mostly in vaporizers, on tissues (for stress, colds and insomnia) and in baths, though it is becoming popular to use them also in a carrier oil for self-application for muscular aches and pains etc.

Education

Those wishing to practise some kind of massage in Switzerland have to learn to do so officially – taking a course of 150 hours in most cantons; the certification has to be given by accredited schools.

Outside the nursing profession, training in aromatherapy is available mostly through German schools in the German sector, each having its own training standards, although everyone would like to see a nationally recognized training for non-medical people.

Long-term education in aromatherapy and aromatology is offered by one or two schools, e.g. Woodtli Schulen, with Martin Henglein, and the Schweizer Schule für Aromatherapie.

Basic training is offered by several organizations, mainly in conjunction with well-known aromatherapy teachers from abroad.

Regarding education in the nursing profession, many changes are under way in order to meet international standards, and the first of two healthcare school training centres started its programme in 2006.

Insurance

The biggest health insurance companies have applied a standard for therapists set by the Erfahrungs Medizinisches Register (EMR) in order for them to be covered. Any therapist requiring insurance has to show a minimum of 150 hours of medical training plus at least 105 hours of aromatherapy training. Without the EMR standard, most health insurance companies will not pay for client treatments.

Use of essential oils in medical establishments

In principle, aromatherapy has begun to be accepted in hospitals, where treatment is carried out only by nurses. Some doctors use essential oils in their private clinics.

No official guidelines for nurses using complementary therapies in a hospital setting have been written, but there is an increasing interest in the possible benefits of aromatherapy, some hospital patients requesting treatment.

The Swiss professional association of nurses (SBK) originally laid down national principles of procedure and basic rules for establishments in which aromatology sanctioned by doctors is allowed. Nurses must be able to justify nursing procedures using essential oils; knowledge must include risks and limitations as well as potential benefits. The patient or relatives decide whether or not therapy with essential oils is to be undertaken.

Use of essential oils

Apart from disinfection of rooms, personal hygiene and hair care, essential oils are used for fear, anxiety, confusion, to give comfort to the dying, and physical problems such as colds, disturbed sleep, fevers, mycosis, pain, relaxation and skin problems, including burns and wounds. They are also used in midwifery. The most common method of application is inhalation (vaporizer, handkerchief, steam), but they are also used in baths, compresses, dressings and swabs, massage and frictions, using neat oils and/or blends. Washing with hydrolats is often used for fevers, and cold compresses with 3% peppermint oil are placed on the forehead for headaches.

No synthetic oils can be used, as they may cause side-effects such as headaches and nausea

Essential oils must be diluted before use (neutral liquid soap, honey, cream, vinegar, vegetable oils etc.). Exceptions are swabs in mycosis.

Essential oils, although natural, are not innocuous. Risks include sensitivity, irritation and possible toxic effects.

Essential oils should never be brought into contact with the eyes.

Oral application is the exclusive domain of medically trained aromatherapists.

A sensitivity test (inside the elbow) should be carried out on those with known allergies before each application of a new oil.

Care should be taken if a homoeopathic remedy is being taken, because of possible interferential action.

Descriptions must be kept of how to store essential oils correctly, and where they can be ordered.

The use of aromatherapy depends to a large extent on the level of acceptance of the medical staff.

Hospitals in the Canton of Bern successfully carry out fever washing for general wellbeing, reduction of fever and healthy sweating in adult patients. The mix used is 1 drop each of bergamot, eucalyptus, lavender and mint (unspecified) emulsified with a dispersant in lukewarm water. For genital and thrush-like ailments, 1–2 drops each of lavender and tea tree are used.

Local massage or compresses with essential oils are also offered/applied to ease insomnia, fear, stress and general pain.

Although aroma lamps cannot be used in hospitals, electric aroma stones or absorbent stones saturated with essential oils are used to help anxiety and sleeplessness etc.

Some psychiatric clinics use aromatherapy regularly and successfully for generalized fear syndrome, psychotic symptoms, depressions, and borderline as well as burn-out syndromes.

The first hospice to use aromatherapy was in Zürich in the 1990s, permission having being given to use essential oils in any external form, with guidelines being written in 1994.

Associations

No association gives standards of training for aromatherapists – each school has its own.

- Oesterreichische Gesellschaft für wissenschaftliche Aromatherapie und Aromapflege (OEGWA) – an Austrian association for scientific aromatherapy and aroma-care, having an occasional conference and newsletter http://cms.oegwa.at
- Aroma Forum Oesterreich – this Austrian association holds an annual conference www .aromaforum-oesterreich.at

- Verein aerztlich gepruefter Aromapraktiker VagA – an Austrian society for medically audited/tested/approved aroma practitioners, which offers insurance, regular newsletters and a yearly conference. www.aromapraktiker.at
- Aroma Forum International – a German association; it holds a yearly conference and has a biannual magazine. www.aroma-forum-international.de
- Forum Essenzia – a German association which has become a more trade-orientated association. It holds a conference once a year and there is a biannual magazine for its members.
- Veroma – a Swiss association, though there has been little activity within it since 2007.

Research/pilot studies

Some studies have been made by Professor Reinhard Saller (in cooperation with his German colleagues) concerning the efficacy of tea tree oil for mycoses, bacterial and viral infections.

He was also involved in proving the antiviral and antiherpetic actions of several essential oils, together with Professor Reichling and his team from the University of Heidelberg in Germany: *Essential oils of aromatic plants with antibacterial, antifungal, antiviral and cytotoxic properties – an overview*

Taiwan

Jen Chang

The general picture

Aromatherapy first appeared around 1990, its development relying mainly on private cosmetic companies selling essential oils. The beauty industry, big business in Taiwan, used the aromas of essential oils to attract consumers without reference to their therapeutic benefits. The key obstacle to development was the lack of knowledge of the English language, thereby limiting access to information. The books *Aromatherapy for the Emotions* (Price S 2000) and *Carrier Oils* (Price L 2006) have been published in Chinese, but now more Chinese publications are available, including those written by people who studied aromatherapy abroad. Aromatherapy knowledge was first encouraged by a few committed people who invited professional aromatherapists from other countries to teach and organize groups. Jen Chang, one of the first to do this, is now the principal of the Penny Price Aromatherapy Academy in Taiwan.

Aromatherapy has currently become more widely used, being appreciated by aromatherapists not only in academic and medical fields, but also in beauty salons, spas and leisure businesses.

Regulation

No aromatherapy regulations have been set as yet. In the early days, when knowledge of aromatherapy was not generally available, a fire occurred when essential oils were being vaporized using a candle. The result was that essential oils containing isopropyl alcohol cannot now be used, to comply with the Taiwan alcohol content law. As aromatherapy has become better known, vaporized air freshener products are no longer confused with therapeutic essential oils.

There are no regulations as yet for practising aromatherapy, even though training has been going on for many years, although in China the government introduced an 'Aromatic Masseurs Qualification Standard' in 2004, which aromatic masseurs have to follow. Training is difficult to achieve in Taiwan because of political issues in China.

Essential oils

Essential oils are sold mostly by aromatherapists and cosmetologists but are also available in some department stores and health shops. The oils and related products are mostly imported from France, the United Kingdom, the United States of America and Germany, but unfortunately there are many low-quality essential oil products available, due especially to dilution and unclear labelling. Many people use the term aromatherapy to sell aromatic oils containing isopropyl alcohol for commercial gain, but those promoting aromatherapy education are selling good-quality essential oils.

Essential oil use

Essential oils are used mainly by aromatherapists and cosmetologists, although some masseurs, holistic therapists and doctors also use them. They are increasingly being recognized in hospitals and care centres.

The main methods of use are by application, massage, inhalation from tissues and vaporization, although because the weather is rather humid in Taiwan, application is less acceptable.

Education

During the 1990s people went to England or Australia to study aromatherapy, returning to promote the knowledge they had learned. At the turn of the century a few universities and private training schools began to offer aromatherapy courses, many inviting members from the International Federation of Aromatherapy (IFA) and the International Federation of Professional Aromatherapists (IFPA) to lecture. In 2004, one school became a branch of the IFPA-accredited Penny Price Academy in the UK. The syllabus covers anatomy and physiology, massage, chemical profiles, the effects of essential oils and methods of use.

In 2000 the Taiwan Institute of Aromatherapy, established in 1996, was invited to lecture in hospitals and schools, also by the Ministry of Education to give an aromatherapy seminar–workshop for professors and teachers from national universities. As a result, several universities have established aromatherapy as elective or required courses. Owing to this increase in knowledge, aromatherapy is now more recognized and accepted by the medical profession, giving people more confidence in essential oils.

More and more education and training institutions come from Australia, Germany, the United States of America and the United Kingdom. The content of these courses is very different: Australian correspondence courses lack technical knowledge, German association courses contain too few hours, and too many institutions with inadequate standards are recognized by an American association. Most people are not aware of the value of belonging to an association, nor do they appreciate the necessity for an aromatherapist to have a recognized qualification.

Use of essential oils in medical establishments

Aromatherapy is used in palliative care hospices, usually on cancer patients. Some educational institutions ask trained aromatherapists to do volunteer work in hospices, which is starting to attract the attention of the medical profession. Since Dr Robert Stephen and Penny Price came to Taiwan in 2005 to give professional training courses related to cancer patients, a team from the Institute of Aromatherapy has been helping terminal cancer patients every week for over 5 years.

People with cancer experience different symptoms of distress, and in 2004 a paper was written[*] on the application of aromatherapy in cancer patients, discussing the following topics:

- The fundamental concept of aromatherapy
- The effectiveness of aromatherapy for cancer patients with distress symptoms
- The principle of essential oil recipes for patients with distress symptoms
- The results of relieving distress symptoms when using aromatherapy
- The method and frequency of using essential oils.

Although focused on the care of cancer patients, the Institute of Aromatherapy team's services also extend to the care of patients' families. Currently five or six hospitals and institutions promote aromatherapy care, and the Penny Price-trained aromatherapists are recognized by the hospitals. In 2009 aromatherapy became part of the supplementary medical outpatients' service.

Associations

There is no independent national organization/association for aromatherapy and each school works individually, which means that at present it is not possible for therapists to gain recognition for their training, as all standards are accepted. It is to be hoped that there will be an independent national organization in the near future, although it may be difficult to establish one because of the political situation in China.

Research

Several academic or medical institutions have in recent years begun to carry out aromatherapy-related research and pilot studies: these include cancer, air quality purification and improving health problems such as depression, dysmenorrhoea, dementia in the elderly, haemorrhoids, asthma, oedema and

---

[*]Jia-Ling Sun, Jen Chang, Mei-Sheng Sung, Mei-Yu Huang, Hsiouh-Hsing Wang, Su-Ching Kuo, 2004. The application of aromatherapy in cancer patients. Taiwan Journal of Hospice Palliative Care.

fatigue. Hopefully, experience in aromatherapy clinics and research can be exchanged internationally, so that every country benefits.

United States of America

Lora Cantele, E Cristina, Pam Conrad

Aromatherapy development

Aromatherapy appeared in California in the mid-1980s, America's first conference being held in Los Angeles in 1990, followed by New York in 1994; several are now held in different states each year.

Healthcare is paid for privately and only a few insurance companies cover complementary therapies, making it difficult for hospitals to provide these services. Nurses belonging to the National Association of Nurse Massage Therapists (NANMT) were among the first to introduce aromatherapy into mainstream hospitals, and many leading healthcare institutions now use aromatherapy. The Massachusetts State Board of Nursing was the first to include aromatherapy in its Nurse Practice Act, an example followed by 25 other State Boards.

Clinical aromatherapy is gaining popularity, with widespread use by nurses throughout the country – nurses in several hospitals have written, or are writing, protocols for their facility, and the medical profession is beginning to show some acceptance. Some nurses have set up trials in medical/hospital settings (see Research/pilot studies below).

Regulations

At present there is no state registration for the practice of aromatherapy – anyone can set up as an 'aromatherapist'.

Education

There are many bogus accreditation claims in aromatherapy education – the only legitimate accrediting bodies in the United States are those approved by the US Department of Education.

The American (formerly Australasian) College of Health Sciences was the first school in the USA to offer this government-approved certificate, although other excellent courses are available (see AIA, AHNA and NAHA websites).

Academic programmes range from study at a university (usually in phytotherapy) to distance learning, including those endorsed by accrediting bodies such as the American Holistic Nurses Association (AHNA) and approved providers offering continuing education units (CEUs) to healthcare professionals. The Aromatherapy Registration Council (ARC) provides an aromatherapy curriculum with a national examination twice a year in 30 states, open to anyone who has completed a minimum of a Level 2 aromatherapy programme (200 hours). Successful candidates qualify for insurance.

In 2008, in an effort to raise the standard of aromatherapy training for clinical settings, the AIA established Level 3 Curriculum Guidelines (minimum 400 hours). These include additional anatomy and physiology, pathologies and chemistry. Schools offering aromatherapy training programmes with less than 400 hours to nurses and other healthcare students can apply for 'advanced placement credit' through the AIA in an effort to bring their students to the 400-hour level.

Essential oils and methods of use

Pure essential oils are not easily available in retail shops, many fragrance oils being labelled 'aromatherapy oils'; this makes it difficult for untrained people to know the difference. Essential oils are often associated with 'new age' stores (not all credible), thereby undermining the true value/properties of essential oils. Nevertheless, a few legitimate essential oil companies are trying to compete against the mass 'aromatherapy fragrance' market.

In the cosmetics industry the term aromatherapy is often misused, with little distinction given between essential oils and fragrance oils. In an attempt to address this problem, the Safe Cosmetics Act 2010 (HR 5786) was introduced into the House of Representatives in July 2010.

Essential oils are used in application, baths, gargles, compresses; an aromatherapy treatment is usually combined with another treatment, e.g. reflexology.

Aromatherapy organizations advise therapists against internal use of essential oils; insurance is not given for the 'European' practice of aromatherapy, because of the likelihood of insurance liability lawsuits.

Use of essential oils in medical establishments

Clinical aromatherapy is recognized and respected by nurses, with successful studies being set up in pain control, cardiology, psychiatry, obstetrics and gynecology, pediatrics, dermatology, oncology, senior care and immunology. Aromatherapy is also gaining acceptance for the care of the chronically and terminally ill, patients now rarely being given hypnotics to regulate sleep patterns. Several hospitals use aromatherapy to aid sore muscles, bruises and vein relief, stress and insomnia. Where essential oils are used on the elderly, the need for antipsychotic drugs has been noticeably reduced. The main methods of use are inhalers, baths, compresses and massage.

Associations

The National Association for Holistic Aromatherapy (NAHA), founded in 1990, is an educational, non-profit organization dedicated to enhancing public awareness of aromatherapy. It offers a quarterly journal and teleconferences, and has established a code of ethics for teachers, practitioners and students. It provides a listing of schools, colleges and educators offering approved Level 1 and 2 syllabi. NAHA offers professional, product and general liability insurance to its professional members.

The Aromatherapy Registration Council (ARC) was established in 1999 as a public benefit, non-profit corporation, independent of any paid membership organization or educational facility, thereby ensuring an impartial and unbiased body. The ARC provides an aromatherapy curriculum and sponsors a national examination (see Education above). Successful candidates may use the letters 'RA' (Registered Aromatherapist) after their name. Registered Aromatherapists, of which there are 449 (2010), have to renew their membership every 5 years and meet continuing education requirements.

The Alliance of International Aromatherapists (AIA) is a non-profit organization, officially launched in 2006 and adopting a code of ethics and standards of practice in 2007. The AIA education committee fosters high standards of safe, ethical and professional practice in the clinical use of essential oils; in 2008 it raised the standard of Level 1 and 2 education and established Level 3 guidelines, assuring the competency of practitioners of clinical aromatherapy and the promotion of essential oil research. Aromatherapy schools can submit their curriculum for AIA recognition. Educational opportunities are developed for the public and members through monthly newsletters/teleconferences and annual conferences.

The Associated Bodywork and Massage Professionals (ABMP) offers membership to aromatherapists who have completed 100 hours or more of training with an institution or educator registered by their own state. Membership includes professional liability insurance.

Research/pilot studies

In early 2010 a pilot programme was conducted by Hope's Circle of Friends, in the children's palliative care facility of the Northeastern Hospice of Illinois, the aim being to improve their quality of life. Many children are exhibiting a significant benefit with regard to agitation, muscle contractures, sadness, alertness and tinea. A second study was started in June 2010.

A successful pilot study was carried out at the San Diego Hospice in California, protocols being included in a guide for physicians and healthcare professionals treating palliative care patients. It is part of the Pal-Med Connect programme created by the Institute for Palliative Medicine.

A research study is currently being conducted in an Indiana hospital to reduce the effects of anxiety and depression in high-risk postpartum mothers.

Summary

In most countries (with the exception of France, Belgium and Germany) aromatherapy has developed from aromatherapy as practised in the UK. Some countries are not yet allowed to practise in hospitals, others can work with the express permission of the nurse or doctor in charge – and still others have advanced further than the UK in their freedom to work in these establishments.

Acknowledgements

The editor (S. Price) would like to thank those who responded to her request for an update to the information on their country, as well as those who sent information for the new countries. Their names appear beside their country. She is disappointed that some countries in the third edition did not respond to her request for an update and are therefore not included in this edition.

Bibliography

Sawamura Masayoshi, Dept. of Agriculture, Kochi University, Active effects of Japanese Yuzu essential oil.

Sei Nobuko, Dept. of Biochemistry, Showa University School of Medicine, 2008. The Effects of Essential Oils to Skin Cells. Aromatopia No. 91, Vol. 17/No. 6.

Tanidagai, Mitsukatu Institute of Wood Technology, Akita Prefectural University, 2009. Regain in the Mountains Effective Usage of Essential oils from Trees. Aromatopia No. 97 Vol. 18/No. 6.

Inoue Shigeharu, ABE Shigeru. Teikyo University Institute of Medical Mycology, 2006. The New Development of Anti-bacterial Aromatherapy. AROMA RESEARCH No. 28 Vol. 7/No. 4.

Sotoike Mitsuo, Graduate School and Faculty of Engineering, Chiba University, 2009. Science of the Human Brain and Aroma. AROMA RESEARCH No. 40, Vol. 10/No. 4.

Glossary

abortifacient inducing an abortion; causing expulsion of the fetus

adaptogenic having a positive general effect on the body, irrespective of disease condition, especially under stress

alcohols group of hydrocarbon compounds frequently found in volatile oils

aldehydes class of organic compounds standing between alcohols and acids

allelopathy a plant exerting an adverse influence over another to protect its environment by the production of a chemical inhibitor, usually a terpenoid or a phenol

allopathy system of medicine which uses drugs with effects opposite to the symptoms produced by the disease (in contrast to homoeopathy)

amenorrhoea absence of menstruation outside pregnancy in premenopausal women

amphoteric capable of functioning in opposite senses, e.g. calming/uplifting according to the dose; having the characteristics of both an acid and a base

analeptic a restorative remedy (in former times smelling salts) for states of weakness that are frequently accompanied by dizziness and fainting

anaphrodisiac of a drug, diminishing sexual drive

anodyne relieving pain; analgesic

anthelmintic destructive of intestinal worms; see vermifugal

antiphlogistic see antipyretic

antipyretic counteracting inflammation or fever

antithermic cooling; antipyretic

antitussive relieving or preventing coughing

anxiolytic relieving anxiety and tension

aperient mildly laxative

aperitive stimulating the appetite

aromachology science of the effects of aromas influencing emotions, feelings and behaviour via the nose/brain system

aromatic organic chemical compound derived from benzene; also called aromatic compound

astringent causing contraction of living tissues (often mucous membranes), reducing haemorrhages, secretions, diarrhoea etc.

balneotherapy treatment by medicinal baths

bitters botanical drugs with bitter-tasting constituents used to stimulate the gastrointestinal tract; also used as anti-inflammatory agents and as relaxants

calmative mildly sedative

cardiotonic having a tonic effect on the heart

carminative: relieving flatulence

cathartic: strongly laxative

chemotype visually identical plants with significantly different chemical components, resulting in different therapeutic properties; abbreviated to ct., as in *Thymus vulgaris* ct. alcohol

cholagogic stimulating gallbladder contraction to promote the flow of bile

choleretic stimulating the production of bile in the liver

cicatrizant promoting the formation of scar tissue and healing

cohobation the operation of repeatedly using the water used in the distillation process of the same or fresh plant material; thus no water is discarded and water-soluble molecules from the plant material are not lost

coumarin a chemical compound, $C_9H_6O_2$, with a high boiling point (290176°C) found within the lactones; hardly volatile with steam, thus hence found mainly in expressed oils and sparingly in some distilled essential oils; characteristic smell of new-mown hay

cultivar cultivated variety: a plant produced by horticulture or agriculture not normally occurring naturally; labelled by adding a 'name' to the species, as in *Lavandula angustifolia* 'Maillette'

cytophylaxis the protection of cells against cytolysis, the dissolution or destruction of a cell

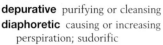

depurative purifying or cleansing

diaphoretic causing or increasing perspiration; sudorific

digestive aiding digestion

dysmenorrhoea painful or difficult menstruation

dyspepsia disturbed digestion

emmenagogic inducing or regularizing menstruation; euphemism for abortifacient

enuresis bedwetting

erethism abnormal irritability or sensitivity

essential oil plant volatile oil obtained by steam distillation or hydrodiffusion

eubiotic brings about conditions favourable to life and healing

eupeptic aiding digestion

febrifuge agent which reduces temperature; antipyretic

fixed oil non-volatile oil; plant oils consist of esters of fatty acids, usually triacylglycerides

forma lowest botanical rank in general use, denoting trivial differences within a species

fruit the ripe seeds and their surrounding structures, which can be fleshy or dry

galactagogic promoting the secretion of milk; lactogenic

genus important botanical classification of related but distinct species given a common name; genera (pl.) are in turn grouped into families; the first word of the binomial botanical name denotes the genus

glycoside sugar derivative found in certain plants (e.g. digoxin, used to treat heart failure)

haemoptysis blood spitting, a symptom possibly indicating serious disease

haemostatic checking blood flow; styptic

hallucinogen agent affecting any or all of the senses, producing a wide range of distorted perceptions and reactions

herb non-woody soft leafy plant; plant used in medicine and cooking

homoeopathy system of medicine using tiny amounts of drugs which in a healthy body would produce symptoms similar to those of the disease (as distinct from allopathy)

hybrid natural or artificially produced plant resulting from the fertilization of one species by another; indicated by 'x', as in *Mentha* x *piperita*

hyperhidrosis excessive sweating

hypermenorrhoea profuse or prolonged menses

hypertensor increasing blood pressure; pressor

hypotensor reducing blood pressure; antihypertensive

immunostimulant stimulating the immune system

lactogenic promoting the secretion of milk; galactagogue

laxative loosening the bowel contents, promoting evacuation

lipid a fat or fat-like substance insoluble in water and soluble in organic solvents

lipolytic breaking down fat

lipophilic having strong affinity for lipids

litholytic breaking down stones

lysigenous breakdown of oil cells forming a cavity not bounded by a definite epithelium as in *Gossypium* species

maceration the extraction of substances from a plant by steeping in a fixed oil

MbOCA symbol for methylenebis (orthochloroaniline); a curing agent for polyurethane and epoxy resins; believed to be carcinogenic

MDA methylenedioxyamphetamine; has hallucinogenic effects; subject to abuse and dependence

menorrhagia excessive periods

metrorrhagia uterine haemorrhage occurring outside menstrual periods

narcotic inducing insensibility (sleep) and relieving pain in small dosage, toxic in high dosage

oestrogenic simulating the action of female hormones

officinalis used in medicine; recognized in the pharmacopoeia

oligomenorrhoea a condition of infrequent menstruation

organic grown without the use of chemical fertilizers, pesticides, etc.

organoleptic concerned with testing the effects of a substance on the senses, particularly taste and smell

parenteral by means other than the gastrointestinal tract; the introduction of substances into an organism by an intravenous, cutaneous, intramuscular or intramedullary pathway

percutaneous applied through the skin

pharmacokinetics study of absorption, distribution, metabolism and elimination of drugs

photosensitization abnormally increased sensitivity of the skin to ultraviolet radiation or natural sunlight; can follow ingestion of or contact with various substances

photosynthesis use of light energy to drive chemical reactions in a plant, which is a photosynthetic organism, whereby carbon dioxide is reduced to carbohydrates and water to free oxygen

phytotherapy treatment of disease by the use of plants and plant extracts; herbalism

polymenorrhoea unusually short menstrual cycles

probiotic favouring the beneficial bacteria in the body while inhibiting harmful microbes; literally 'for life' as distinct from antibiotic, 'against life'

prophylactic preventing disease

psoralens polycyclic molecules whose structure gives them the ability to absorb ultraviolet photons

psychopharmaceutical pertaining to drugs affecting the mind or mood

psychotropic of a drug, affecting the brain and influencing behaviour

purgative strongly laxative

rhizome underground stem bearing roots, scales and nodes

rubefacient increasing local blood circulation causing redness of the skin

schizogenous secretory cavities or sacs arising by separation of cells followed by formation of a secretory epithelium – as in eucalyptus

schizolysigenous type of oil cavities which occur in the Rutaceae and Burseraceae

spasmolytic relieving convulsions, spasmodic pains and cramp

stomachic agent which stimulates the secretory activity of the stomach

styptic arresting haemorrhage by means of an astringent quality; haemostatic

subspecies subdivision of a species, often denoting a geographic variation; structure or colour are peculiar to subspecies and are more definite than characteristics identifying varieties; subspecies can interbreed; abbreviated to subsp.

sudorific inducing sweating

synergy increased effect of two or more medicinal substances working together

taxonomy an ordered, scientific classification of living things

thymoleptic antiseptic

tonic producing or restoring normal vigour or tension (tone)

trichome hairlike structure on the epidermis of a plant

variety indicates a botanical rank between subspecies and forma; abbreviated to var., as in *Citrus aurantium* var. *amara*

vermifugal expelling intestinal worms; see anthelmintic

vesicant producing blisters (therapeutically, to induce counterirritant serosity)

vulnerary agent promoting healing of wounds

Useful Websites and Addresses

Education

National Occupational Standards with
Skills for Health
www.skillsforhealth.org.uk

Penny Price Academy of Aromatherapy
Tel: 01455 25 10 20
Fax: 01455 25 10 65
Email: info@penny-price.com
Website: www.penny-price.com

The Institute of Traditional Herbal Medicine &
Aromatherapy (ITHMA)
Email: gm@aromatherapy-studies.com

Products

Penny Price Aromatherapy
Tel: 01455 25 10 20
Fax: 01455 25 10 65
Email: orders@penny-price.com
Website: www.penny-price.com

Associations

IAM (Institute of Aromatic Medicine)
Email: aromed@hotmail.com

IFA (International Federation of Aromatherapy)
Tel/Fax: 0208 992 5095
Email: office@ifaroma.org

IFPA (International Federation of Professional
Aromatherapists)
Tel: 01455 637 987
Fax: 01455 890 956
Email: admin@ifparoma.org
Website: www.ifparoma.org

Aromatherapy Council (AC)
Email: info@aromatherapycouncil.org.uk
Website: www.aromatherapycouncil.org.uk

Aromatherapy Trade Council (ATC)
Email: info@a-t-c.org.uk
Web site: www.a-t-c.org.uk
Email: info@a-t-c.org.uk
Website: www.a-t-c.org.uk

Regulatory bodies:

Medicines & Healthcare products Regulatory Agency
[MHRA] www.mhra.gov.uk
UK Cosmetic Products (Safety) Regulations 2008
www.opsi.gov.uk/si/si2008/uksi_20081284_en_1

Other interesting or useful websites

Alzheimer's:
www.alzheimers.org.uk
Autism:
www.autism.org.uk/dhstrtegy

Cancer:
www.cancerbacup.org
www.helpthehospices.org.uk
www.learnzone.macmillan.org.uk
www.mariecurie.org.uk
www.pennybrohncancercare.org
www.suerydercare.org E-mail: info@suery
dercare.org

Dementia
www.dementia2010.org
Learning difficulties
www.mencap.org.uk
Palliative and supportive Care
www.ncpc.org.uk

Index

Note: Page numbers followed by *b* indicate boxes, *f* indicate figures and *t* indicate tables.